EMERGENCY MEDICINE

Case Studies

A Compilation of 47 Clinical Studies

By

JAMES T. McRAE, M.D.
Assistant Professor of Surgery
Section on Emergency Medical Services
Department of Surgery
Bowman Gray School of Medicine
Wake Forest University
Winston-Salem, North Carolina

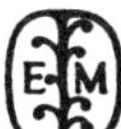
Medical Examination Publishing Co., Inc.
an Excerpta Medica company

969 Stewart Avenue • Garden City, New York 11530

Library of Congress Card Number
79-88721

ISBN 0-87488-002-5

August, 1979

Printed in the United States of America

SIMULTANEOUSLY PUBLISHED IN:

Brazil	:	GUANABARA KOOGAN Rio de Janeiro, Brazil
Europe	:	HANS HUBER PUBLISHERS Bern, Switzerland
Japan	:	IGAKU-SHOIN Ltd. Tokyo, Japan
Mexico, Central America, and South America (except Brazil)	: ;	EDITORIAL EL MANUAL MODERNO Mexico City, Mexico
South and East Asia	:	TOPPAN COMPANY (S) Pte. Ltd. Singapore
United Kingdom	:	HENRY KIMPTON PUBLISHERS London, England

preface

The field of emergency medicine, like so many other medical fields, is changing so rapidly that anyone who ventures to write a book about it is either very brave or very foolhardy. In no other area of medicine are rapid diagnosis and treatment so necessary as in the emergency medical services setting. This book is written primarily for the physician or nonphysician who is working in that setting, whether it is called an emergency department (ED), an emergency ward (EW) or an emergency room (ER).

It has often been said that the first clinician who sees a patient plays a critical role in the outcome of his medical care. That certainly applies to the emergency department physician. He is the person who decides whether the patient has a condition requiring urgent treatment, consultation or possible hospitalization. The physician working in an emergency department has to gain an idea quickly of what the patient's problem is and where in the course of his illness or injury he is at the moment of arrival. The traditional methods of making a diagnosis are often impossible in the emergency department, and thus, the practice of medicine in that setting requires the highest form of detective work.

The approach in this book is that the clinical evaluation, however brief and incomplete, should give the physician a working diagnosis on which to base his request for further studies. Those studies should then be done concurrently, insofar as is possible, in order to decrease the waiting time for the patient. Inevitably, that means ordering some screening laboratory studies that might not be indicated if the physician were in an office where the patient may have been seen in the past and can usually be seen in the future for follow-up.

One basic assumption of the book is that the physician has ready access to consultants in the various specialty areas of medicine and that he can admit or transfer patients for more appropriate or long-term care than he can render in the emergency department.

The book is not encyclopedic, in the sense of covering all of the clinical conditions seen in the average emergency department. Nor is it a manual of emergency medical care, the question and answer format almost completely precluding that approach. It is, rather, a review of certain information and approaches to emergency patients and some of their problems. Few techniques and procedures are given, since many books on technique are already available. This book is designed to supplement those rather than to replace them or even to build on them.

Most of the case studies were taken from the files of the North Carolina Baptist Hospital. Their selection was not easy, but was based upon my desire to include some of the most frequently seen problems in the emergency setting. I have made an effort to summarize the outcome of each case, even when most of the care of the patient took place in some area other than the emergency department.

I did not attempt to formulate the questions on a par with those used in actual examinations. Rather, my goal was to stimulate interest in the subject as well as in the care of the patient as illustrated by the case study.

I made no effort to address or resolve the broad issue of the appropriateness of general patient care in the emergency department setting. Although I do not believe in converting emergency departments into walk-in clinics, I am aware that the public has already done that to a large extent, and that hospitals and physicians are trying to learn to live with that situation and still render consistently good care in the emergency department setting. Unfortunately for good public relations, many emergency departments have a policy against follow-up in the same setting even for the same condition, such as removal of sutures. That is a policy that many patients are unaware of when they take advantage of the convenience of emergency department care.

I have not attempted to cover pediatric cases adequately here, a coverage that would require a separate book. What I have done, whenever possible, is to bring out the points relating to children in each case study, although, admittedly, I have done so rather inadequately, and at times even haphazardly.

Most of the case studies did not seem to require documentation of the statements made, since most of the statements are common knowledge. However, in a few case studies, I thought it wise to list the articles that I had found especially useful. The general reference section that appears at the end of the book lists sources that cover, in much greater detail, the problems described in this book, as well as the many clinical problems that were excluded because of space limitations.

The opinions expressed and the statements made in this book are entirely my own and do not necessarily reflect the official opinion or the recommended treatment protocol of any official body.

James T. McRae, M.D.

To my wife
Inez
who showed infinite patience
and rendered valuable assistance
during the preparation of this book.

contents

acknowledgments

I would like to thank the faculty and residents in Emergency Medicine at Bowman Gray School of Medicine, North Carolina Baptist Hospital and Forsyth Memorial Hospital, all of Winston-Salem, North Carolina. They have offered helpful suggestions on which clinical problems to include in this book and the particular points to bring out that will be helpful to others working in emergency departments.

My thanks also go to Mrs. Judith T. MacMillan, editor in the Department of Surgery at Bowman Gray School of Medicine, and her assistant, Mrs. Frances H. Casstevens, both of whom did far more than the usual work in typing, re-typing, revising and general editing of this material.

My special appreciation goes to my family for waiting patiently for me once more to have time available for them.

notice

EMERGENCY MEDICINE

CASE 1: SEVERE MID-ABDOMINAL PAIN IN A 42-YEAR-OLD MAN

HISTORY: A 42-year-old man reported to the emergency department with severe mid-abdominal pain and vomiting of two days' duration. He had previously experienced several similar, although less severe, episodes of pain. He had consumed one pint of alcohol daily for several years. He denied having had alcohol withdrawal symptoms in the past, but had been tremulous for two days before admission. He had been shot in the abdomen two years before; the wound had been "just sewed up" and there were no complications. His appendix had been removed sometime in the past without sequelae.

Examination revealed a tremulous, agitated man in moderate distress. His pulse was 120 per minute; blood pressure, 160/120 mm Hg. There was moderate tenderness in the epigastrium and right upper abdominal quadrant. Liver was palpable 2 cm below the right costal margin. There were no other abnormal findings.

LABORATORY DATA:

Hemoglobin: 14.3 gm/dl
Hematocrit: 43.6%
White blood cell count: 9,600/mm^3 with 87 segmented neutrophils and 5 bands
Urinalysis: negative except for trace of protein
Electrolytes: within normal range
Serum amylase: 600 Somogyi units/100 ml (normal range: 50 to 150 Somogyi units/100 ml); six hours later - 450 Somogyi units/100 ml
Serum creatinine: 1.1 mg/dl
Serum calcium: 11.8 mg/dl (normal range: 8.5-10.5 mg/dl)
Serum phosphorus: 4.1 mg/dl

Total bilirubin: 1.07 mg/dl
Alkaline phosphatase: 116 I.U. (normal range: 30 to 110 I.U.)
Lactic dehydrogenase: 225 I.U. (normal range: 60 to 220 I.U.)
Serum glutamic oxaloacetic transaminase: 62 I.U. (normal range: 0 to 40 I.U.)
VDRL: Nonreactive
X-rays: Chest: bilateral atelectasis, lower lobes. Abdomen: ileus in transverse colon and splenic flexure; no calcification in the region of the pancreas.

QUESTIONS:

1. Your main working diagnosis in this patient is:
   A. Alcohol withdrawal syndrome
   B. Acute alcoholic hepatitis
   C. Acute alcoholic gastritis
   D. Penetrating peptic ulcer
   E. Acute pancreatitis

2. TRUE OR FALSE: There is more than one clinical type of pancreatitis.

3. Which of the following are related etiologically to the development of acute pancreatitis?
   A. Trauma
   B. Gallstone disease
   C. Alcoholism
   D. Recent abdominal operation
   E. All of the above

4. The most important historical features in diagnosing acute pancreatitis are:
   A. Abdominal pain, usually upper
   B. Back pain opposite the epigastrium
   C. Nausea and vomiting, usually severe
   D. Fever
   E. All of the above

TRUE OR FALSE (Questions 5-9):

5. Serum amylase elevation has been known to be pathognomonic of acute pancreatitis since 1929.

6. Urinary amylase excretion is a useful test for diagnosis of acute pancreatitis.

7. Elevated serum lipase is specific for acute pancreatitis.

8. It is usually possible to accurately predict the course of pancreatitis once the diagnosis is made.

9. Nasogastric intubation with suction is indicated in all cases of acute pancreatitis, regardless of the severity.

10. This patient was admitted to the hospital and treated with bed rest, nasogastric suction for 55 hours, intravenous fluids, and pain medication. Would any narcotic have been satisfactory for pain relief?
    A. Yes
    B. No

11. The complications of acute pancreatitis are:
    A. Paralytic ileus
    B. Hypocalcemia
    C. Pseudocyst
    D. Abscess
    E. Hypovolemic shock
    F. All of the above

TRUE OR FALSE:

12. Operation is almost never indicated in uncomplicated acute pancreatitis.

13. It is not particularly important to differentiate alcoholic pancreatitis from gallstone pancreatitis.

14. The role of anticholinergics and antibiotics in acute pancreatitis is clearly defined and they should always be used.

COURSE: This patient's serum calcium level was 10.3 mg% on the day of discharge. Blood pressure was 140/100 mm Hg on his return visit to the clinic, one month later. Further studies were planned to investigate his biliary system and the cause of his hypertension. He was advised to stop drinking. He failed to return for further follow-up visits.

ANSWERS AND COMMENTS:

1. (E) Acute pancreatitis. The others are possibilities and any of them, or any combination of them, could explain this patient's symptoms and signs. He probably does have early and mild alcoholic withdrawal symptoms (A), precipitated by decreased intake of alcohol from vomiting. However, unless fullblown delirium tremens develops, treatment can be deferred until

more important diagnostic and therapeutic steps are taken.

Acute alcoholic hepatitis (B) is suggested by both the history and the finding of an enlarged liver. However, it is unlikely that all of the patient's symptoms are related to liver derangement. Acute alcoholic gastritis (C) could have caused some of his findings, but the abdominal tenderness in this condition is usually less severe. One must always be aware of penetrating or perforating peptic ulcer (D) in this clinical setting, and the studies ordered should reflect that awareness.

The diagnosis of acute pancreatitis is often very difficult, even with the best history-taking, examination, and ancillary studies. A high index of suspicion is one of the most valuable diagnostic tools. The clinical picture of pancreatitis varies considerably from one patient to the next, and even in the same patient from one attack to the next and during each attack.

2. (True) Of the acute forms, the range of severity is from mild acute edematous (or interstitial) pancreatitis to hemorrhagic (or necrotizing) pancreatitis. Edematous pancreatitis can progress to hemorrhagic pancreatitis, although the mechanism of that progression is unknown. Acute relapsing pancreatitis is that form of the disease in which there are multiple attacks that leave no permanent pancreatic scarring. This is the picture most often associated with biliary (gallstone) pancreatitis.

Chronic pancreatitis is usually associated with alcoholism. With this form, intraductal and parenchymal calcification appears within the pancreas and usually progresses over a period of years. Most patients with chronic pancreatitis have severe chronic abdominal and back pain.

3. (E) All. About 40% of cases are associated with biliary tract disease, and 40% with acute or chronic alcoholism. The pathophysiological mechanisms in these 80% are poorly understood. Five percent of cases are associated with trauma (usually blunt abdominal), operation (usually, but not necessarily, upper abdominal), hyperparathyroidism, hyperlipidemia, or hereditary causes (often beginning in childhood). The remaining 15% of cases are classified as idiopathic.

4. (E) All. It is most unusual for a patient with acute pancreatitis not to have abdominal pain. The pain may last only a few hours and not be very severe, but it is usually present. In most instances, it is quite severe and steady, is of a boring character, and is usually located in the epigastrium and corresponding

portion of the back. If true board-like rigidity of the abdominal muscles is present, the patient is more likely to have a perforated duodenal ulcer than acute pancreatic disease.

Nausea and vomiting are almost invariably present, beginning at the same time as the pain, and are usually quite severe.

Fever is variable but frequently present, along with other symptoms suggesting inflammation in the upper abdomen.

5. (False) Although in 1929, Elman and associates[3] reported an elevation in serum amylase in most patients with acute pancreatitis, it has never been thought to be pathognomonic of this condition, and it may not even be present at a particular time in patients with known acute pancreatitis. It is one of the signs in too wide a spectrum of diseases[2] to be of definitive diagnostic value alone in acute pancreatitis. In a series of 519 patients with acute pancreatitis, Jacobs, et al.,[6] found the degree of elevation of serum amylase to be unhelpful in prognosis.

6. (True) Excretion of amylase, via the kidneys, is speeded up in the presence of acute pancreatitis. The cause is not well understood, since the increased rate of excretion persists longer than the elevation of serum amylase in patients with acute pancreatitis; in many of these patients, the level of serum amylase may be only slightly elevated or normal.[9]

The specimen to be checked should be a timed specimen, if possible, since checking a urine sample collected at random may not give definitive results. A one- or two-hour specimen is most commonly used.

7. (False) Hyperlipasemia occurs in acute pancreatitis but is not specific for it, as it does occur in other conditions, sometimes alone and sometimes concomitantly with hyperamylasemia.[2] In other words, it is no more specific for acute pancreatitis than an increased serum amylase, although it persists longer. This may be useful diagnostically in patients seen late in an acute episode, since the elevated serum amylase usually returns to normal after 24 to 72 hours.

To repeat, no one of the three usual tests, serum amylase, timed urinary amylase excretion, serum lipase, is specific for acute pancreatitis. At least one, and frequently all three, modalities are elevated early in the course of an attack and may serve as diagnostic guides. Because the diagnosis is often so elusive, it is wise to check all three in any patient with severe upper abdominal pain and tenderness, unless some other diagnosis is obvious. If some, or all, are normal initially, they should be rechecked at least daily, because in some patients with acute pancreatitis, the levels may not be elevated at all, while in other such patients, they are elevated only transiently. In this patient, the diagnosis of acute pancreatitis was obvious and additional tests were not required.

The patient who has recently ingested alcohol or other drugs presents a special problem, not only in the differential diagnosis but in the extent to which the alcohol can mask pain and tenderness. In such a patient, screening tests, such as the ones described previously, are mandatory. Repeated evaluation is also essential, including key laboratory tests.

Even when all laboratory tests for acute pancreatitis are negative, it is wise not to abandon this diagnosis in the patient who has upper abdominal pain and tenderness, with associated vomiting, when no other diagnosis seems acceptable. Such patients should be hospitalized for observation and further diagnostic studies.

In summary, the following are pitfalls in the diagnosis of acute pancreatitis: (1) failure to consider pancreatitis in the differential diagnosis; (2) failure to determine enzyme levels early enough and frequently enough; (3) failure to remember that other diseases may elevate the serum amylase; and (4) labelling upper abdominal pain "functional", because it does not fit nicely into any other diagnostic category.

8. (False) The initial evaluation is often very misleading, in that the patient may become progressively sicker, or he may improve rapidly, even though he was moderately ill when first seen. Because of this unpredictability, it is safest to hospitalize the patient with acute pancreatitis and to start treatment as soon as possible.

9. (True) It relieves pain, rests the pancreas, and relieves or prevents the recurrence of ileus. Relief of pain is frequently used as the signal for removal of the nasogastric tube, provided the bowel sounds have returned to near normal.

10. (B) No. It is far better to avoid narcotics known to produce severe spasm of the sphincter of Oddi, since such spasm may make both the pain and the pancreatitis worse. The narcotic that is both effective and least likely to cause such spasm is meperidine (Demerol®), usually given in doses of 100 mg or more,

every three to four hours.

The pain usually subsides after one to two days, as it did in this patient. Persistent pain suggests the presence of very severe disease or a complication (see answer 11).

11. (F) All. One of the early roentgenographic signs is paralytic ileus (A), usually localized.[1, 10] It may become quite severe, unless the stomach is kept empty by nasogastric suction. Serum calcium levels below 8 mg/dl (B) are usually an indication of hemorrhagic pancreatitis, but may occur in the less severe forms. Levels of serum calcium below 7.5 mg% are associated with a high mortality rate. Any degree of hypocalcemia should be treated with calcium ion, given intravenously, usually 10 ml of 10% calcium gluconate. Serial measurements of serum calcium levels should be used to determine whether additional doses are needed.

Pseudocyst formation (C) is a potentially serious complication. Surgical drainage is usually required, but occasionally, a pseudocyst regresses spontaneously. These pseudocysts can grow until they displace adjacent organs and erode into hollow viscera and blood vessels, producing obstructive and hemorrhagic complications. In acute pancreatitis, if serum amylase levels fail to subside toward normal within a few days, pseudocyst or abscess is probably present.

Abscess (D) is more common with hemorrhagic or necrotizing pancreatitis. It requires immediate operative intervention; even so, the mortality rate is from 40 to 60%.[5, 7]

As for shock (E), the fluid loss in severe pancreatitis is similar to that in extensively burned patients. Moderate sequestration of blood in and around the pancreas often occurs with hemorrhagic pancreatitis. Pancreatic ascites, which is not uncommon; hydrothorax, usually on the left side but sometimes bilateral; and sequestered fluid in the intestine, further deplete blood volume. Rapid fluid replacement is indicated, sometimes of large volumes. This replacement therapy should be started in the emergency department without delay. It is usually guided by central venous pressure monitoring and may later require Swan-Ganz catheter monitoring (pulmonary capillary wedge pressure). In addition to electrolyte and fluid replacement, albumin or whole blood may be indicated.

12. (False) When it is impossible to make a definitive clinical diagnosis, exploratory celiotomy may be required in the early

stages of the illness to differentiate among acute pancreatitis, perforated peptic ulceration without demonstrable free air in the peritoneal cavity, and strangulation of a loop of bowel. Contrary to earlier thinking, it does not presently appear to be harmful to operate upon a patient with acute pancreatitis.

Definitive treatment of acute pancreatitis is sometimes possible at such an early operation, especially if gallstones appear to be an etiologic factor.

13. (False) In general, alcoholic patients with pancreatitis do well when treated conservatively, unless there is also biliary tract disease, especially the calculous type. In patients with unusually high serum levels of amylase (more than 1500 international units), gallstone pancreatitis is usually present, especially when serum bilirubin and alkaline phosphatase levels are also elevated. These patients usually do better with early operative intervention.[8] Early in acute pancreatitis, cholangiography is not very helpful because of false-negative results, but it is useful in the recovery phase.

14. (False) There is no question that pancreatic secretions need to be suppressed, and clinicians who use anticholinergic agents for this purpose believe that their patients improve more rapidly. Controlled studies have not unequivocally confirmed these results. Besides, the relatively large doses required to suppress pancreatic secretions decrease patient comfort and may precipitate or complicate paralytic ileus.

Antibiotics used prophylactically in the absence of overt infection are also highly controversial. The consensus is that they should be reserved for patients with pancreatitis related to biliary calculi and those with hemorrhagic or necrotizing pancreatitis.[4] They are, of course, indicated when abscess formation exists as a complication of pancreatitis.

REFERENCES

1. Benson, G. N.: Plain film findings in acute pancreatitis. _J. Nat. Med. Assoc._ 66:148-151, 159, 1974.

2. Bishop, R. P.: The diagnosis of pancreatic disease. _Amer. J. Gastroenterol._ 49:112-119, 1968.

3. Elman, R., et al.: Value of blood amylase estimation in the diagnosis of pancreatic disease. A clinical study. _Arch. Surg._ 19:943-967, 1929.

4. Finch, W.T., et al.: A prospective study to determine the efficacy of antibiotics in acute pancreatitis. Ann. Surg. 183:667-671, 1976.

5. Gliedman, M.L., et al.: Acute pancreatitis. Curr. Probl. Surg. 7(Aug.):3-52, 1970.

6. Jacobs, M.L., et al.: Acute pancreatitis: analysis of factors influencing survival. Ann. Surg. 185:43-51, 1977.

7. Kraft, A.R. and Saletta, J.D.: Acute alcoholic pancreatitis: current concepts and controversies. Surg. Annual 8:145-171, 1976.

8. Paloyan, D. and Simonowitz, D.: Diagnostic considerations in acute alcoholic and gallstone pancreatitis. Am. J. Surg. 132:329-331, 1976.

9. Saxon, E.I., et al.: Comparative value of serum and urinary amylase in the diagnosis of acute pancreatitis. Arch. Intern. Med. 99:607-621, 1957.

10. Stone, L.B., et al.: Inflammatory disease of the pancreas. Curr. Probl. Radiol. 5:3-43, 1975.

::

CASE 2: LOWER ABDOMINAL PAIN IN A 30-YEAR-OLD WOMAN

HISTORY:

A 30-year-old woman noted anorexia and gradual onset of pain in the right lower abdominal quadrant 14 hours before reporting to the emergency department. At no time was the pain present in any other area of the abdomen nor did it radiate. It was steady and progressive. Three hours after onset, she vomited once, a greenish material, with no relief of her pain. She passed a formed stool, with no blood or mucus, ten hours after onset of pain.

The patient's medical history was negative. She had never had any operations or pregnancies. Her last menstrual period had started 11 days earlier, and had lasted the usual six days. Her menstrual interval was 26 days. She denied recent exposure to venereal disease and had noted no leukorrhea. She had no urinary symptoms.

QUESTIONS:

1. Which of the following are true regarding right lower abdominal pain?
   A. It is the location of pain in many patients seen in emergency departments.
   B. In any patient who has not had an appendectomy, it should be considered a symptom of acute appendicitis until proved otherwise.
   C. The internal genital organs are often the source of such pain in young adult females.
   D. Several diseases present with pain in the right lower quadrant and require examination and laboratory studies to distinguish among them.
   E. All of the above

EXAMINATION:

Her oral temperature was 98.8°F. (37°C.). General examination revealed no abnormalities, except for moderate tenderness and muscle guarding just superior to McBurney's point, and slight tenderness in the right flank. Peristalsis was normal. Pelvic and rectal examinations were negative.

LABORATORY DATA:

Hemoglobin: 13.5 gm/dl
Leukocytes: 13,500/mm^3; segmented neutrophils: 73%; nonsegmented neutrophils: 5%
Urinalysis: (clean-voided) negative, except that the sediment contained three to five white blood cells per high power field; no bacteria
Chest x-ray: negative
Abdominal x-ray: not considered necessary

TRUE OR FALSE (Questions 2 and 3):

2. Pain which begins in the right lower quadrant, as in this patient, rules out acute appendicitis.

3. The two essential features of appendicitis are pain and tenderness in the area of the appendix, usually the right lower quadrant.

4. The basis for the pain of appendicitis usually appearing first in the mid-abdomen or epigastrium and then moving to the right lower quadrant is:
   A. Location of the mobile appendix more toward the midline than usual, at the time of onset
   B. Association of early pain with vomiting
   C. Malrotation of the colon
   D. The initial pain is a referred visceral type

5. At this point, which of the following seems most likely?
   A. Mesenteric lymphadenitis
   B. Acute appendicitis
   C. Right ureteral calculus
   D. Right tubal pregnancy with rupture
   E. Acute salpingitis or pelvic inflammatory disease (PID)
   F. Mittelschmerz

COURSE:

The patient was operated upon, and acute suppurative retrocecal appendicitis was found. Appendectomy was followed by a smooth convalescence.

6. The appendix may be located in which of the following areas of the abdominal cavity?
   A. The left lower quadrant
   B. The right upper quadrant

C. The true pelvis
D. The left upper quadrant
E. The right lower quadrant
F. All of the above

TRUE OR FALSE:

7. Appendicitis is a disease of teenagers and young adults, but it can occur at any age, even in the very young and the very old.

8. Appendicitis almost never occurs in pregnant patients.

9. The most likely complication of appendicitis is perforation and abscess formation.

ANSWERS AND COMMENTS:

1. (E) All of the statements are true. The one that should be emphasized here is B, since appendicitis is a common problem and delayed diagnosis, for any reason, is dangerous.

2. (False) The pain of acute appendicitis usually begins in the epigastrium or periumbilical region, but not always. Also, it may be so short-lived in that area as to pass unnoticed.

3. (True) Pain and tenderness are almost invariably found, except that both are attenuated or otherwise difficult to elicit in small children and in the elderly, as well as in the emotionally disturbed or mentally retarded patient.

4. (D) The initial pain is a referred visceral-type pain. Although the exact mechanism of referred pain remains obscure, it is common in abdominal disease. The small intestine and the appendix are supplied by spinal nerves nine through eleven. The discomfort caused by distention of the appendiceal wall, or contraction of the muscles of the appendix, is felt in the portion of the abdominal wall supplied by the corresponding spinal nerves. In the case of acute appendicitis, this means the epigastrium or periumbilical region.

The subsequent pain is located in the area of the appendix and is somatic in type. It is due to peritoneal irritation from the inflamed appendix. Typically, the pain of appendicitis has these two components. Whenpresent, this sequence is helpful in making the diagnosis.

5. (B) Acute appendicitis. The flank tenderness suggests that the tip of the appendix may be lateral to the cecum or that the appendix may be retrocecal.

Mesenteric lymphadenitis (A) is difficult to distinguish from appendicitis, and a period of observation may be required to differentiate them. Usually, mesenteric lymphadenitis gradually improves over a period of hours, whereas appendicitis fails to improve or becomes worse.

If ureteral calculus were suspected (C), an x-ray of the abdomen would be indicated. In the absence of microscopic hematuria, it is unlikely that a stone would be blocking the ureter in this patient. Intravenous pyelography is needed to detect a small calculus or a non-opaque calculus.

Right tubal pregnancy in the early stage, after rupture (D), can present as in this patient. However, the 14-hour duration and the negative pelvic examination rule against this diagnosis.

Acute pelvic inflammatory disease (E) usually presents with bilateral pain and tenderness, although unilateral symptoms and signs are not unusual. In any case, there should be tenderness on pelvic examination.

Mittelschmerz, or rupture of a graafian follicle of one ovary (F), can be confused with appendicitis. However, usually, but not always, there is tenderness on pelvic examination with mittelschmerz. The pain is due to peritoneal irritation from bleeding, and it is most unusual for this to last more than a few hours. A period of observation, as in the case of mesenteric lymphadenitis, will usually allow the distinction to be made.

6. (F) All. Largely due to incomplete rotation of the colon, the appendix, which is always attached to the cecum, can be located in any portion of the abdomen. This should be kept in mind when diagnosing abdominal pain and tenderness in any patient whose appendix has not been removed. Any doubt as to whether the appendix is inflamed requires surgical consultation and may require exploratory celiotomy. Roentgenographic examination is usually helpful in determining the location of the cecum in such patients.

7. (True) It is rare before the age of two years, but there is no upper age limit. The patients at either extreme are much more prone to develop complications, because of inability or failure to report the symptoms early or because the physician

is not suspicious enough of appendicitis.

8. (False) Appendicitis occurs in the presence of pregnancy and even during labor. In each of these instances, it is particularly dangerous to both mother and fetus, largely because of delayed diagnosis and delayed operation. Any pregnant patient with pain and tenderness suggestive of appendicitis, even though atypical, should be referred immediately for surgical consultation.

9. (True) The abscess can be in the retrocecal position, in the true pelvis or almost anywhere in the abdomen. Localization occurs if the omentum and adjacent bowel loops are able to wall off the leakage of fecal and purulent contents. The omentum is not well-developed in the young and the elderly, or it may be adherent in some other part of the peritoneal cavity. If the tip of the appendix remains free or if an appendiceal abscess ruptures secondarily, generalized peritonitis is produced, a truly life-threatening condition.

CASE 3: VAGINAL BLEEDING IN A 15-YEAR-OLD PREGNANT GIRL

HISTORY:

A 15-year-old girl, who was 12 weeks pregnant, began bleeding vaginally, developed lower abdominal cramping pain, and passed some tissue from the vagina. She reported to the emergency department six hours later. She was unmarried and had been scheduled for a therapeutic abortion three days later. She had had no previous pregnancies.

There was some blood, but no tissue, in the vagina; the cervix was dilated, and the uterus was slightly enlarged and soft. No other abnormalities were noted.

QUESTIONS:

1. TRUE OR FALSE: The most likely diagnosis in this patient is incomplete, spontaneous abortion.

2. When a patient presents in the emergency department with spontaneous abortion, which of the following constitute proper treatment?
   A. Obtain a complete blood cell count, hematocrit, and blood typing
   B. Start an intravenous infusion
   C. Discharge the patient after she stops bleeding
   D. Administer Rh_O (D antigen) immunoglobulin if the patient has an Rh negative blood group
   E. Do a dilatation and curettage of the uterus if the abortion is incomplete
   F. Submit all tissue to the pathologist
   G. Administer oxytocin or ergonovine
   H. All of the above

3. Which of the following characterize ectopic pregnancy (usually tubal)?
   A. One or two menstrual periods missed, then vaginal spotting or bleeding
   B. Lower abdominal pain and adnexal tenderness
   C. Pelvic findings of a unilateral pelvic mass
   D. Signs of serious blood loss, even if no vaginal bleeding occurs
   E. A positive urine pregnancy test
   F. All of these

4. Which of the following are also causes of significant vaginal bleeding during pregnancy?
   A. Placenta previa
   B. Abruptio placentae
   C. A and B

TRUE OR FALSE:

5. Pelvic examination should always be done in the emergency department on any pregnant patient in the third trimester who has painless vaginal bleeding.

6. Abruptio placentae is reliably diagnosed by pain and rigidity over the uterus and profuse vaginal bleeding.

ANSWERS AND COMMENTS:

1. (True) Although there are other complications of pregnancy, many of them serious, the ones associated with bleeding are the ones most likely to be seen in emergency departments.

The history and findings in this patient are typical of incomplete abortion, and since there was no evidence of a specific cause, they are typical of incomplete, spontaneous abortion. That is the most common emergency occurring during the early weeks of pregnancy.

By definition, abortion is termination of gestation before the fetus becomes viable, usually before the twentieth week after the first day of the last menstrual period. In addition to the incomplete, spontaneous type, types of abortion include intentionally produced abortion, which is "criminal" if illegal or "therapeutic" if legal; threatened abortion, characterized by lower abdominal pain but with little or no bleeding and no tissue being passed; inevitable abortion, in which the fetus cannot be saved; "missed" abortion, in which the fetus dies but is not passed; habitual abortion, which is the occurrence of three or more consecutive spontaneous abortions; and septic abortion, the type accompanied by chills, fever and purulent uterine discharge, usually with bacteremia. The overwhelming majority of abortions are the type this patient had, although some of them are "complete", meaning that all tissue has been passed.

2. (A, B, D, E, F, G) (A) The complete blood cell count and hematocrit determination are useful for ruling out significant anemia

and infection. Blood typing is essential, in case the patient bleeds sufficiently to require a blood transfusion. The Rh typing is necessary, so the patient can be given Rh_O (D antigen) immunoglobulin, if the patient has an Rh negative blood group (D).

(B) An intravenous infusion should be started in every patient for administration of both fluid and drugs.

(C) The patient may be discharged from the emergency department under certain circumstances, but not just because she has stopped bleeding. Unless the uterus is emptied by artificial means, or unless the abortion has been complete, she will almost certainly have recurrent, often profuse, bleeding. In most instances, it is better to do a dilatation and curettage (D and C) either in the emergency department, under intravenous analgesia (as was done in this patient), or in the operating room (E). Regardless of where the D and C is done, all tissue must be removed and all of it submitted to the hospital pathologist (F).

(G) It is very important to begin an infusion of oxytocin (20 units in 1000 ml of Ringer's lactate intravenously) or ergonovine (0.2 mg intramuscularly) as soon as the diagnosis of incomplete abortion is made. That promotes contraction of the uterus, which helps to expel more of the tissue and clots, and stop the bleeding. The drug should be given before and during the D and C and should be continued postoperatively for at least a few hours of observation. If blood loss has been large, another hemoglobin measurement may be indicated. All patients undergoing abortion with moderate to severe hemorrhage should be admitted to the hospital, as should all patients with septic abortion, regardless of the amount of bleeding.

3. (A, B, D) (A) One or two missed periods are typical in 75% of patients with unruptured ectopic pregnancy. However, about 25% of patients will have had no amenorrhea. A small amount of vaginal bleeding is usually present and may be the earliest clue to the presence of an ectopic pregnancy. A pelvic mass will not be palpable in almost half of the patients (C), but pain and tenderness (B) are present in almost all patients. Those symptoms and signs are accentuated in patients who have ruptured ectopic pregnancy. Also, in the latter group, significant, usually rapid, hemorrhage is present, with signs of hypovolemic shock (D).

The pregnancy test (E) is positive in only 50% of patients with ectopic pregnancy, making the test of no real value. In general, a pregnancy test is of greatest value when it is negative, but, in this instance, a negative test obviously does not rule out ectopic pregnancy.

The diagnosis is usually made by the combination of the clinical features listed, but it must then be confirmed by culdocentesis (unclotted blood recovered if rupture has occurred), laparoscopy or culdoscopy (suitable for diagnosis of both nonruptured and ruptured tubal pregnancy), or laparotomy (celiotomy). If there is evidence of significant blood loss, the diagnostic confirmatory step must be taken immediately and must always be abdominal, never vaginal. Salpingectomy, usually of only the involved tube, is almost always the indicated procedure.

It should be added that a negative culdocentesis does not rule out intraperitoneal bleeding from either ectopic pregnancy or ruptured ovarian cyst. If the diagnosis of either one is still suspected, it must be confirmed by laparoscopy or culdoscopy in the operating room, or by immediate laparotomy if the situation is urgent.

4. (C) Both of those conditions occur in the third trimester of pregnancy. They are discussed in the next two answers.

5. (False) Such a patient is very likely to have placenta previa. The cardinal rule is that a pelvic examination of a painfree, bleeding patient in the third trimester of pregnancy should never be done unless the physician is prepared to deliver the baby. The reason for that precaution is that the manipulation of even the most gentle pelvic examination may cause the bleeding to recur and to be very profuse. Pelvic examination in the previously mentioned circumstances must be deferred to an obstetrician who can do the examination in an operating room.

6. (False) Although rigidity and tenderness of the uterus are the most reliable signs of the diagnosis, vaginal bleeding, without pain, does not exclude the diagnosis. On the other hand, the bleeding may be "concealed," that is, retained within the uterine cavity. The latter type of bleeding carries the same hazard for the fetus and for the patient, that hazard depending upon the extent of the separation and the amount of bleeding.

Treatment is by amniotomy, done in the hope of immobilizing the detached portion of the placenta, thus controlling or slowing the bleeding and improving the chance of fetal survival. Oxytocin, 10 units in 1000 ml of Ringer's lactate, should be started by intravenous infusion, in the hope of stimulating uterine contractions. Delivery should be accomplished rapidly by the vaginal route or by cesarean section. Hypofibrinogenemia and disseminated intravascular coagulation are serious dangers and must be anticipated in every patient with abruptio placentae. Fibrinogen, given intravenously, 2 to 10 grams, may be necessary, along with transfusions of fresh whole blood.

::

CASE 4: HEAT SYNDROMES

HISTORY:

A 61-year-old brick mason was brought to the emergency department after he had collapsed while working in the sun on a very hot and humid day. For no apparent reason, he had been feeling tired for two or three days. There was no history of injury, nor of alcohol or drug abuse. His only medication was hydrochlorothiazide, 50 mg each morning, for mild hypertension.

Examination revealed a comatose patient who responded only to painful stimuli, the response being movement of all extremities. He was not obese. His rectal temperature was 108.6°F (42.5°C); pulse, 150 per minute and regular; respirations, 30 per minute; blood pressure, 150/50 mm Hg. He was not perspiring, and his skin was hot but not particularly dry. He had no nystagmus or other ocular abnormality. Neurologic examination revealed no other abnormalities. There was no evidence of injury.

LABORATORY DATA:

Hemoglobin: 12.7 gm/dl
Hematocrit: 38.4%
White blood cell count: 7,700 with normal differential and normal platelets
Urinalysis: within normal limits
Serum sodium: 142 mEq/l; CO2 combining power - 30 mEq/l; chloride - 102 mEq/l; potassium - 4.0 mEq/l
Blood urea nitrogen (BUN): 21 mg/dl
Glucose: 117 mg/dl
Calcium: 9.9 mg/dl
Phosphorus: 5.6 mg/dl
Prothrombin time: 12.4 seconds with control 11.4, partial thromboplastin time - 29.4 seconds with control 21.7
Lumbar puncture: was not done
Stool examination (guaiac) for blood: was negative

Chest, skull and spine x-rays showed no evidence of trauma or other abnormalities. Central venous pressure (CVP) was 10 cm H_2O. Arterial blood showed normal pH and gases. Electrocardiogram was within normal limits.

The clinical impression was heat stroke and essential hypertension.

Treatment consisted of (1) endotracheal intubation and administering of 100% oxygen; and (2) removing all of his clothing and cooling his body with ice packs, a cooling blanket and a fan, until his rectal temperature dropped to 102°F (38.8°C). His extremities were massaged gently. By the end of the first hour, he was beginning to talk coherently and drink liquids. Glucose, 5% in 0.45% saline, was administered intravenously, 1000 ml in the first two and one-half hours, with no evidence of pulmonary edema. He had no seizure. The concentration of inhaled oxygen was gradually reduced when it was shown that his arterial blood gases and pH were within normal limits. There was no evidence of vomiting with aspiration. He was admitted to the intensive care unit, where he continued to improve. He was discharged four days later and seen in the clinic four days after that. He was doing quite well and was allowed to return to work one week after his clinic visit. He was advised to avoid working in direct sunlight for the remainder of the summer because of increased susceptibility to heat stroke.

QUESTIONS:

1. The heat syndromes include which of the following?
   A. Heat cramps
   B. Heat exhaustion
   C. Heat stroke
   D. All of the above

2. TRUE OR FALSE: Heat stroke almost never affects teenagers and young adults.

3. Which of the following are among the additional predisposing and precipitating causes of heat stroke?
   A. Obesity
   B. Alcoholism
   C. Use of anticholinergic drugs
   D. Heart disease
   E. Chronic disabling disease
   F. Previous heat stroke
   G. All of the above

4. Which of the following characterizes the circulatory abnormalities in severe heat stroke?
   A. Tachycardia
   B. Wide pulse pressure
   C. Cardiovascular collapse
   D. Right-sided heart failure
   E. All of the above

5. Which of the following characterizes acclimatization to a high-temperature, high-humidity environment?
   A. Increased maximal cardiac output
   B. Decreased peak heart rate
   C. Decreased stroke volume
   D. Decreased sodium concentration of sweat
   E. Decreased volume of sweat in response to a given work load
   F. Enhanced metabolic efficiency
   G. All of the above
   H. None of the above

6. Therapeutic management for heat stroke should consist of which of the following?
   A. Immediate cooling by removal of clothing, application of a cooling blanket, and a fan or ice bath
   B. Intravenous fluids
   C. Massage of the skin
   D. Oxygen
   E. Careful and frequent monitoring of rectal temperatures, vital signs, central venous pressure, urinary output, arterial blood gases and pH
   F. Norepinephrine, epinephrine and stimulants, as needed
   G. All of the above

ANSWERS AND COMMENTS:

1. (D) All. (A) Heat cramps, also called miner's cramps or stoker's cramps, are painful spasms of voluntary muscles following strenuous exercise. They occur in persons whose physical condition is good and who are acclimatized to heat. This syndrome must be differentiated from tetany, which is due to hyperventilation, a common condition with exposure to high environmental temperature (see B). The cause of muscle cramps is probably an acute deficiency of sodium in a person who drinks an adequate amount of water for the amount lost in perspiration. Therefore, there is hyponatremia, although not all who develop hyponatremia will have heat cramps. The cramps are relieved promptly by ingestion of sodium.

(B) Heat exhaustion, or heat prostration, is the most common heat syndrome, and it may occur in epidemic proportions during a heat wave which is prolonged for several days or weeks. One type is that due to predominant water depletion in a person who perspires in excess of water replacement. This happens when one does not usually replace the total volume of water lost by sweating and maintains a negative water balance of 1% or 2% of of his total body weight. It is much more likely to occur when the water supply is limited or when the person, such as an infant or an elderly person, is unable to express thirst. The symptoms are intense thirst, fatigue, weakness, anxiety and impaired judgment. Heat exhaustion is frequently associated with hyperventilation, and the symptoms and signs of tetany, due to respiratory alkalosis, must be differentiated from the remainder of the syndrome. However, this is not the usual hyperventilation syndrome due to anxiety, but rather a syndrome due to central nervous system dysfunction, which also manifests itself by agitation, muscular incoordination and even frank psychosis. It is a mistake for an emergency physician to jump to the conclusion that the hyperventilation caused by heat exhaustion requires treatment only with paper bag rebreathing and reassurance. The tip-off is the usual presence of dehydration and hyperpyrexia, which can progress to frank heat stroke. This progression can be very rapid when circulatory failure or a convulsion supervenes.[1]

Another variation of heat exhaustion is that due predominantly to salt depletion. Here, large volumes of thermal sweat are replaced by adequate water, but no additional salt is taken. Symptoms of this condition are profound weakness, fatigue, severe frontal headache, nausea, vomiting, diarrhea, and skeletal muscle cramps. Thus, this form of heat exhaustion differs from heat cramps in that it is accompanied by systemic symptoms; it also tends to occur in unacclimatized persons. The cramps of heat exhaustion are usually made worse by giving large quantities of water without giving salt as well. The patient is rarely intensely thirsty. He may have hypotension and tachycardia, but his body temperature usually remains normal, unless dehydration occurs secondary to vomiting. Treatment consists of administering normal saline, although hypertonic saline may be used cautiously if the hyponatremia is of sufficient magnitude to be symptomatic.[1] Such severe salt depletion is extremely rare.

(C) Heat stroke, also called sunstroke or heat pyrexia, is a life-threatening emergency characterized by severe central nervous system disturbances, hyperpyrexia and hot, dry skin which is pink or ashen, depending upon the circulatory state. It is caused by excessive heat storage that develops when high ambient temperature prevents heat dissipation by radiation or convection, and sweat evaporation is limited by humidity. As indicated previously, heat stroke is presumed to be an extension of the pathophysiological changes and associated clinical symptoms of heat exhaustion.

Heat stroke also occurs in epidemic proportions, and carries a mortality rate of up to 80%. The highest mortality is in small infants and the elderly, especially those with debilitating diseases. Severe persistent disability occurs in many survivors.[1] Emergency department physicians can expect to treat many such patients whenever there is a major and prolonged heat wave. Since heat stroke is life-threatening and requires immediate recognition and treatment, the remainder of this study will be devoted to it.

2. (False) Each year, an alarming number of young persons die from heat stroke in the United States. Usually, they are unacclimatized teenagers or young adults who are engaging in strenuous physical activity, such as military drilling or football practice. The setting is usually outside, in the summer sun, and in the presence of high relative humidity, although it may be inside, as in a gymnasium. Some victims have predisposing or associated illnesses but many have no known or detectable health problems. Frequently, they fail to replace lost fluid and salt, either because they are not thirsty, or because they are under the impression that conditioning and acclimatization develop faster with minimum fluid intake. Therefore, they may take salt tablets avidly, with little or no liquid. This is a dangerous practice, since it may precipitate a severe water-depletion type of heat exhaustion, which may culminate in frank heat stroke. Fatal heat stroke can also occur in perfectly healthy, fully acclimatized and physically conditioned individuals whenever the physical means of dissipating heat is exceeded by endogenous heat production.[1]

3. (G) All. (A) A person who is obese is much more likely to develop heat stroke under the same working conditions than a lean person. The cause is probably the added strain on the cardiovascular system, as discussed in D.

(B) Alcoholism in both the acute and chronic forms is a predisposing factor to heat stroke. An incidental point is that the comatose or delirious patient who has the odor of alcohol on his breath must not be shunted aside in the emergency department setting, especially if his skin is hot and dry, and his rectal temperature is high. Such a patient may die if he is not cooled promptly. Heat stroke must be recognized and treatment started; then studies to rule out concomitant infection and delirium tremens can be done.

(C) Anticholinergic drugs decrease sweating and thereby contribute to the development of heat stroke. These include atropine and its derivatives, as well as the phenothiazines, since most of these major tranquilizers have an anticholinergic effect.

(D) Since the prevention of heat stroke is directly related to the sustained response of the cardiovascular system to the stress of heat, it is logical that any compromise in this response would predispose to heat stroke. Also, any cardiovascular disease in a patient who suffers a heat stroke could jeopardize his survival.

In one series of 100 patients with heat stroke and over 12 years of age, 84% of patients had cardiovascular disease, and 30% admitted an alcoholic intake prior to onset of their heat stroke.[2]

(E) Diabetes mellitus and malnutrition are notable among the other chronic diseases that can predispose a person to heat stroke. Any chronically ill person who becomes hyperpyretic must be suspected of having a heat stroke. Any condition with fever, acute or chronic, predisposes the patient to heat stroke. Barbiturate poisoning in the patient's past may have damaged the sweat glands sufficiently to predispose to heat stroke.

(F) A previous heat stroke predisposes a person to heat stroke. The mechanism may be sweat-gland injury, even necrosis, at the time of the previous attack.[1]

4. (E) All. Both tachycardia (A) and wide pulse pressure (B) are usually present, as in this patient. They are due to high cardiac output (high circulatory demand) and low peripheral vascular resistance, problems that also occur in conditions involving tissue injury, such as trauma and sepsis.[3]

(C) Acute circulatory failure has preceded death in more than 80% of fatalities from heat stroke. Survival depends upon an adequate and sustained response of the cardiovascular system.

(D) Dilatation of the right side of the heart has been found regularly at autopsy. This enlargement accounts for the elevated CVP in patients with heat stroke, but whether the right-sided heart failure is due to a myocardial defect, or to elevated pulmonary vascular resistance, is not known.[3]

5. (A, B, D, F) (C) There is an increase in stroke volume, not a decrease. This increase, plus increased maximal cardiac output (A) and decreased peak heart rate (B), means more efficient delivery of heated blood from muscles and viscera to the body surface, where heat can be dissipated to the environment.[1]

(D) The sodium concentration of sweat is decreased by the action of aldosterone, which is produced and excreted into the urine in large amounts during acclimatization. Decreased sodium concentration in the sweat and increased aldosterone production are also seen in persons living in tropical environments; and there is evidence that increased production of aldosterone is necessary for the acclimatization process to occur.[1] These two changes, in addition to an increased (not decreased) volume of sweat (E), are physiological hallmarks of the heat-acclimatized state. However, there may be a reduction in the volume of perspiration after pronounced acclimatization, as a result of enhanced metabolic efficiency (F). This is a reflection of a lesser quantity of endogenous heat production under basal, as well as working, conditions.

One further change leading to acclimatization is an increase in the volume of extracellular fluid and plasma. These volumes may return to original values once complete acclimatization has occurred, probably as a result of the improved metabolic efficiency.

6. (A, B, C, D, E) Any delay in beginning the cooling of such a patient may be fatal. Thus, excuses for delay, such as the need to make a firm diagnosis, fear of damaging the patient's heart, the need to gather equipment or to get an ice bath ready, are intolerable. While necessary preparations are being made, a large fan can be directed at the almost totally exposed patient, cold water and ice can be applied to his trunk and extremities (A), and the skin of his trunk and extremities can be massaged to improve the peripheral circulation. As soon as possible, the patient should be placed in an ice water bath until his rectal temperature drops to 102°F (38.8°C) or 103°F (39.2°C). The cooling from that point on should be done more slowly to prevent making the patient hypothermic, since a further decrease in rectal temperature may not reflect a more rapid decrease in core temperature.

If shivering becomes a problem during the initial cooling process, the patient may be given a small dose of a phenothiazine, such as prochlorperazine, 10 to 15 mg intramuscularly for an adult and even smaller doses for the elderly and for a child.

(B) Cool intravenous fluid, usually Ringer's lactate, should be given cautiously, as it is possible for pulmonary edema to develop even without fluids having been given. The amount of intravenous fluid required to replace fluid lost in perspiration is approximately 1000 to 1500 ml in the first three to four hours.

This administration will contribute to core cooling, as will the administration of cold liquids by mouth, as soon as the patient is able to take them without the risk of vomiting.

(C) Massage of the skin is helpful in overcoming the stasis of dermal circulation that is usually present.

(D) Oxygen is mandatory in any patient who is unconscious due to heat stroke, to prevent anaerobic metabolism with accumulating lactic acid and to improve tissue oxygenation. It should be administered initially in high concentrations through a cuffed endotracheal tube, the tube having been inserted for this purpose, as well as to protect the airway in the event the patient vomits or has a seizure.

Usually, patients with heat stroke recover from coma within a few hours of prompt cooling if the circulation is well maintained.[4] The oxygen can then be administered by mask or nasal prongs at a lower concentration. Oxygen may improve cardiovascular function, which is vital to the cooling process; it may also protect vital organs from damage.

(E) All of the factors listed here should be monitored first, since all heat stroke patients, when first seen, are critically ill.

(F) Epinephrine, norepinephrine and all other stimulants are contraindicated, since they interfere with heat loss. These drugs cause peripheral vasoconstriction, which further decreases blood flow to the skin, where vasoconstriction is already preventing heat dissipation. They may also decrease blood flow to the already underperfused kidney and liver, and possibly to the brain. In short, such treatment is not only of no value, it will very likely make the patient worse. For failing circulation, isoproterenol may be titrated in a continuous intravenous infusion at the rate of 1 to 5 micrograms/minute (1.0 mg in 500 ml of 5% dextrose, in sterile water, produces a concentration of 2 micrograms/ml).

REFERENCES

1. Knochel, J.P.: Environmental heat illness. An eclectic review. Arch. Intern. Med. 133:841-864, 1974.

2. Austin, M.G. and Berry, J.W.: Observations on 100 cases of heat stroke. JAMA 161:1525-1529, 1956.

3. O'Donnell, T.F., Jr. and Clowes, G.H.A., Jr.: The

circulatory abnormalities of heat stroke. N. Eng. J. Med. 287:734-737, 1972.

4. Clowes, G.H.A., Jr. and O'Donnell, T.F., Jr.: Heat stroke. N. Eng. J. Med. 291:564-567, 1974.

::

CASE 5: STATUS EPILEPTICUS

HISTORY:

A 47-year-old woman was transferred from another general hospital, where she had had 30 convulsions during the previous 24 hours. She had progressed from postictal drowsiness to failure to regain consciousness between seizures. There was no known precipitating cause for this episode of seizures. She had had a seizure two and one-half years earlier. A fairly comprehensive work-up had been done with the following relevant information: negative physical findings; negative neurologic findings, except for an expressive aphasia and mental confusion, which gradually cleared; normal brain scan; electroencephalographic evidence of a focal left temporal slowing of uncertain significance; no abnormality on cerebral arteriography, done by bilateral common carotid injection; electrocardiography was within normal limits, except for sinus tachycardia of 120 per minute of unknown cause; and no evidence of infection or hyperthyroidism. She was placed on maintenance therapy of phenytoin and phenobarbital. The discharge diagnosis was probable thrombosis of the distribution of the left middle cerebral artery, with expressive and receptive aphasia and seizure disorder.

She did quite well for ten months and then developed ataxia. Phenytoin and phenobarbital levels were in the therapeutic range. Computerized cranial tomography showed a lucent area in the right frontal lobe, with contrast enhancement consistent with infarction in the area of the right anterior cerebral artery. The patient was unable to cooperate when a repeat of the test was tried; it was finally done under general anesthesia and showed no abnormalities.

Thereafter, she did well, although her ataxia continued, and she had no seizures until the beginning of the present illness. The present episode of seizure activity began with a chewing movement and twitching in the right side of the face, progressed to tonic and clonic movements of the right upper extremity and then to generalized seizures. As far as could be determined, she had not missed any doses of her anticonvulsant medication.

On admission to the first hospital, her temperature was 98.6°F (37.0°C) rectally; blood pressure, 170/94 mm Hg; pulse, 100 beats per minute; respirations, 20 per minute. General and neurologic examinations were negative, except for the postictal state. Her hemoglobin was 15.7 gm/dl and her white blood cell count, 15,700. Her blood glucose was 106 mg/dl. Despite the administration of diazepam, 5 mg intravenously every 4 hours, her seizures gradually became more frequent. The total intravenous dose of diazepam over the four hours preceding her transfer to the second hospital was 15 mg; that of intramuscular phenobarbital was 320 mg. Her temperature rose to 102.4°F (39.1°C) rectally, during those four hours. Nasal oxygen was started as soon as she failed to regain consciousness between convulsions.

Examination on arrival at the emergency department of the second hospital revealed an obese woman who was unconscious and having seizures, as described, about every 5 minutes, lasting 20 to 60 seconds each. Blood pressure was 150/100 mm Hg; temperature, 101.6°F (38.6°C) rectally; pulse, 110 per minute and regular; respirations, 20 per minute. She did not respond to painful stimuli. Plantar reflex was equivocal bilaterally. Otherwise, neurologic examination was within normal limits.

The initial impression was status epilepticus, focal right, of uncertain etiology. Treatment in the emergency department consisted of (1) diazepam, 10 mg by slow intravenous administration and repeated twice at 20-minute intervals; and (2) phenobarbital sodium, a total of 390 mg given intramuscularly in 2 divided doses. The result was control of most of her seizure activity. Although her blood glucose was normal (Dextrostix®), she was given 50 ml of 50% glucose intravenously, without noticeable improvement in her coma. Bag-valve-mask ventilation had been substituted for the nasal prongs as soon as she arrived. Endotracheal intubation, with cuffed tube, was accomplished promptly after the glucose was given, and there was no evidence that she had aspirated. She was admitted to the intensive care unit within one hour after her arrival.

LABORATORY DATA:

Urinalysis: negative
Hemoglobin: 18.2 gm/dl
Hematocrit: 52.6%
White blood cell count: 18,400/mm^3
Phenytoin blood level: 15 micrograms/ml
Arterial blood:
  PO_2: 95 torr (while on nasal oxygen, five liters/minute)
  PCO_2: 35 torr
  pH: 7.35

HCO_3^-: 18.9 mEq/1

Computerized axial tomography of the head, with infusion of contrast medium, showed no abnormalities.

Electroencephalography was technically unsatisfactory, but did show a left central spike and diffuse slowing, which suggested subclinical seizure activity, possibly on the basis of toxic encephalopathy.

Electrocardiography showed a sinus tachycardia of 114 beats per minute and no other abnormalities.

QUESTIONS:

TRUE OR FALSE (Questions 1-4):

1. There is no difference in the terms <u>seizure</u> and <u>convulsion.</u>

2. Status epilepticus refers only to generalized (tonic-clonic) convulsions.

3. Status epilepticus is more common in children than in adults.

4. In older children and adults, the most frequent cause of status epilepticus is abrupt discontinuation of anticonvulsant medication.

5. Which of the following statements are also true of status epilepticus?
   A. It is a true medical emergency.
   B. It occurs in 5 to 10% of children who have idiopathic epilepsy.
   C. It is more common with epilepsy of demonstrable cause than with idiopathic epilepsy.
   D. It may be the initial manifestation of certain diseases.
   E. Death or permanent neuronal damage may result if it is untreated or uncontrolled.
   F. Death occurs in approximately 15% of patients.
   G. All of the above

6. During repetitive seizures or status epilepticus, which of the following are potential causes of physical harm to the patient?
   A. Physical trauma, such as from falls
   B. Cerebral hypoxia
   C. Cardiac dysrhythmias, with or without heart failure

D. Metabolic acidosis, especially lactic acidosis
E. Exhaustion
F. Hyperpyrexia
G. All of the above

7. The initial pharmacologic approach to control of status epilepticus should consist of which of the following?
   A. Diazepam intravenously
   B. Phenytoin intravenously
   C. Phenobarbital intravenously or intramuscularly
   D. All of the above

8. Which of the following statements about diazepam are true, making it the drug of choice for treatment of status epilepticus?
   A. It is effective in stopping seizure activity.
   B. It can be given intravenously.
   C. It can be used safely for all ages.
   D. Given orally, it is a good anticonvulsant.
   E. Its anticonvulsant effect lasts for six to ten hours after intravenous administration.
   F. It can be given as an intravenous infusion after being mixed with 5% dextrose in water.
   G. All of the above

9. Which of the following characterizes phenytoin for its use in status epilepticus?
   A. Given intravenously, phenytoin sodium can achieve therapeutic blood levels in 15 minutes.
   B. In usual therapeutic doses, phenytoin causes little or no drowsiness.
   C. Given intramuscularly, phenytoin sodium's absorption is unpredictable.
   D. Phenytoin sodium may be given to patients with heart disease without concern for adverse reactions.
   E. Up to 1000 mg (15 mg/kg) may be given intravenously over a period of 25 to 45 minutes in most patients.
   F. All of the above

10. Which of the following statements about phenobarbital sodium for treatment of status epilepticus are true?
   A. It is superior to diazepam for initial control.
   B. It requires 15 to 20 minutes to reach peak blood concentrations when given intravenously.
   C. It may be used intravenously or intramuscularly.
   D. The usual total adult dose is 200 to 320 mg.
   E. The intramuscular dose for children in status epilepticus

is 3 to 5 mg/kg.

F. If combined with diazepam for control of status epilepticus, preparation must be made for airway and ventilation control, as well.

G. The therapeutic blood levels are 1 to 2 micrograms/ml.

H. All of the above

11. Which of the following laboratory studies are to be done as soon as possible after the patient in status epilepticus arrives?

A. Arterial blood gases and pH

B. Blood glucose

C. Electrolytes, especially sodium, calcium, and blood urea nitrogen

D. Drug screen, if there is clinical suspicion of drug abuse

E. Blood alcohol concentration, if there is suspicion of alcohol abuse

F. Urinalysis

G. Skull x-rays

H. Chest x-rays

I. Blood levels for anticonvulsants

J. Lumbar puncture with examination of cerebrospinal fluid

K. All of the above

ANSWERS AND COMMENTS:

1. (False) Convulsion implies a motor component, whereas a seizure may occur without movement. However, in practice, they are commonly used interchangeably.

In the emergency department, one should try to be as specific as the clinical situation permits, the term used being subject to confirmation by further clinical and laboratory evaluation, observation, and response to treatment.

Petit mal and grand mal are terms that are too broad to be clearly understood. Under the terminology recommended by the International League Against Epilepsy, the terms are now, respectively, simple absence seizures and tonic-clonic seizures.

About 90% of all seizures are of the tonic-clonic type.

2. (False) The term status epilepticus refers to the occurrence of at least two seizures, between which the patient fails to regain at least his former level of consciousness. The term is not restricted to tonic-clonic convulsions, but it is most serious

when it is of this type. The occurrence of two or more seizures in which the patient regains consciousness, following the usual postictal state, is termed serial or repetitive seizures, not status epilepticus.

3. (True) The pathophysiology of status epilepticus is not understood, but it is clear that the immature nervous system is particularly vulnerable to status epilepticus. In some series, as many as half of the children reported were less than three years of age.

4. (True) In the emergency department setting, the seizures seen, including status epilepticus, are usually in patients who have epilepsy and have abruptly discontinued their anticonvulsant medication. Other causes are intercurrent infection, not necessarily confined to the nervous system; metabolic disorders, such as hypoglycemia, hypocalcemia and hyponatremia; drugs, such as alcohol and phenobarbital, withdrawal from which causes status epilepticus; toxins, such as lead encephalopathy; occlusive cerebrovascular disease, which this patient probably had; hypertensive encephalopathy; hepatic and renal disease; head trauma; subarachnoid hemorrhage; and rarely, cerebral tumor.

5. (G) All. (A) Even in the busiest emergency department, very few emergencies take precedence over a patient having status epilepticus, regardless of his age. The patient is in coma, by the very definition of the disease, and has all the problems of the patient in coma, as well as the hazards of almost continuous seizures. The following steps to be taken (drug therapy will be discussed in a separate answer) are mostly self-explanatory and are the steps that are carried out in almost any comatose patient. They are listed more or less in order, but the team approach used in most busy emergency departments allows many of them to be carried out simultaneously:

a) Establish and maintain an airway
b) Prevent aspiration
c) Start at least one intravenous line, if one is not already running
d) Insert a padded tongue blade or other object between the patient's teeth to protect his tongue, lips, and teeth or dentures
e) Use restraints cautiously, to prevent injury to the patient and personnel
f) Assist ventilation by means of bag-valve-mask unit and intubate the trachea as soon as possible

g) Administer oxygen in high concentration
h) Establish adequate cardiovascular monitoring
i) Insert a Foley catheter to measure urine output every 30 to 60 minutes
j) Monitor vital signs every 15 to 30 minutes
k) Do a brief physical examination to determine possible causes of status epilepticus and other possible contributory, or associated, conditions
l) Administer 50 ml of 50% glucose intravenously
m) Correct any fluid and electrolyte imbalances
n) Recheck the neurologic status every 30 to 60 minutes
o) Do arterial blood gases and pH, and repeat as often as necessary

Airway control refers to whatever steps are necessary to prevent obstruction once the airway is opened. This control can be difficult while the patient is having a seizure, and in the interictal phase, any manipulation inside the mouth causes increased irritability and may actually precipitate another seisure. However, an oropharyngeal airway is usually suitable and is a must for the patient who is to be ventilated with a bag-valve-mask unit, preparatory to endotracheal intubation. It obviates the need for the traditional padded tongue blade, which may not be as helpful as we have always thought it to be. Aspiration is a constant threat, until the cuffed endotracheal tube is in place. High concentrations of oxygen, given by whatever means, are mandated by the invariable presence of lactic acidosis and hypoxemia. Monitoring of central venous pressure, urinary output and vital signs is required, and a Swan-Ganz catheter is indicated if serious dysrhythmias, or other evidence of cardiovascular or renal disease or fluid or electrolyte imbalance, are present.

The physical examination during status epilepticus is, of necessity, cursory, but it may provide leads to further studies or treatment procedures. One such procedure that should be done in any comatose patient is the administration of at least 50 ml of 50% glucose intravenously. One of the most common causes of seizures and of status epilepticus in the emergency department is hypoglycemia. It is curable by this harmless maneuver, which should never be omitted, since the penalty, if hypoglycemia is present, is permanent brain damage and possible death. Specific fluid and electrolyte abnormalities suspected or confirmed on initial screening tests should be corrected as rapidly as possible, since the seizure may not otherwise be controllable by any means.

Careful re-evaluation, from the clinical standpoint, should be noted on a flow sheet designed for this purpose. All too often, only the initial examination is reflected on the emergency department record, even when the patient spends one to four hours in the unit. This is inadequate guidance for the physicians who will continue the care of the patient and is of almost no medicolegal value. Serial determinations of arterial blood gases and pH are mandatory for monitoring the patient in status epilepticus.

(D) Two such conditions in which status epilepticus can be the earliest sign are meningitis and subarachnoid hemorrhage.

(E, F) The mortality rate in status epilepticus is about 15%, although in some series, including the very young and the very old, the rate is much higher. In those who survive, there is great likelihood of permanent brain damage because of anoxia, especially in the patients whose status epilepticus is not brought under control for several hours.

6. (G) All. (A) Much of the literature states that physical injuries are uncommon during convulsions, but this is not the situation as seen by most emergency department physicians. Patients are brought in with various injuries, from significant lacerations of the tongue (see Case 17) to head injuries that include extensive lacerations of the face, nose, ears and scalp, and injuries to other parts of the body. Fractures of the skull and facial bones, including the nasal bone, are not uncommon. Physical injuries are more likely to occur when convulsions are associated with drug abuse or withdrawal, including alcohol, but they occur in patients who have idiopathic epilepsy, as well. Falls from heights or other dangerous circumstances can cause serious injury or death.

(B) Cerebral hypoxia occurs in any patient who has an obstructed airway during a seizure. This is much more likely to happen in status epilepticus than in a single seizure or serial seizures. Such obstruction can be caused by accumulation of mucus or blood in the mouth, hypopharynx or glottis, or by regurgitation and aspiration (the latter especially when the seizures are associated with withdrawal from alcohol or other drugs, including poisoning or overdose).

(C) Cardiac dysrhythmias tend to occur in any seizure patient who has underlying cardiac disease, especially during the metabolic acidosis (D) that is common with most seizures. Certain drugs, such as tricyclic antidepressants, are known for their tendency to cause both cardiac dysrhythmias and seizures of the tonic-clonic type. Some children accidentally poisoned by these and similar drugs have life-threatening dysrhythmias with prolonged seizures; such children usually respond promptly to physostigmine salicylate. Heart failure and death may occur in older patients, or in those with underlying heart disease, if status epilepticus is prolonged for one or more hours. Exhaustion (E) and hyperpyrexia (F) occur when status epilepticus cannot be controlled or when the patient is not found within hours or days after the start of his seizures.

7. (D) All, if they are needed to control a single episode of status epilepticus or to prevent recurrence of isolated seizures or status epilepticus.

8. (A, B, C) Diazepam is not very effective in abolishing the focus of seizure activity, but it suppresses the propagation of the seizure impulse, itself, and thus very quickly stops the seizure activity. Diazepam is now the drug of choice for all types of status epilepticus. Used alone and in the proper dosage, it seldom causes any untoward effects, although respiratory depression, even apnea, and bradycardia with hypotension have been reported. These adverse effects can almost always be prevented if the diazepam is given no faster than 1 to 2 mg per minute, although an amount up to 5 mg per minute is usually safe. Diazepam acts rapidly and is the only presently available drug that can stop a seizure in its incipient stage of motor hyperexcitability. It will not prevent future seizures and its anticonvulsant effect lasts for only 30 to 60 minutes. If seizures recur after diazepam administration, there is some evidence that they will be harder to control. In any case, diazepam should always be followed by longer-acting drugs, either phenytoin sodium or phenobarbital, the former being preferred, since it is less likely to cause central nervous system and respiratory depression.

Diazepam should be given as an intravenous bolus, not placed in aqueous intravenous fluids to be used as a drip, since the solvent for the commercial parenteral preparation is a propylene glycol-ethanol-water mixture that does not disperse well. If intravenous administration is impossible, the same dose may be given intramuscularly, but the onset of action may therefore be delayed, an unacceptable alternative in status epilepticus. Diazepam is definitely not a good anticonvulsant when administered orally, and the side effect of drowsiness would make it prohibitive.

For patients who have been taking barbiturates regularly in

large doses, diazepam should be used with caution and possibly not at all, because the combination of drugs causes a dangerous depression of the central nervous and respiratory systems. If this combined use is necessary, the patient should probably be intubated first; all preparations should be made for controlled ventilation, possibly for hours.

For children up to 5 years of age, the intravenous dose is 0.3 mg/kg or 2 to 5 mg, or 1 mg/year of age in the 5- to 10-year age group. The adult dose is 5 to 10 mg; the injection is to be stopped in both children and adults as soon as control is achieved. However, there is something to be said for giving enough the first time, and 5 mg may not be enough for certain patients, as it was not for this patient. The dose may be repeated twice at 10- to 15-minute intervals, if necessary, for control of status epilepticus, with not more than 30 mg being given in the first hour. In some patients, 50 mg may be required in the first 12 to 24 hours, depending upon the cause of the status epilepticus. Some reports suggest that relatively larger doses are required if the patient has been taking phenytoin and phenobarbital regularly.

Although diazepam is metabolized in the liver and excreted in the kidneys, there are no significant hepatic or renal complications from its use in therapeutic amounts. No serious hematologic or other adverse effects have been noted. However, caution should be used in the administration of all anticonvulsant drugs in the presence of hepatic or renal disease.

9. (B, C, E) (A) Given intravenously, phenytoin can achieve therapeutic blood levels in one hour, but not in 15 minutes. Given orally, it takes effect too slowly (days are required to achieve therapeutic levels); given intramuscularly (C), it is unreliable due to poor water solubility and definitely is not satisfactory for control of status epilepticus.

Phenytoin has no hypnotic effect and does not interfere with further studies in a patient admitted to the hospital following an episode of status epilepticus (B). However, it must be administered intravenously, very cautiously, to patients with heart disease (D), as it may cause cardiovascular collapse and central nervous system depression when given too rapidly, even in normal patients.

It is difficult to decide how much phenytoin sodium to give a patient emerging from status epilepticus. The maximum rate is 50 mg/minute given in saline solution, not in water. The optimal blood level is from 10 to 20 micrograms/ml, and the concentration should be checked at least daily for several days to be certain that the maintenance dose is adequate to prevent any further seizures. If the patient is not already taking phenytoin, he should be given it intravenously in a full loading dose (E) as soon as the seizure activity is brought under control, either with diazepam, phenobarbital or both. However, if the history indicates, as in this patient, that phenytoin has been used for chronic control of seizures, the full loading dose may not be required as such; rather, supplementation in increments of 250 mg intravenously may be preferred until it is certain that control is adequate. Even for these smaller doses, the rate should not exceed 50 mg/minute.

10. (C, D, E, F) Phenobarbital eradicates the focus of seizure activity, which diazepam is not capable of doing. However, it is inferior to diazepam (A) for immediate control of status epilepticus, because it crosses the blood-brain barrier more slowly (20 minutes) and causes more sedation and more central nervous system and respiratory depression in the doses required to be effective. It also requires 30 to 45 minutes (not 15 to 20 minutes as stated in B) to reach peak blood concentrations, even when given intravenously. This allows enough overlap with the first dose of diazepam to prevent recurrence of seizure activity in most patients, but it does require nearly simultaneous administration of the two drugs. If initial control with diazepam is prompt, and provided phenytoin can be started immediately, it is best not to give phenobarbital at all during the acute episode. In that case, a second dose of diazepam may be required if the patient begins to show signs of agitation again, that is, before phenytoin has its full protective effect at about one hour after administration.

(G) The therapeutic blood levels are 5 to 15 (not 1 to 2) micrograms/ml. To obtain those levels, the adult dose of phenobarbital is 200 to 320 mg (D), given either intravenously or intramuscularly (C), or divided between the two routes. It must be given slowly (not exceeding 100 mg/min) when given intravenously. In children, because it depresses the respiratory and central nervous systems, phenobarbital is best given intramuscularly at 3 to 5 mg/kg (E). A full anticonvulsant dose should be used initially, since fractional doses may result in the paradoxical situation of drug-induced depression with continued status epilepticus in both children and adults. This is very likely the mechanism in the patient described. In any case, if phenobarbital has been used for chronic seizure control and if it is used in controlling the episode of status epilepticus and diazepam is also being used, the patient's ventilation may need to be controlled. It is assumed that the airway is being kept open at all times.

11. (K) All. Laboratory tests are difficult, if not impossible, to do while the patient is having a seizure. But, for that matter, so are the procedures needed for treatment, such as intravenous injections, endotracheal intubation, and restraining the patient to prevent self-injury or iatrogenic injury. Regardless of the difficulties involved, certain laboratory tests must be started as soon as the patient arrives. As discussed in answer 5, status epilepticus is a true medical emergency and a diagnosis must be made as quickly as possible. One of the main responsibilities of an emergency department physician is to anticipate the worst and prepare for all eventualities. One such eventuality is the possibility that a particular patient in status epilepticus will not respond to the usual treatment procedures, either because of an incorrect working diagnosis of the precipitating cause(s) or because of the incorrect treatment, such as the wrong drug or the wrong amount of a drug given, the wrong combination of drugs given or even the right drugs given in the wrong order. The most important aspect of using laboratory data early in status epilepticus is to prevent a treatable condition from being overlooked. Some of these treatable conditions include hypoglycemia, nonketotic hyperosmolar coma, hyponatremia, and hypocalcemia, as well as lead poisoning and other toxic encephalopathies, although these last ones are admittedly harder to treat. In infants and small children, pyridoxine dependency and certain aminoacidurias must be ruled out. The taking of insulin is not a prerequisite to hypoglycemic convulsions, since other causes of hypoglycemia are common, and hypoglycemic attacks often precede the onset of clinical diabetes mellitus. Convulsions resulting from hypocalcemia require prompt treatment. Convulsions may herald the onset of hypoparathyroidism; they may also accompany acute pancreatitis through the mechanism of hypocalcemia. Amylase in serum and urine should always be measured if the patient has a history suggestive of pancreatitis or has any upper abdominal tenderness. Hyponatremia usually occurs with water intoxication, which is very likely to cause seizures, including status epilepticus if the hyponatremia is severe (serum sodium less than 120 mEq/l).

Certain other tests should be done in most or all patients with status epilepticus, provided they have not been done recently. These include chest and skull x-rays, electroencephalography, radionuclide brain scan, and when a structural lesion is strongly suspected, cerebral arteriography and pneumoencephalography.

Where available, computerized cranial tomography (CCT scan) should be done on any patient who has a focal aspect to his seizure, although probably not on all patients with epilepsy. All patients over age 20 years who present with a first seizure should be evaluated by CCT scanning. As soon as it becomes more widely available, CCT scanning will replace many of the tests that are necessary now. However, in this patient, all tests, including CCT scan, failed to yield a definite diagnosis, even when combined with the history and physical findings.

Blood levels for anticonvulsants are useful, not only in chronic seizure control but also in the acute situation, to determine how much more medication is required to maintain control after the episode of status epilepticus has ended. Just how useful they will be depends upon the time required to receive a report. New methods of providing quicker results are becoming available, and these will certainly make the tests more helpful in clinical care.

Lumbar puncture, with examination of the spinal fluid, is necessary (if not contraindicated as by increased intracranial pressure) to rule out both meningitis and subarachnoid hemorrhage.

In patients who fail to respond to diazepam, phenytoin or phenobarbital, to any combination of these drugs, or to other measures, general anesthesia may be necessary to control status epilepticus. Definitive correction of the precipitating cause of the status epilepticus should be undertaken at the same time, if this is feasible.

COURSE:

The patient's temperature gradually subsided to normal over the next five days. No definitive cause of the fever was found. Lumbar puncture was done and the cerebrospinal fluid was clear, with 63 fresh red blood cells and 4 mononuclear white blood cells per cubic millimeter. Cerebrospinal fluid culture was negative. Her expressive aphasia appeared again as she gradually regained consciousness. Also, right-sided weakness was again noted, but gradually cleared over the next few days. She was discharged home, much improved, to continue her anticonvulsant therapy and with arrangements having been made for careful follow-up. Her final diagnosis was seizure disorder with status epilepticus of uncertain cause and mild hypertension.

::

CASE 6: FEVER IN A 5-YEAR-OLD BOY

HISTORY:

A 5-year-old boy was brought to the emergency department complaining of fever, sore throat, headache, and loss of appetite of 12 hours' duration. Otherwise, history was noninformative.

EXAMINATION:

His rectal temperature was 104°F (40.0°C); his pulse, 120/minute. There was hyperemia and enlargement of his tonsils with exudate present. Enlarged, tender regional lymph nodes were noted. The results of the remainder of the physical examination were negative.

QUESTIONS:

1. The most likely diagnosis in this patient is:
   A. Pharyngitis due to Group A beta hemolytic streptococcus
   B. Upper respiratory disease due to a virus
   C. Infectious mononucleosis
   D. Meningitis
   E. None of the above

2. Which of the following infections are due to Group A beta hemolytic streptococcus?
   A. Scarlet fever
   B. Erysipelas
   C. Impetigo contagiosa
   D. All of the above

3. TRUE OR FALSE: The most important noninfectious complications of streptococcal infections are rheumatic fever and glomerulonephritis.

4. Which of the following are infectious or pyogenic complications of Group A beta hemolytic streptococcus infections?
   A. Otitis media
   B. Pneumonia
   C. Meningitis
   D. Osteomyelitis
   E. Septicemia
   F. All of the above

ANSWERS AND COMMENTS:

1. (A) The reason that pharyngitis, due to Group A beta hemolytic streptococcus, is the most likely diagnosis is the presence of fever, exudate on the tonsils and regional adenopathy. However, one or more of those signs may be present in a patient five years of age with viral pharyngitis (B), although the combination of all three rules in favor of a bacterial cause. His having an elevated white blood cell count (above 10,000/mm^3) would have added to the assurance of a bacterial cause, but, again, in young children, leukocytosis can be present with viral infections, especially of the upper respiratory tract.

The definitive test is a throat culture. Controversy still exists as to whether a throat culture should be done routinely in patients such as this one, and if it is done, whether antibiotic treatment (see answer 3) should be delayed until the results are obtained, usually in 24 hours or less.

My own opinion is that the culture should be done in most instances. Whether treatment should be started immediately should probably be individualized. Even without a white blood cell count, it was the opinion of the pediatrician who saw this patient that treatment should be started immediately, and the patient was given a prescription for penicillin V potassium, 250 mg orally every six hours for a total of 10 days. The plan was to contact the patient's family and have the medication discontinued if the culture proved negative. Obviously that approach would not have been appropriate if long-acting penicillin was to have been administered, since the decision to start that drug must be made before the culture report is available or the patient must be called back for treatment to begin.

The throat culture from this patient was positive for Group A beta hemolytic streptococcus. His recovery was complete from the clinical standpoint, although no attempt was made to grow a second culture. Indeed, such a repeat culture is almost never justified if clinical recovery occurs.

Group A beta hemolytic streptococcus is the one to be concerned about in pharyngitis, since Group C and Group G only rarely produce symptoms. Other bacteria probably do not cause significant infection of the upper respiratory tract. In order words, if the culture from a patient with pharyngitis grows other gram-positive or gram-negative organisms, they probably are not causative and the infection, in most such instances, is of viral origin. One exception is Corynebacterium diphtheriae, which causes diphtheria, now rare in the United States. Another exception is Neisseria gonorrheae, an increasingly common organism in older children and adults. Gonococcal pharyngitis should be treated according to the guidelines of the Center for Disease Control (CDC), which are the same as those for treatment of genitourinary and anal gonococcal infection: aqueous procaine penicillin G, 4.8 million units intramuscularly, and probenecid, 1.0 gram orally. However, the schedules for ampicillin and spectinomycin are not adequate for gonococcal pharyngitis, which is usually more difficult to cure than gonorrheal infection at other locations.

(B) Virtually all known viruses can cause acute respiratory disease, and many of them have an effect mainly, or only, on the respiratory tract. The most common viral cause of pharyngitis is adenovirus, most often type 3.

(C) Infectious mononucleosis is not mutually exclusive with streptococcal pharyngitis, since many patients have both diseases. However, there was no clinical evidence of infectious mononucleosis in this patient.

(D) Meningitis must be considered in any patient with these findings, and it is a possible complication of any streptococcal infection. However, there was no clinical indication of that condition in this patient. Group B streptococcus is a cause of meningitis as well as of sepsis in neonates (the first month of life).

Meningitis should be ruled out in any child who has a fever without obvious cause and without localizing signs. The disease is not manifested in children by the usual classical physical signs found in older patients. If there is any doubt about the diagnosis, spinal tap is indicated. If the tap is negative and the symptoms persist, the tap may need to be repeated after 24 to 36 hours. Diagnosis is made and treatment dictated by the examination of the spinal fluid.

2. (D) Scarlet fever (A) represents Group A beta hemolytic streptococcal pharyngitis, plus a skin rash. The rash is due to susceptibility to the erythrogenic toxin and appears 12 to 48 hours after the onset of fever. Treatment is the same as for streptococcal pharyngitis (see answer 3).

(B) Erysipelas is a rapidly spreading cellulitis caused by Group A beta hemolytic streptococcus. Diagnosis can be made by gram stain and culture of material swabbed or aspirated from the leading edge of the involved area of skin.

(C) Impetigo contagiosa is caused by either Group A beta hemolytic streptococcus or staphylococcus. In neonates, staphylococcus is usually the cause. In children over one month of age, it is safer to assume streptococcal origin until proved otherwise by culture, because the complications are more severe in most instances. Treatment consists of washing and rupturing all lesions and giving a systemic antibiotic, preferably penicillin or erythromycin. A topical antibiotic is not usually necessary, and there is considerable risk of causing sensitization. For suspected or proved staphylococcal cause, treatment with a semisynthetic penicillin derivative that is penicillinase-resistant is advisable.

3. (True) The Group A beta hemolytic streptococcus is the only organism that results in those two complications, the full discussion of which is beyond the scope of this case study.

Rheumatic fever is relatively common even now, in that there are approximately 100, 000 new cases diagnosed each year in the United States alone. The prevention of rheumatic fever requires eradication of the organism, not simply suppression of the symptoms. Eradication requires continuation of the medication for at least ten days if given orally, or the administration of a long-lasting penicillin in sufficient dosage to maintain a therapeutic level for a minimum of ten days (e. g., penicillin G benzathine, administered intramuscularly in the amount of 600, 000 units for children weighing less than 60 pounds, and 1, 200, 000 units for all persons weighing 60 pounds or more).

For patients who are sensitive to penicillin, erythromycin or cephalexin, 250 mg of either, every six hours for ten days, should be prescribed. Tetracycline and sulfonamides should not be used.

Contacts within the family should be treated if they are symptomatic, since at least 25% of them will contract a streptococcal infection. Confirmation by culture again is desirable but not mandatory, provided the primary patient had a culture-proved diagnosis.

Only about one in twenty-five untreated patients with streptococcal pharyngitis develop rheumatic fever. Rheumatic fever may be dependent upon repeated infection, in contrast to glomerulonephritis, which may follow a single streptococcal infectious episode.

4. (F) All require early diagnosis and treatment, if possible.

::

CASE 7: SALICYLATE POISONING

HISTORY:

A 26-month-old girl was seen in the emergency department with a history of having taken adult aspirin, possibly as many as 15 tablets (4.5 grams). She had vomited six times at home, but the parents could identify no tablets in her vomitus, a finding that suggested that all tablets had been dissolved, if not absorbed.

EXAMINATION:

The patient weighed 28 pounds (12.8 kg). Her rectal temperature was 100.2°F (39°C); her pulse, 126 per minute; her respirations, 40 per minute. She was hyperpneic, perspiring, and appeared drowsy. No other abnormalities were noted.

LABORATORY DATA:

<u>Serum acetylsalicylic acid</u>: 65.1 mg/dl (therapeutic level: 2-10 mg/dl)
<u>Complete blood cell count</u>: normal (WBC - 12,500 with 66 neutrophils and 3 bands)
<u>Urinalysis</u>: normal except for large amounts of ketones and a positive ferric chloride test
<u>Serum electrolytes</u>:
Sodium: 148 mEq/l
Chloride: 104 mEq/l
Potassium: 3.6 mEq/l
Bicarbonate: 14 mEq/l
<u>Blood urea nitrogen</u>: 12 mg/dl
<u>Blood glucose</u>: 120 mg/dl

QUESTIONS:

1. Which of the following statements about salicylates are true?
   A. They comprise four compounds: salicylic acid, methyl salicylate (oil of wintergreen), sodium salicylate, and acetylsalicylic acid (aspirin).
   B. Aspirin is the most extensively used analgesic, antipyretic and anti-inflammatory agent on the market.
   C. Aspirin has a wide margin of safety and may be used by both children and adults, with little or no supervision by physicians.

D. Chronic excessive dosage, or acute overdosage of aspirin, can endanger life.
E. All of the above

2. TRUE OR FALSE: Generally, the correlation between the serum level of salicylate and the clinical picture is excellent.

3. Which of the following symptoms and signs are likely to be present in salicylate toxicity?
A. Hyperpnea
B. Fever
C. Sweating
D. Dehydration
E. Vomiting
F. Restlessness, irritability, delirium and convulsions
G. Tetany
H. Drowsiness or coma
I. All of the above

4. TRUE OR FALSE: Any patient seen shortly after ingestion of massive doses of salicylates will be hyperventilating with respiratory alkalosis.

5. The dangerous metabolic acidosis seen in intoxicated patients is produced by which of the following mechanisms?
A. Derangement of carbohydrate metabolism
B. Displacement of plasma bicarbonate by salicylic acid derivatives
C. Impairment of renal function
D. Inadequate ventilation with a rise in PCO_2 and fall in pH
E. All of the above

6. TRUE OR FALSE: Administration of the specific antidote for salicylate intoxication is the first step in treatment.

7. Additional emergency measures that might be useful include which of the following?
A. Intravenous fluids
B. Monitoring of arterial blood pH and gases
C. Sodium bicarbonate
D. Artificial ventilation and oxygen
E. Glucose in all intravenous fluids
F. Activated charcoal orally
G. Sponging the child with tepid water
H. Forced alkaline diuresis
I. Potassium administration
J. All of the above

8. In patients who fail to respond to the measures listed in question 7, extrarenal clearance measures that have proved useful include:
   A. Exchange transfusion
   B. Hemodialysis
   C. Peritoneal dialysis
   D. Hemoperfusion
   E. All of the above

ANSWERS AND COMMENTS:

1. (A, B, D) (A) Salicylic acid is very irritating and is normally used only externally, mainly as a keratolytic agent. Methyl salicylate (oil of wintergreen) is normally used only as a cutaneous counterirritant in the form of salves and liniments. It is highly toxic when used in excess, the ointment having produced 13 known deaths by percutaneous absorption.[1] It is also highly toxic when ingested, one teaspoonful being equivalent to 21 aspirin tablets. Unfortunately, it has a sweetish odor that children love, and they will eat or drink it if given the chance. Methyl salicylate may remain in the stomach for hours and continue to be absorbed for days or until it is removed. As little as 4 ml taken orally may be fatal in small children. Goodman and Gilman[2] state that, "Hospitalization is particularly advisable in the case of methyl salicylate poisoning, because children have been known to succumb within a few hours after the parents had been informed that recovery seemed assured or that the intoxication was inconsequential." Sodium salicylate and aspirin are the two most commonly used salicylate preparations for systemic effects.

Besides being the most extensively used agent for the purposes listed in B, aspirin is the most common offender in accidental poisoning. The incidence of this tragedy has decreased considerably in the last decade, with the advent of safety closures and the limitation on package size of baby aspirin, but it is still far too high. Aspirin is <u>not</u> safe to use without careful supervision by a physician and considerable patient education as to what it can do and what its dangers are (C, D). For example, most patients who take aspirin for chronic conditions, such as arthritis, do not seem to know the risks involved in a self-prescribed increase in daily dosage. Renal excretion does not increase proportionately, and toxic symptoms appear after a few days. In infants, this approach on the part of the parents has accounted for acute toxicity; and the cumulative effect of a slightly higher-than-usual dose has caused at least one death in a two-week-old child.[1]

2. (False) It is possible to have high blood levels of salicylate and relatively few symptoms and signs of toxicity. On the other hand, it is possible to have severe toxicity with salicylate levels as low as 15 mg/dl, especially in infants and small children, and especially with chronic overdosage. Frequently, there may be a relatively good correlation; for instance, in this patient, there were a slight to moderate elevation in the salicylate blood level and relatively few symptoms or signs.

The average toxic dose of sodium salicylate and of aspirin is 150 to 200 mg/kg (or 1.92 to 2.56 grams in a patient this size). From 10 to 30 grams have caused death in adults, with the mean lethal dose being 20 to 30 grams. On the other hand, Goodman and Gilman[2] have reported the ingestion of up to 130 grams by one patient, without a fatal outcome.

3. (I) All. The hyperpnea (A) of even mild salicylate intoxication occurs early, due to direct stimulation of the respiratory center with resultant respiratory alkalosis (low PCO_2 and higher than normal arterial blood pH). In younger children and in all patients with severe intoxication, this hyperpnea is replaced by a secondary or compensatory hyperpnea caused by a severe metabolic acidosis, as described in the answers to questions 4 and 5.

Fever (B) is frequently quite high. It accelerates dehydration, and dehydration potentiates hyperpyrexia. A vicious cycle is set up in small children who have chronic overdosage and are given more aspirin to reduce fever that was caused or made worse by the aspirin in the first place. The fever in acute salicylate intoxication results from an increase in heat production, coupled with a decrease in the efficiency of the normal cooling mechanisms. Severe hyperthermia is a common cause of death in salicylate intoxication.

Sweating (C) is not only a useful sign in making the diagnosis, but it is the mechanism used by the body to attempt to maintain the delicate balance between heat production and heat dissipation. The evaporation of water from the skin augments the cooling process, but for the mechanism to work, sweat must be available, and this may not be the case in the patient severely dehydrated by fever. Thus, dehydration (D) is a serious threat to the life of the patient (particularly a child) who has taken a moderately large dose of salicylate. Shock and acute renal failure can occur. Maintenance fluid therapy should be increased by 25 to 50% to correct the dehydration and to allow enough urine formation to promote diuresis.

Vomiting (E) tends to occur early, and this may be life-saving in many patients. However, the electrolytes and fluid lost must be replaced as soon as possible, even in the emergency department, while more vomiting is being produced with syrup of ipecac or more fluid is being removed by gastric lavage.

Restlessness, irritability, delirium, and convulsions (F) may be quite a problem in the management of these patients, both adults and children. The central nervous system stimulation is a direct effect, as was mentioned in connection with the initial hyperpnea. It later changes to central nervous system depression and coma (H); in the presence of metabolic acidosis, coma is a dangerous complication.

Tetany (G) is a manifestation of hyperventilation and of the administration of alkali. If it appears, it is easily treated with calcium gluconate, given intravenously.

4. (False) While this is true of adults (although a metabolic acidosis soon overwhelms the respiratory alkalosis), this early alkalosis is so short-lived in children that it will rarely be seen. Therefore, most children brought to the emergency room with salicylate intoxication will be hyperventilating but will be in a metabolic acidotic state. The hyperventilation (Kussmaul respiration) at this stage is essential to life. If it decreases spontaneously or is reduced by ill-advised administration of bicarbonate, the PCO_2 will rise, and the blood pH will drop to levels incompatible with survival. The guidance of arterial blood pH and gases is vital for management of patients with severe toxicity.

5. (A, B, C) It is important to understand the mechanism of acidosis, since it results in a shift of salicylate from plasma into the brain and other tissues. Death may result from the high concentrations of salicylate in the brain, so avoidance or correction of the salicylate-induced metabolic acidosis must be a primary therapeutic goal. Derangement of carbohydrate metabolism (A) is the primary cause of this acidosis. Synthesis of carbohydrates decreases and utilization of glucose increases because of the vomiting and the increased metabolic rate; the result is depletion of liver glycogen, which, in turn, results in fat mobilization and conversion to ketone bodies for energy utilization. As they are formed in excess of tissue utilization and renal excretion, these acetoacetic acid ions represent unmeasured acids in the extracellular fluid. In addition, pyruvic and lactic acids accumulate because of faulty aerobic carbohydrate metabolism.

Salicylate, itself, is an acid, and at the pH of plasma, it displaces up to 2 to 3 mEq/l of bicarbonate (B). This acidosis is further augmented by impairment of renal function (C), which is caused by dehydration, direct vasomotor depression, and a direct toxic effect of salicylate on the kidney. Renal impairment can result in the accumulation of sulfuric and phosphoric acids; the result of all of these mechanisms is the increased production of various acids in a patient whose defenses against acidosis are impaired by pre-existing depletion of his buffering capacity and impairment of his renal function. Small children are more likely to experience these deleterious effects than are older children and adults. Respiratory acidosis, not metabolic acidosis, is caused by inadequate ventilation (D).

6. (False) Unfortunately, there is no specific antidote for salicylate intoxication. Treatment is largely supportive, with first attention being paid to removal or elimination of the poison from the body. This is best accomplished, in most instances, by syrup of ipecac given orally, followed by one to three cups or glasses of water. The syrup of ipecac may be repeated once in 20 minutes, if necessary. The water is important, since syrup of ipecac will not work as well on an empty stomach. Ten to fifteen milliliters is the correct dose for children, although a smaller amount may be used for infants. Fifteen to thirty milliliters is the correct dose for adults. If the patient fails to vomit after the second dose (and he may if he has also taken an overdose of an antiemetic drug, such as a phenothiazine or an antihistamine), the syrup of ipecac should be recovered by gastric lavage. It is usually advisable to follow this emesis routine even if the patient has already vomited, since the history of vomiting at home or en route to the emergency department may not be entirely accurate. If syrup of ipecac cannot be administered for some reason, gastric lavage is preferable to giving apomorphine to a patient who may already be drowsy and is becoming even drowsier. If the patient is comatose, endotracheal intubation, with a snug-fitting tube for children under eight or nine years of age and with a cuffed endotracheal tube for older children and adults, must be done to prevent aspiration of the vomitus.

This patient was given ipecac syrup 7.5 ml orally, which caused three additional episodes of vomiting starting within 15 minutes; again, no pills were visible.

7. (J) All. These are given for the following purposes: (A) to correct dehydration and electrolyte imbalance; (B) to detect and (C) to correct severe metabolic acidosis; (D) for respira-

tory depression; (E) to correct or prevent hypoglycemia and to correct ketosis, which may clear only very slowly; (F) to bind any salicylate remaining in the gastrointestinal tract; (G) to reduce fever; (H) to speed up renal excretion of salicylate; and (I), along with (C) and (E), to prevent further depletion of intracellular potassium. Most patients will improve and survive even massive poisoning if these procedures are carried out promptly. But this care is still mainly supportive and best carried out in an intensive care unit. The guidance of an excellent laboratory is mandatory, specifically one that can provide arterial blood pH and gases at any hour of the day and night for the most severe cases of salicylate poisoning.

8. (E) All. It has been said that any poisoned or intoxicated patient who lives long enough to arrive in an emergency department should ultimately recover. Though this may be somewhat optimistic, it is true that patients are presently recovering from a severity of poisoning or overdosage that would have been fatal a few years ago. The techniques listed in the question form the basis for this optimism.

Exchange transfusion (A) works best in infants less than one year of age and with salicylate or barbiturate intoxication of severe degree.

Hemodialysis (B) is reserved for patients who are not responding to lesser measures, except for patients who have ingested ethylene glycol, methanol or heavy metals; for these, hemodialysis should be considered as a primary or early method of treatment. This emphasizes, again, the importance of identifying the type and amount of drug or other substance that the patient has taken, or otherwise been exposed to, as soon as possible. Hemodialysis is especially helpful in patients with renal failure or serious impairment of liver function.

Each year it is being found that more and more drugs and substances can be removed from the body by the newer techniques available. The lists vary according to the experience of the dialysis unit, but up-to-date information is available on any identified or suspected drug or substance from your nearest Poison Control Center.

Peritoneal dialysis (C) is available in many more locations than hemodialysis and should be used if transfer to a hemodialysis unit is not possible. However, peritoneal dialysis is far less effective in most of the severe cases of poisoning. Salicylate poisoning usually responds to the treatment regimen outlined in question 7, but if complications, such as renal failure, develop, dialysis may be life-saving, especially in a small child with a serious degree of poisoning.

Hemoperfusion (D) is a new concept and technique for removing drugs early in the course of an intoxication. It may be effective for some of the drugs that do not respond to present techniques of dialysis.

COURSE:

This particular patient's response was prompt, and supportive therapy allowed rapid removal of the salicylate. Intravenous fluid, 5% dextrose in 0.2% saline, was started and continued at a calculated 2500 ml/m^2/day. The first liter of this fluid contained 30 mEq of potassium chloride, as well. No sodium bicarbonate was administered, since the plasma bicarbonate concentration was down to only 14 mEq/l. Within one hour, the test for ferric chloride in the urine was negative. No record can be found on the chart of arterial blood pH and gases having been measured, or of a second measurement of serum levels of salicylate. The patient became more alert shortly after admission and by the following day was back to her usual mental alertness and activity. Her temperature was 100.4^{o}F at 24 hours after admission, but was normal thereafter, and she was allowed to return home 40 hours after she was first brought to the emergency department.

REFERENCES

1. Arena, J.M.: Poisoning, Toxicology, Symptoms, Treatments, 3rd Edition. Springfield: Charles C Thomas, 1974.

2. Goodman, L.S. and Gilman, A.: The Pharmacological Basis of Therapeutics, 5th Edition. New York: Macmillan Publishing Co., 1975, p. 336.

::

CASE 8: CHEST PAIN, DYSPNEA, BLOODY SPUTUM

HISTORY: A 30-year-old woman reported to the emergency department with chest pain on the left side and dyspnea of three days' duration. She had noted a small blood clot in her sputum the day before.

The patient had had two episodes of pulmonary embolism in the past. The first had occurred 14 months before and she had been started on long-term warfarin therapy. The second one occurred seven months later; there was some question about whether she had been taking warfarin as regularly as instructed.

She had had asthma since childhood and had frequently had similar chest pain during asthmatic attacks.

She had been taking oral contraceptives intermittently for eight years. She had taken medication in the past for mild hypertension, but had not recently renewed her prescription.

She had never experienced documented acute thrombophlebitis but usually had calf pain and tenderness at the onset of her menstrual period. The last period had started one day before admission.

Physical examination revealed an obese woman in no distress. Her blood pressure was 144/84 mm Hg; pulse, 96/minute and regular; respirations, 20/minute and not labored; temperature, 98.6°F (37.0°C). There was bilateral expiratory wheezing, with some rhonchi. Both calves were tender but not swollen, and Homan's sign was absent bilaterally.

QUESTIONS:

1. The most likely diagnosis in this patient is:
   A. Pulmonary embolism
   B. Acute asthmatic attack
   C. Pleural effusion
   D. Pneumonitis
   E. Spontaneous pneumothorax
   F. Pulmonary edema
   G. Myocardial infarction
   H. Air embolism

2. In addition to the findings in this case, which of the following

are common with pulmonary embolism?
- A. Cough and syncope
- B. Peripheral venous thromboembolism
- C. History of recent operation, trauma, pregnancy, or prolonged bed rest
- D. Chills and fever
- E. Cardiac signs, such as tachycardia, accentuation of the second pulmonic sound, protodiastolic gallop, loud systolic murmur, hypotension
- F. Pulmonary signs, such as rales, pleural friction rub, signs of consolidation
- G. All of the above

3. For confirmation, what laboratory tests may be necessary for this patient?
   - A. Electrocardiogram
   - B. Arterial blood gases and pH
   - C. Pulmonary radionuclide scan
   - D. Pulmonary arteriography
   - E. Bronchoscopy
   - F. All of the above

TRUE OR FALSE (Questions 4-6):

4. Pulmonary embolism is the most common lethal pulmonary disorder.

5. Sudden chest pain and dyspnea are common in patients with pulmonary embolism.

6. Hemoptysis is common in patients with pulmonary embolism.

7. Which of the following statements are true about venous thrombosis as it relates to pulmonary embolism?
   - A. Less than 50% of deep venous thrombi in the lower extremities are clinically detectable.
   - B. Phlebothrombosis is much more dangerous than thrombophlebitis.
   - C. The most dangerous emboli arise from the veins of the thigh.
   - D. Pelvic veins are a common site of origin of massive pulmonary embolism.
   - E. The upper extremities contribute substantially to the problem of pulmonary embolism.
   - F. Significant embolic phenomena frequently arise from thrombophlebitis of the superficial veins of the legs.
   - G. All of the above

8. Immediate management of this patient should entail:
   A. Inferior vena caval interruption
   B. Pulmonary artery embolectomy
   C. Heparin therapy
   D. Isoproterenol therapy
   E. Dopamine therapy
   F. Oxygen therapy

ANSWERS AND COMMENTS:

1. (A) Pulmonary embolism is the most likely diagnosis. It is possible that an acute exacerbation of her asthma (B) could account for the symptoms, especially since she had experienced substernal or lateral chest pain with most of her attacks. However, there was no history of a flare-up of her asthma during the three days of her present illness. Other factors making pulmonary embolism the most likely diagnosis are the history of two previous episodes of pulmonary embolism, her use of oral contraceptives, and her obesity. The main point against this diagnosis is the fact that she was taking warfarin. However, she had already experienced one documented pulmonary embolus while taking the drug.

The next three conditions (C, D, E) are less likely, although pneumothorax is a condition that must always be considered in patients with chest pain. The infiltrate of pneumonitis is often difficult to differentiate from that of pulmonary infarction or the congestive atelectasis that is sometimes present with pulmonary embolism. This patient's chest roentgenogram was normal.

(F) Pulmonary edema must be differentiated from pulmonary embolism, but it must be remembered that pulmonary embolism may be the underlying cause of pulmonary edema. One must be careful not to do a phlebotomy on a patient whose pulmonary edema might be secondary to massive pulmonary embolism, since the procedure may cause a fall in blood pressure sufficient to be disastrous.

(G) Acute cor pulmonale develops within a few minutes of a massive pulmonary embolism and must be differentiated from inferior myocardial infarction. Marriott's aphorism is helpful at times: If you find yourself diagnosing inferior myocardial infarction from the limb leads, and anteroseptal infarction from the chest leads, think of pulmonary embolism (see question and answer 3A). CPK isoenzymes may be helpful in distinguishing myocardial infarction from pulmonary embolism, since, in the latter, CPK isoenzymes are usually not elevated unless there is associated myocardial damage.

(H) Air embolism is a complication of surgical procedures or an accident occurring any time an intravenous line is left open, allowing ingress of air. It can sometimes be distinguished from thromboembolism by precordial Doppler monitoring, but it does not show up well, if at all, on roentgenograms.

2. (A, B, C, E, F) (A) Cough occurs in at least half of all patients who are found to have pulmonary embolism. Syncope is the initial event in some patients with massive emboli, but is rare with smaller emboli.

(B) History and findings of peripheral venous thromboembolism should always be sought, but their absence does not rule out pulmonary embolism (see question and answer 7).

(C) Any patient who has recently undergone a major operation, has sustained trauma, is pregnant or early postpartum, or has been confined to bed is much more likely to develop peripheral thrombosis and complicating pulmonary embolization.

(D) Fever usually occurs at the time the pulmonary embolus develops but usually subsides promptly. If infection supervenes, several days are usually required before it becomes manifest clinically. Chills are not common with this disease unless complicated by extensive infarction of lung parenchyma with secondary infection (pneumonitis).

(E, F) Careful search usually reveals cardiopulmonary evidence of an acute process, Increased loudness of the pulmonic second sound and a pulmonic insufficiency murmur are related to acute pulmonary hypertension, which may develop in association with pulmonary embolism. Hypotension occurs in massive pulmonary embolization; these are the patients who die within one to two hours despite treatment (see question and answer 4). Pulmonary signs are absent unless pulmonary infarction has occurred. Since the infarct is usually located peripherally, there is frequently a pleuritic type of pain and an associated pleural friction rub. Rales can frequently be heard in areas of congestive atelectasis, as well as signs of consolidation if the infarct is fairly large.

3. (A, B, C, D) Routine admission laboratory studies should also be done, as well as prothrombin time and activated partial thromboplastin time. Both of these tests were in the low therapeutic range of the oral anticoagulant this patient was taking,

findings that rule against pulmonary embolism as the diagnosis but that do not rule it out. Her blood platelet count was also normal, as were her blood enzyme studies.

(A) An electrocardiogram should be done so that acute and chronic myocardial disease can be ruled out or detected, and changes suggestive of pulmonary embolism can be looked for. These changes are those of acute cor pulmonale: (1) a deep S wave in lead I, prominent Q wave in lead III, and inverted T waves in leads III and V_{1-4}; (2) occasional P-wave changes, usually in the form of a tall P wave in lead II; (3) right axis deviation with moderate to large embolism, and prominent R waves over the right precordium; and (4) transient right bundle branch block. Despite these changes, the electrocardiogram is diagnostic in only about 25% of patients with pulmonary embolism. Therefore, it, alone, is not a reliable test for this disease entity, but is useful only as an adjunct to other tests. This patient's electrocardiogram was noninformative, showing only nonspecific S-T and T-wave changes.

(B) Arterial blood gases and pH should be measured in every patient such as this. Hypoxemia is a characteristic finding, although it is not invariably present. This patient's PaO_2 was 74 torr, definitely lower than the normal level for her age. Her $PaCO_2$ was 33 torr and arterial pH was 7.46, findings of mild respiratory alkalosis caused, in this instance, by hyperventilation. These changes are also found in patients having an asthmatic attack. It is not known why patients with pulmonary embolism have hypoxemia, but the finding is very helpful, indicating that further studies should be done.

(C) Pulmonary radionuclide scanning should be done at this point. In this patient, it showed patchy, non-segmental, bilateral perfusion defects with no corresponding infiltrates on the chest roentgenogram. As this could have represented either obstructive airway disease or pulmonary emboli, a ventilation scan was then in order, but, for technical reasons, could not be done at that time. Four days later, pulmonary radionuclide scanning was repeated and ventilation scanning was done. The perfusion scan revealed no defect on the right side and only a small defect in the left middle lung field, compatible with pulmonary embolism. The ventilation scan was normal.

A positive perfusion scan only indicates that an area is avascular; a negative scan rules out most pulmonary emboli. A positive scan in a patient whose chest roentgenogram is negative is highly suggestive of embolism. The same is true in the patient whose chest roentgenogram shows increased radiolucency in an area of positive scan.

(D) If further testing is required, pulmonary arteriography is the definitive test. In this patient, it was not considered necessary.

(E) Bronchoscopy was not indicated in this patient, and is not necessary for the diagnosis of pulmonary embolism, although it may be useful in detecting the site of bleeding in a patient with hemoptysis. The small amount of blood in this patient's sputum was thought to come from her gingivae, which sometimes bled while she was taking warfarin.

4. (True) Death, if it is to occur from pulmonary embolism, occurs rapidly. Large embolization of the pulmonary artery is usually fatal within a few minutes to a few hours. In fact, two-thirds of the deaths due to massive pulmonary embolism occur within the first hour. However, repeated minor embolization to the lungs occurs and is usually not diagnosed in life, as evidenced by autopsy series.

5. (True) Chest pain occurs in 75%, and dyspnea occurs in 80% of all patients with pulmonary embolism. These were the chief symptoms in this patient. The chest pain may be pleuritic, but only in patients with pulmonary infarction; it may be anginal, with no definite relation to pre-existing coronary disease. It is usually a vague, poorly localized discomfort, and it may be transient.

Sudden dyspnea in the absence of obvious evidence of cardiac or pulmonary disease is characteristic of pulmonary embolism. Thus, it is a diagnostic clue, provided emotional causation can be ruled out. Mild wheezing may be all that is noted, unless pulmonary edema is precipitated by the pulmonary embolus. Any patient with sudden onset of pulmonary edema should be suspected of having single or multiple pulmonary embolization.

Dyspnea in the patient who has obvious cardiac disease or pulmonary disease, or both, is much less informative. In these patients, special studies are always required when pulmonary embolism is suspected.

6. (False) Hemoptysis occurs in only about one-third of patients with pulmonary embolism - that third who also have pulmonary infarcts. Therefore, one should never rule out the possibility of pulmonary embolism in a patient with sudden onset of dyspnea solely because hemoptysis is not present.

7. (A, C) (A) With more sophisticated techniques for demonstrating venous thrombosis, such as impedance phlebography, Doppler ultrasound testing, radioactive fibrinogen testing and venography, it is now obvious that physical examination fails to reveal at least 50% of the venous thrombi of the lower extremities. In practical terms, then, even if tests for venous thrombi of the lower extremities are negative, it must be remembered that the lower extremity veins are still the most likely embolic source.

(B) Formerly, it was thought that emboli were much more likely to arise from phlebothrombosis (or bland thrombus) than from thrombophlebitis, which is thrombosis associated with inflammation. The inflammation, it was thought, tended to anchor the clot firmly to the intima of the veins, preventing it or any part of it from breaking loose. Now, we believe that the inflammation is secondary to the thrombus and that there is little, if any, significant difference in the types of thrombosis, insofar as their embolic potential is concerned.

(C) The thrombi that develop in the large veins of the thigh are indeed the most dangerous. The reasons are not clear, except that these thrombi are large, and thus are more likely to cause death upon lodging in the pulmonary artery or its major branches. It may be that since they are larger, they are also more likely to fragment or break loose. Conversely, it is possible that thrombi in the leg veins, besides being smaller and less dangerous, are less likely to embolize or more likely to resolve.

(D) The pelvic veins, formerly thought to be a common source of pulmonary emboli, are now known to be an uncommon source, possibly for the reasons given in (C), mentioned previously.

(E) For reasons not known, the veins of the upper extremities, although subject to thrombosis, rarely contribute to the problem of pulmonary embolism.

(F) Although thrombophlebitis of the superficial leg veins is a common problem, emboli arising in such veins are uncommon. If they do arise, they are probably small and hence, less dangerous. However, extension of thrombosis from the superficial to the deep veins does occur, which then enhances the potential for embolization.

8. (C, F) (A) Inferior vena caval interruption (partial or complete) is carried out under very limited circumstances nowadays, although it was once the procedure of choice for recurrent pul-

monary embolism. Although 90% of all such emboli originate in the deep veins of the lower extremities, it was found that this operation did not prevent recurrences, probably because large collaterals develop and are capable of transporting moderately large emboli to the lungs.

(B) Pulmonary artery embolectomy is a "last resort" procedure with a high mortality. It certainly would not be applicable in this patient with few symptoms and signs. It should never be undertaken unless the size and extent of the pulmonary embolus, as demonstrated by pulmonary arteriography, are obviously life-threatening.

(C) Heparin is the cornerstone of therapy for pulmonary embolism. It is given initially as 10, 000 to 15, 000 units intravenously, as a bolus. There should be no hesitation in giving this first dose on suspicion that pulmonary embolization has occurred, provided there are no absolute contraindications, such as active bleeding, central nervous system lesions that may bleed, or active gastrointestinal lesions that may bleed. The follow-up doses should be 5, 000 units as an intravenous bolus, given every four hours, although an intravenous infusion of 1, 000 units per hour seems to be equally satisfactory. Although intravenous heparin therapy is being done in some areas on an outpatient basis (and in some instances, by the patient himself), in most areas, this form of treatment is best done in the hospital.

(D, E) Isoproterenol or dopamine is used to support the circulation in a patient in shock from massive pulmonary embolism, but was not needed in this patient. Of the two drugs, dopamine is preferred, although isoproterenol has bronchodilatory and vasodilatory effects that make it useful, along with its inotropic effects. However, isoproterenol produces dysrhythmias, lowers systemic blood pressure and may re-establish pulmonary blood flow to non-ventilated areas of the lung with resultant worsening of hypoxemia, at least temporarily.

(F) Oxygen is certainly indicated in all such patients.

COURSE:

This patient was discharged on the fifth hospital day, much improved. She was instructed to continue her warfarin therapy, with prothrombin times maintained at two to two and one-half times the control (20-25% of normal), to discontinue the oral contraceptives and to lose weight. She refused any special tests to determine the source of the emboli, but they were presumed to be coming from the deep veins of her lower extremities.

::

CASE 9: ACUTE ASTHMATIC ATTACK

HISTORY:

A 47-year-old woman presented at the emergency department with an acute asthmatic attack of nine days' duration. Because she had failed to maintain initial improvement on epinephrine and aminophylline therapy, she was transferred from her local hospital to the medical center. She had received steroids early in this attack, but it was uncertain whether the amount and duration were adequate. Her arterial blood gases and pH one hour before transfer were: PO_2, 40 torr; PCO_2, 68 torr; and pH, 7.16. She was given oxygen by nasal cannulae at 6 liters/minute during the one-hour transfer by ambulance. No other medication had been administered for approximately four hours before she arrived at the medical center.

She had had intermittent asthmatic attacks for 9 years, and also had chronic bronchitis of moderate degree.

Examination revealed that she was slightly cyanotic, in moderate respiratory distress, and complained of marked fatigue. Her pulse was 120/minute; respirations, 48/minute; blood pressure, 140/90 mm Hg; and rectal temperature, 100°F (37.8°C). There were diffuse, marked expiratory wheezes. The results of the remainder of the examination were normal. Her arterial blood gases on arrival: PO_2, 48 torr; PCO_2, 30 torr; pH, 7.44.

QUESTIONS:

1. TRUE OR FALSE: The most likely diagnosis in this patient is status asthmaticus.

2. Treatment failure should be considered in terms of possible missed diagnosis, as well as in terms of inadequate treatment. The differential diagnosis of acute asthmatic attack involves which of the following:
   A. Congestive heart failure with pulmonary edema
   B. Pneumonitis
   C. Partial airway obstruction due to foreign body
   D. Pulmonary embolism
   E. Bronchitis
   F. Pneumothorax
   G. All of the above

3. Which of the following statements about status asthmaticus are true?
   A. It is a true medical emergency.
   B. The physical signs are often misleading.
   C. Bronchopulmonary infection is frequently the triggering event.
   D. Many of the patients can be treated and sent home from the emergency department.
   E. It occurs only in adults who have heart trouble.

4. Which of the following initial laboratory studies should be ordered for the patient having a severe attack of asthma?
   A. Determination of arterial blood gases and pH
   B. Complete blood count
   C. Chest roentgenogram
   D. Pulmonary radionuclide scan
   E. Blood electrolyte determinations
   F. Electrocardiogram and continuous monitoring
   G. Sputum smear (Gram's stain), culture and sensitivities
   H. All of the above

5. What is the proper treatment for this patient?
   A. Continued oxygen therapy
   B. Adrenal corticosteroid therapy
   C. Antihistamine administration
   D. Intravenous fluids
   E. Sedation
   F. Slow-release epinephrine
   G. Antibiotic therapy
   H. Aminophylline intravenously
   I. Epinephrine subcutaneously

6. Which of the following are true about aminophylline and its use in acute asthmatic attacks?
   A. It is one of the most effective bronchodilating agents.
   B. It inhibits phosphodiesterase, resulting in an increase in cyclic adenosine - 3', 5'-monophosphate (cAMP).
   C. It potentiates beta-stimulators, increasing their action.
   D. It often relieves severe asthma that is resistant to adrenergic drugs, such as epinephrine.
   E. It is the drug of choice when it is difficult to distinguish between bronchospasm and pulmonary edema.
   F. It is satisfactorily administered intramuscularly.
   G. It should be given first in an intravenous loading dose over a 20-minute period and then by infusion.

H. It has no significant side effects
I. All of the above

ANSWERS AND COMMENTS:

1. (True) This patient had status asthmaticus, which, by definition, is a severe asthmatic attack that fails to respond to treatment with epinephrine (or isoproterenol) and aminophylline in adequate doses. However, it is sometimes difficult to assess the adequacy of the treatment given before a patient arrives in the emergency department.

Although it is difficult to explain the discrepancy in this patient's arterial blood gases since they were done within 2 hours of each other, it is obvious that most of her acid-base abnormality was in the form of respiratory acidosis. Better ventilation en route to the second hospital allowed correction of this acidosis, although her arterial oxygen tension remained dangerously low and her pulse rate remained rapid without adrenergic drugs having been given. Her condition improved somewhat in the two hours before arrival, but the $PaCO_2$ of 68 torr and the pH of 7.16 indicated CO_2 retention of severe degree, or acute respiratory failure, a serious complication of status asthmaticus. Her extreme fatigue was also a danger signal; usually the severity of the asthmatic attack increases as the fatigue increases.

Patients die from such attacks, often at times when they seem, from the clinical standpoint, to be improving. The mortality in recurrent attacks runs as high as 30% if treatment is inadequate or is started late.

2. (G) All. Although the diagnosis of severe asthma is usually quite easy to make, there are certain conditions that must be differentiated from it. Also, associated conditions and complications are frequent in patients who have severe and prolonged or recurrent attacks, as this patient had, and these conditions must be detected.

(A) In most patients, the differentiation between pulmonary edema (see Case 10) and acute severe asthmatic attack is not too difficult. The presence of basal rales and other signs of congestive heart failure would point toward pulmonary edema. It is important that a differentiation between the two conditions be made, since the drugs used in the treatment of one may not be effective or even safe if the other is present. For example, morphine may be administered intravenously to a patient with pulmonary edema, whereas this would be dangerous in a patient with status asthmaticus. However, it is entirely appropriate to give aminophylline intravenously to a patient in whom you are unable to make this differentiation, since it is the correct treatment for both.

(B) Roentgenological changes and the absence of fever usually allow pneumonitis to be differentiated. However, pulmonary infiltration may be difficult to detect in a patient who has emphysematous changes.

(C) Airway obstruction due to aspiration of a foreign body is somewhat more difficult to differentiate in many patients. The history of possible aspiration is helpful, but it is often negative, even in older children and adults. The foreign body may be radiolucent. Therefore, more informative is evidence of changes in the lung secondary to the obstruction, such as atelectasis and pneumonitis. Detection of these changes requires bronchoscopy for detection of a foreign body in any patient at high risk of foreign body aspiration.

(D) Pulmonary embolism is very difficult to differentiate from acute asthma at times, especially since the chest roentgenogram is frequently normal in both of these conditions. In the former, wheezing should be minimal or absent and basal rales are often present, especially if pulmonary edema has been precipitated by the embolization.

(E) Acute bronchitis or exacerbation of chronic bronchitis is sometimes difficult to differentiate from acute asthma. Both types of bronchitis are frequently accompanied by wheezing, and both frequently occur together, as in this patient. If only one or the other is present, the history should be helpful in this differentiation.

(F) Pneumothorax is sometimes difficult to rule out by clinical examination, but is relatively easy to detect on chest roentgenogram. It is often a complication of an asthmatic attack, especially if positive pressure ventilation has been used.

3. (A, B, C) (A) Asthma is a reversible form of diffuse obstructive lung disease, characterized by paroxysmal episodes of wheezing respiration and difficult breathing. Patients of all ages may be affected by asthma; mortality is much higher in adults than in children. Even a seemingly minor attack of asthma must be treated early and vigorously to prevent a more serious episode, such as status asthmaticus, from developing.

Bronchospasm is the predominant cause of the obstruction, but edema of the mucosa and hypertrophy and hypersecretion of the mucosal glands also contribute to the obstruction.

(B) The physical signs of acute severe asthma are not difficult to recognize, consisting, as they do, of tachypnea, labored breathing, coughing (usually with whitish sputum in the absence of infection), tachycardia, pulsus paradoxus, and wheezing. Wheezing is present in most asthmatics during an attack, but it may be absent if bronchospasm and mucus plugging are severe. This can be a serious pitfall in the initial evaluation of the patient. Also, one can be lulled into a false sense of security if the patient under treatment develops less wheezing, misinterpreting this as improvement. The key to response to treatment is whether the patient is moving air in and out of the chest better. Pulsus paradoxus is an exaggeration of the normal drop in arterial pressure on inspiration. The normal decrease is 5 to 7 mm Hg or less. In a patient with a severe asthmatic attack, the drop is usually more than 10 mm Hg and is often 20 mm Hg or more, and is correlated fairly well with the degree of airway obstruction. With adequate treatment of the respiratory problems, the pulsus paradoxus should decrease, giving an additional clinical variable for monitoring response to treatment. Surprisingly, pulsus paradoxus was not present in this patient.

(C) Infection often accompanies an attack of asthma and may be difficult to recognize as such. The sputum usually becomes purulent, indicating acute bronchitis. Such an infection is often the triggering event, occurring in about 40 per cent of cases, most commonly in the very young, the elderly, and those with the most serious disease. At times, the infection seems to be confined to the upper respiratory tract, but there is usually some extension into the tracheobronchial tree in the patients whose asthma is precipitated or made worse by it.

(D) The best criterion for admission to the hospital is treatment failure. And, by definition, the patient in status asthmaticus has failed to respond to vigorous and normally adequate treatment. If this failure to respond persists for a reasonable period - say from four to ten hours - the patient should almost always be hospitalized. In many hospitals, immediate admission to the intensive care unit is arranged as soon as the emergency department physician and consultant agree that the patient's attack is indeed refractory to the usual measures.

(E) Status asthmaticus occurs at any age. Most of the younger patients and many of the older ones have no health problems other than their asthma.

4. (A, B, C, E, F, G) (A) If possible, arterial blood should be used for blood gas and pH determinations, even in small children, in whom it is sometimes difficult to obtain arterial blood immediately. Serial determinations are required if the patient fails to respond to the initial treatment procedures. In any case, even if clinical improvement is dramatic, arterial blood gases and pH should be measured again before the decision is made whether to send the patient home.

(B) If at all possible, blood for the complete blood count should be drawn before epinephrine is administered, since epinephrine causes a leukocytosis that may be misinterpreted as a sign of infection. This patient's white blood cell count was 15, 000 with a slight shift to the left.

(C) The chest roentgenogram in a patient with severe asthma shows hyperventilation with widened intercostal spaces, horizontal ribs, depressed or inverted diaphragm and radiolucency. However, the clinical history and findings must determine whether the condition is acute or chronic. One should search for evidence of atelectasis, pneumonitis, blebs and bullae, as well as pneumomediastinum and pneumothorax. The latter is dangerous, because it can quickly lead to tension pneumothorax, especially if intermittent positive pressure ventilation is used as treatment. If tension pneumothorax occurs, it, in turn, can quickly lead to cardiac arrest. The physician suspecting tension pneumothorax should relieve it promptly by needle aspiration or insertion of a small pleural catheter without waiting for a roentgenological examination.

This patient's chest roentgenogram showed minimal left pleural effusion, as well as increased lucency in both lung fields, suggestive of air trapping. There was no evidence of pneumonitis.

(D) Radionuclide scanning of the lungs is not necessary in a patient with severe bronchial asthma. However, as previously indicated, a patient with acute pulmonary edema may have pulmonary embolization as the precipitating event. If this is suspected, and the chest roentgenogram is normal except for the presence of interstitial edema and alveolar fluid accumulation, that patient may require radionuclide scanning to rule out pulmonary embolism.

(E) Blood electrolyte determination should be done initially for better assessment of the patient's ability to respond to the drugs.

Blood urea nitrogen will give some indication of renal function. The serum potassium concentration is useful, especially in elderly patients prone to develop cardiac dysrhythmias.

(F) Electrocardiography, with continuous monitoring, is always advisable for a patient having a severe asthmatic attack, regardless of his age. Even if the attack is not severe, it is advisable to establish cardiac monitoring if isoproterenol or another adrenergic drug is being administered. All adults who have coexisting cardiac or pulmonary problems should be on continuous cardiac monitoring. Cardiac dysrhythmias are prone to occur because of hypoxemia or acid-base derangements. Cardiac arrest is a constant threat in status asthmaticus, and it is usually caused by a combination of severe hypoxemia and metabolic or respiratory acidosis.

(G) Sputum is not as useful for bacteriological study as a transtracheal aspirate or endotracheal suction specimen. However, the former is relatively contraindicated in a patient in status asthmaticus, as it may increase the bronchospasm, and the latter is best postponed until controlled ventilation is begun. In the meantime, the predominant organism of any bronchopulmonary infection present may be obvious on a gram stain of the sputum.

5. (A, B, D, H, I) (A) Humidified oxygen therapy was started by face mask in a concentration of 50-60% (assisted ventilation). This promptly raised the patient's arterial PO_2 to 60 torr, so it was decided to postpone endotracheal intubation and controlled ventilation, at least temporarily. Her hypoxemia was thought to be due to ventilation/perfusion ($\dot{V}/\dot{Q}$) imbalance, that is, alveoli being perfused with blood but not being ventilated.

(B) The immediate start of corticosteroid therapy was indicated in this patient. Approximately 4 mg/kg or 250 mg (or the equivalent if other steroids are used) of hydrocortisone sodium succinate, given intravenously over one to two minutes, is the standard dose for adults with status asthmaticus. Even in children with status asthmaticus, as much as 100 mg should be administered intravenously. The initial dose should be repeated every four to six hours for several doses (at least 100 mg each dose for adults), but oral therapy, as well as a reduction in dosage, can probably be substituted by 12 to 24 hours, depending upon the patient's condition.

Corticosteroid therapy may be life-saving when used early in any severe asthmatic attack. It may potentiate the effect of epinephrine, thereby preventing failure of this treatment; it may also prevent respiratory failure in a patient whose condition seems to be deteriorating. Corticosteroids activate adenyl cyclase to produce cyclic 3', 5'-adenosine monophosphate (cAMP), which leads to bronchial dilatation. They also reduce inflammation and edema, and suppress allergic responses. In a patient who has been taking steroids systemically on a long-term basis, a steroid must always be given, even if the last dose was given three to six months earlier. The maximum beneficial effect in status asthmaticus may not be apparent for up to six hours.

(C) Antihistamines should not be given because of their atropine-like effect with drying of tracheobronchial secretions and worsening of mucus plugging of bronchi. Further, their sedating effect may cause respiratory depression and recurrence of carbon dioxide retention. In this patient, the assisted ventilation started on arrival would probably have prevented the latter effect.

(D) Hydration is essential, since most patients with status asthmaticus are dehydrated, due to failure of adequate intake, as well as increased loss through the respiratory tract and other insensible loss, such as sweating. The intravenous route is preferred, using 5% dextrose in water or in 0.5 normal saline (or 0.2 normal saline in small children). Underhydration is more common in treatment than overhydration, so one should not hesitate, unless there is some contraindication, to give one to two liters to an adult over the first four hours and up to four liters in the first 24 hours. Careful monitoring is necessary to prevent pulmonary edema, although this is unlikely to occur in an asthmatic patient without cardiac disease. The rehydration is vital to liquefaction and loosening of secretions in the tracheobronchial tree.

(E) As mentioned under answer C, sedation is dangerous in asthmatic patients having a severe attack. It masks the severity of the bronchospasm and may actually depress respirations to a dangerously low level, with a drop in arterial PO_2. Also, an increase in carbon dioxide retention with narcosis may result and may be difficult to distinguish clinically from the sedating effect of the drug. Finally, sedation is not usually necessary if the bronchospasm and associated hypoxia can be relieved fairly promptly.

(F) Slow-release epinephrine (1:200 or 1:400 aqueous suspension) should not be used in status asthmaticus, as its effect is unpredictable and the dose cannot be repeated in less than four hours. It is satisfactory to use in mild attacks of asthma, when the patient has shown a good response to aqueous epinephrine and needs a longer-acting dose before being discharged home. The 1:200 aqueous suspension lasts four to eight hours and may be used for children in a maximum dose of 0.15 ml; for adults, in a dose of 0.15 to 0.3 ml. It is only for subcutaneous administration.

(G) Antibiotics are not usually indicated initially in status asthmaticus, unless the examination and laboratory results indicate significant pulmonary infection. This patient had a history of chronic bronchitis and her sputum had changed to a more purulent type over the previous few days. Therefore, ampicillin was started immediately, 500 mg by mouth every six hours.

(H) See question and answer 6 for discussion of aminophylline.

(I) Ordinarily, epinephrine would not be administered to such a patient, on the assumption that adequate doses had already been given. However, this patient was treated with epinephrine subcutaneously, along with oxygen, in adequate concentrations and aminophylline to full therapeutic levels. At times, this combination seems to break the unresponsiveness to epinephrine that sometimes develops in these patients. That seemed to be the case with this patient, since she improved initially. However, she then became worse, and after several hours, terbutaline was substituted for epinephrine, with further improvement.

6. (A, B, C, D, E, G) (A) Aminophylline is theophylline ethylenediamine, and theophylline is the keystone of the treatment of both acute and chronic asthma. Aminophylline is the only theophylline derivative that can be administered intravenously. It is a methylxanthine, not an adrenergic drug, such as epinephrine, isoproterenol, terbutaline and metaproterenol. In general, only one of the last four drugs should be used at one time, along with aminophylline, in order to accomplish a combined effect, since the two classes of drugs work to reduce bronchospasm by different mechanisms. Aminophylline is certainly one of the most effective bronchodilating agents. Every physician who works in emergency departments should be thoroughly familiar with its use.

(B, C) Aminophylline inhibits phosphodiesterase, resulting in an increase in the intracellular concentration of cAMP by preventing its conversion to 3', 5'-AMP. It also stimulates beta receptors and potentiates beta stimulators, increasing their action in relaxing bronchial musculature.

(D) Aminophylline, either alone or in combination with epinephrine, frequently relieves bronchospasm that has failed to respond to epinephrine alone. For this reason, it is wise to administer both drugs to a patient whose bronchospasm is severe.

(E) At times, acute pulmonary edema is difficult to distinguish from acute severe bronchospasm. While the differential diagnosis is being pursued, aminophylline should be used. However, morphine should be reserved until the diagnosis of pulmonary edema is definite, since it may harm a patient with severe asthma.

(F) The intramuscular route is not justified, as it may cause severe, persistent pain.

(G) A loading dose of aminophylline intravenously is 5.6 (4 to 6) mg/kg, diluted to 100 ml and administered over a 20-minute period. It should be followed by an infusion of 1 mg/kg/hour. This dose gives a plasma concentration of 10 micrograms/ml, which is satisfactory in most patients, since the therapeutic range is 10 to 20 micrograms/ml. The total dose in 24 hours should not exceed 16 mg/kg.

Before the loading dose is administered, it is important to determine how much theophylline or other xanthine derivative the patient has had in the previous 12 to 24 hours. If the history in this regard is not dependable or available, it is helpful to have a plasma theophylline determination, if such a test is available. If the test is unavailable, a reduced amount should be administered as a loading dose, as was done for this patient.

(H) Aminophylline can cause toxic manifestations, including irritability, severe vomiting, cardiac dysrhythmias, hypotension, convulsions, coma and death.

Too rapid an intravenous injection may stimulate the vagus nerve, causing bradycardia and possibly asystole. Thus, aminophylline is not an innocuous drug and must be used cautiously, with careful cardiac monitoring. There is some indication that children tolerate combinations of xanthines and sympathomimetics in the presence of hypoxemia and acidosis better than adults, but even in children, careful monitoring is required, and the approach should be conservative.

Aminophylline has a diuretic action and will tend to increase dehydration unless intravenous fluids are administered at the same time and in adequate amounts.

Since there is great individual variation in the plasma levels of theophylline from the same dosage, the plasma concentration should be measured, where possible, until the individual patient's optimal dosage schedule is determined. This is true even for the patient with an acute attack.

COURSE:

This patient was treated with aminophylline, 3 mg/kg, as a reduced loading dose, then 1 mg/kg/hr as an infusion. Epinephrine was also tried, on the assumption that she may not have had the full dosage. Hydrocortisone sodium succinate was given in a 250-mg dose intravenously, and there was some initial improvement. She was admitted to the hospital and shortly thereafter required nasotracheal intubation with controlled ventilation, because of increased carbon dioxide retention. Three days later, she was so much improved that weaning and extubation were carried out. Twenty-four hours later, reintubation was considered advisable, and this time, controlled ventilation was continued for two days. She had no further problems and was discharged on the fifteenth hospital day. She was advised to continue corticosteroid therapy by mouth, with alternate-day doses to be started after one more week.

::

CASE 10: PROGRESSIVE DYSPNEA AND PITTING EDEMA

HISTORY:

A 71-year-old woman reported to the emergency department because of progressive shortness of breath of five months' duration. At first, this was only on exertion, but for the previous two weeks, it had occurred at rest, as well. She had been unable to lie flat because of breathing difficulty and had begun having paroxysmal nocturnal dyspnea one week earlier. Since her last medical evaluation five months before, she had gained three to four pounds per month, with increasing leg and ankle edema. One hour before this visit, after she had swept her porch, she had developed extreme dyspnea and sweating, and moderate cough without sputum production.

She had a 15-year history of hypertension and a two-year history of diabetes mellitus. Medication consisted of methyldopa, hydrochlorothiazide, and chlorpropamide, as well as digoxin, 0.25 mg daily for chronic congestive heart failure.

Examination revealed a faintly cyanotic woman in moderate respiratory distress. Blood pressure was 210/120 mm Hg; pulse, 160/minute on admission but decreased to 110/minute after initial treatment; respiration, 30/minute. There was moderate distention of the neck veins and a positive hepatojugular reflex at 45 degrees. Rales were noted throughout both lung fields. Moderate cardiac enlargement was noted. The liver was palpable 1 cm below the right costal margin. There was 2+ pitting edema of the legs and feet. The results of the remainder of the physical examination were normal.

QUESTIONS:

1. TRUE OR FALSE: The most likely diagnosis in this patient is congestive heart failure with pulmonary edema.

2. The pathophysiology of pulmonary edema due to cardiac disease is which of the following?
   A. Dysfunction of the left ventricle
   B. Increased hydrostatic pressure in the left atrium and left pulmonary venous system
   C. Transudation of fluid into the interstitium of the lungs
   D. Accumulation of fluid in the alveoli
   E. All of the above

3. Initial treatment for pulmonary edema due to heart disease is which of the following?
   A. Oxygen, with positive pressure ventilation
   B. Morphine sulfate
   C. Trunk-up, legs-down position
   D. Rapid digitalization
   E. Potent diuretics
   F. Aminophylline
   G. Rotating tourniquets
   H. Phlebotomy
   I. Intravenous fluids
   J. Tracheostomy

4. Pulmonary edema of noncardiac origin is associated with which of the following?
   A. High altitude
   B. Inhalation of toxic substances
   C. Drugs, especially heroin
   D. Fluid overload
   E. Central nervous system injury
   F. Pulmonary embolism
   G. Pericarditis
   H. All of the above

ANSWERS AND COMMENTS:

1. (True) The patient had chronic heart failure, with acute pulmonary edema of the alveolar type. The dyspnea on exertion, that had developed some months earlier, was probably due to interstitial pulmonary edema (see answer 2).

This case is presented to illustrate the most common cause of pulmonary edema, namely, congestive heart failure. Noncardiac causes of pulmonary edema will be discussed only in question and answer 4.

Pulmonary edema is a complication of other disease processes, not a disease itself. It is life-threatening, particularly when acute, or when the acute form is superimposed on a chronic pulmonary condition, as in this patient. However, it need rarely be the cause of death today, since very effective means of emergency treatment are available.

2. (E) All, and approximately in that order. The causes of ventricular dysfunction leading to congestive heart failure are many and are beyond the scope of this discussion. This patient's left ventricle was not functioning at maximum efficiency, due

largely to the fact that her long-standing hypertension was not under control. Hypertension is the cause of pulmonary edema in a large proportion of patients. Very often, cardiac failure improves with the reduction of diastolic pressure.

It should be noted that frequently the only clinical evidence of pulmonary edema in its interstitial phase is the presence of tachypnea and exertional dyspnea. However, a chest roentgenogram made at this stage shows evidence of increased fluid in the interstitium, namely, hilar prominence with distended pulmonary veins, especially in the upper lung fields, along with constriction of the arteries and veins of the lower lung fields in many patients. Kerley B lines, which are horizontal lines at the lung bases, represent dilated lymphatics from long-standing elevation of pulmonary venous pressure. The roentgenographical picture of alveolar pulmonary edema is an extension of these findings, with "bat-wing" mottling and prominence of the hilar regions. Pleural effusion may be present.

As fluid collects in the alveoli, they begin to collapse, thus preventing the ingress of air. The result is a right-to-left intrapulmonary shunt, so that blood flowing to these collapsed alveoli is not oxygenated. This blood is then mixed with well-oxygenated blood from other parts of the lungs, and the partial pressure of oxygen in the pulmonary venous blood is reduced.

The accumulation of fluid around the small vessels and bronchioles causes some of them to be compressed. This causes obstruction and wheezing in some patients. Such wheezing may be hard to differentiate from that of asthma, although patients with pulmonary edema in the alveolar stage usually also present with rales throughout the chest, as this patient did.

3. (A, B, C, D, E, F, G, H) (A) Oxygen is needed because of the degree of hypoxemia that develops as soon as right-to-left shunting takes place. Administered by mask of the Venturi type at 24%, 28%, or 35%, supplemental oxygen will frequently raise the arterial PO_2 enough to relieve the patient's dyspnea. This method of oxygen administration should be changed to positive pressure ventilation as soon as possible, for the added amelioration of the alveolar pulmonary edema.

(B) Morphine sulfate is the single most important medication for a patient with acute pulmonary edema. In most adults, it should be administered intravenously in a 4-mg dose, the dose to be repeated after 15 to 20 minutes if needed. The mechanism of action of morphine is to decrease peripheral vascular resistance, thus allowing blood to pool in the veins. The sedative effect of morphine allays anxiety and decreases tachypnea, thus helping to break a vicious cycle. If respiratory depression occurs, it can be corrected by intravenous administration of small doses of naloxone.

(C) When first seen, the patient may be sitting up, trying to improve his breathing. If he is recumbent, he should have his head and trunk raised and his feet lowered, unless he is hypotensive.

(D) If the patient is not taking a digitalis preparation, he should be digitalized by the slow intravenous administration of 0.25 to 0.5 mg of digoxin initially. The effect is apparent within 30 minutes, but does not reach its peak for approximately two hours. Then, a 0.25 mg dose of digoxin may be repeated one or two times at four- to six-hour intervals as required. This patient had been taking digoxin, but there was some question of whether she had missed daily doses or not. In such an instance, determination of the digoxin blood level may be helpful, although the correlation between an effective blood level and the therapeutic effect is poor. A reduced dose of digoxin (0.25 mg) was given this patient with no evidence of toxicity.

(E) Furosemide, in an intravenous dose of 40 mg, or ethacrynic acid, in an intravenous dose of 50 mg, is very useful in treating pulmonary edema. It allows mobilization and elimination of the fluid in the lungs, thus giving rapid relief of the dyspnea, as well as the hypoxemia, in most patients.

(F) If bronchospasm is a prominent feature, aminophylline should be used for control, just as it is in patients with asthma. For most adults, 250 mg of aminophylline added to 100 ml of fluid and infused into the vein over 20 minutes is effective.

(G) The use of three tourniquets, rotated every 15 minutes, helps reduce the amount of intravascular volume by trapping blood in the extremities. The tourniquets should be tight enough to occlude venous return, but not so tight that they occlude arterial inflow.

(H) Phlebotomy (100-500 ml) is another means of decreasing the intravascular volume, but must not be used in patients with anemia or hypotension. Usually the previously mentioned measures (A-G) are adequate, and phlebotomy is not required.

(I) Intravenous fluid is contraindicated in patients with pulmonary edema, except for the small amounts needed to keep the intravenous line open and to dilute the medications.

(J) Tracheostomy is not indicated, except in the most unusual circumstances.

4. (A, B, C, D, E, F) All of these agents and conditions are causes of acute pulmonary edema, and many of the patients affected by these agents and conditions have normal cardiovascular and pulmonary systems. The pulmonary edema seems to be due to adrenergic overactivity, which causes a shift of blood from the systemic to the pulmonary circulation.

(A) The mechanism of high-altitude pulmonary edema is obscure, although nonuniform increases in precapillary resistance may be responsible. High-altitude pulmonary edema is characterized by dry cough, dyspnea, and lower substernal discomfort; it is more apt to develop at altitudes above 9000 feet, and it develops 6 to 36 hours after the patient arrives at those altitudes. It is precipitated or made worse by exertion. Treatment is return to lower altitudes, if possible. If this is not feasible, bed rest and oxygen therapy are all that are required in most instances. Adaptation to the higher altitude usually occurs within a few days, if no underlying pulmonary or cardiac disease exists.

(B) Inhalation of toxic substances, such as smoke, causes pulmonary edema in many, although not all, patients so exposed. The edema seems to result from a direct injury to the alveolar membrane cells, which alters permeability. The pulmonary edema of near-drowning appears to develop on the same basis.

(C) Heroin and drugs such as nitrofurantoin, paraldehyde (intravenous) and salicylates, taken in excess, cause pulmonary edema, presumably by altering pulmonary capillary permeability, although other, presently unknown, mechanisms may be responsible. In any patient with pulmonary edema of obscure origin, the emergency department physician should always consider heroin overdosage, confirmed by the presence of needle tracks on the upper extremities, and administer naloxone if the patient is mentally obtunded.

(D) Excessive administration of fluids sometimes causes pulmonary edema by diluting plasma proteins and raising intravascular hydrostatic pressure. Fluid overload is also involved in an increased production of antidiuretic hormone. This occurs occasionally in patients with pneumonia and in some patients on a ventilator.

(E) Head injury is followed in some instances by pulmonary

edema, which seems to be neurally mediated. In such instances, blood is shifted from the systemic to the pulmonary circulation.

(F) As mentioned in Case 8, pulmonary embolism is occasionally accompanied by pulmonary edema.

(G) Pericarditis is not likely to precipitate pulmonary edema.

Treatment for most of these types of pulmonary edema is the same as that outlined in question and answer 3. However, morphine should be administered with caution, if at all, and digitalis is not likely to help, unless there is concomitant cardiac failure.

COURSE:

This patient was admitted to the hospital one hour after arrival at the emergency department and remained for six days. Initial arterial blood gases while she was receiving oxygen at four liters flow by nasal cannulae were: PO_2, 137 torr; PCO_2, 30 torr; pH, 7.32. Chest roentgenograms confirmed the clinical impression of extensive alveolar pulmonary edema, as well as moderate left ventricular enlargement. She gradually improved with the treatment outlined in question and answer 3. A regular follow-up program was arranged so that the development of such a serious complication could be prevented in the future.

CASE 11: SPONTANEOUS PNEUMOTHORAX WITH TENSION

HISTORY:

A 30-year-old woman reported to the emergency department with "difficult breathing" of 30 minutes' duration. She was sitting at home, recovering from a recent episode of coryza with bronchitis, when she coughed and stood up. At that moment, she experienced sudden onset of pain in her left hemithorax with subsequent shortness of breath. Both symptoms progressed as she continued to cough, producing yellowish sputum, as she had for four days.

She had suffered asthmatic attacks since childhood, but none for the previous four years. She had smoked one package of cigarettes per day for ten years. There was no history of pneumonia or tuberculosis.

Examination revealed moderate respiratory distress, diminished breath sounds on the left side of the thorax, slight deviation of the trachea to the right, and moderate cyanosis. Her skin was cool and clammy. Pulse was 132/min; temperature, 97°F (36.0^{o}C); blood pressure, 130/80 mm Hg. The results of the remainder of the examination were normal.

Portable chest roentgenography revealed pneumothorax, with 90% collapse of the left lung and a fluid level at the base, which was thought to represent hemothorax. No shift of the mediastinal structures was noted.

QUESTIONS:

1. Which of the following are true about spontaneous pneumothorax?
   - A. It most often affects young adult males.
   - B. It is rarely asymptomatic.
   - C. The diagnosis can almost always be made by careful physical examination.
   - D. Onset is sudden and usually associated with strenuous activity.
   - E. The most frequent cause is rupture of a subpleural bleb.
   - F. It usually causes at least 50% collapse of the lung.
   - G. Simultaneous bilateral spontaneous pneumothorax is almost unheard of.

2. Which of the following characterizes tension pneumothorax?
   A. It is a dangerous complication of pneumothorax.
   B. It occurs only in patients with chest injury.
   C. A ball-valve action allows air to enter the pleural cavity but prevents its escape.
   D. The mediastinum usually shifts to the opposite side.
   E. All of the above

3. Which of the following is the proper treatment of this patient?
   A. Wait for consultation by the surgical/thoracic service.
   B. Repeat the chest roentgenograms in one hour.
   C. Insert a needle into the left hemithorax and evacuate the the excess pleural air.
   D. Allow the pneumothorax to correct itself by resorption of the pleural air.
   E. Insert a thoracostomy tube with underwater seal suction.

ANSWERS AND COMMENTS:

1. (A, B, E) (A) It is much more frequent in young adults, although it can occur at any age. Males are more frequently affected than females.

(B) Most patients have symptoms, usually chest pain of sudden onset, often pleuritic in nature. They also complain of dyspnea and may have a dry, hacking cough. If acute or chronic pulmonary disease is present, these symptoms may be explained on that basis and the diagnosis of pneumothorax missed. Beyond the first few minutes after onset, the symptoms depend upon the extent of lung collapse, which is usually expressed in percentage of normal lung size.

(C) Physical examination fails to reveal pneumothorax in many patients when the degree of lung collapse is small (5 to 10%). Even larger collapse can be difficult or impossible to detect without roentgenography, which is definitive for diagnosis, especially if the film is exposed with the patient in expiration. Diminished or absent breath sounds, decreased tactile and vocal fremitus and decreased excursion of the hemithorax may be present and suggest the diagnosis.

(D) Onset, as in this patient, is sudden but is not associated with strenuous activity in most instances.

(E) The most frequent cause is spontaneous rupture of a bleb, which is a small outpouching of the visceral pleural. Any time a patient presents with spontaneous pneumothorax, a search should be made on the chest roentgenogram for subpleural blebs. They are usually small (a few millimeters to 3 centimeters in diameter) and are usually situated over the apex of one or both lungs or over the superior portion of the other lobes, frequently in or near the fissures. They are difficult to see because of their small size, as well as their location. On the side of the pneumothorax, the ruptured bleb is no longer distended and therefore usually cannot be seen. If other nearby blebs can be seen, their presence furnishes a clue to the etiology of the pneumothorax. Blebs may be bilateral, and this has implications for treatment. If blebs are seen at both apices or elsewhere, but in both sides of the chest, one would be more inclined to do a definitive, open thoracotomy procedure at the time unilateral pneumothorax occurs. Otherwise, the patient is at risk to develop simultaneous bilateral pneumothorax (G) at some future time, a potentially fatal complication.

(F) The degree of lung collapse varies widely, but it is usually from 15 to 50% by the time the patient is seen.

2. (A, C, D) (A) Tension pneumothorax, which this patient had, is a complication of pneumothorax of any of the usual types. These types are, in addition to spontaneous, traumatic, iatrogenic, and secondary (to pulmonary disease). However, tension pneumothorax is more frequently due to trauma (B) than to the other types. If unrecognized and untreated, it can be fatal, especially in the patient who develops it while receiving positive pressure ventilation. The mechanism is a ball-valve action of the ruptured visceral pleura (C), which allows air to enter the pleural cavity but prevents its escape. As the intrapleural pressure builds up gradually (or rapidly, as in this patient), the mediastinum tends to shift to the opposite side (D), interfering with venous return to the heart. Also, expansion of the contralateral lung is interfered with because of direct pressure, increasing the hypoxemia that is usually present.

3. (C, E) (A, B) Treatment of spontaneous pneumothorax is urgent, but treatment of tension pneumothorax is an emergency. Tension pneumothorax is life-threatening, but death from it is preventable if the patient is seen in time. Thus, no delay can be countenanced in the initial treatment, particularly in a patient like this one, whose symptoms were progressing.

(C) For confirmation of the diagnosis and for correction of the tension pneumothorax, it is always a good idea to insert a needle or small plastic catheter first, preferably at the site proposed for the thoracostomy tube. This will prevent the occasional confusion as to which side the patient's pneumothrax is on, the confusion resulting from misleading physical findings or mislabelled roentgenograms.

A thoracostomy tube is always indicated for treatment of tension pneumothorax. However, while it is being readied for insertion, or during delay for any other reason, the tip of the finger of a sterile glove may be passed over the head of the needle or catheter to serve as a flutter valve. This allows air to egress from the pleural cavity but does not allow air to enter it.

Any type of tube is satisfactory, although the newer plastic (Silastic™) type is easiest to insert and is least likely to become obstructed by blood clots. The tube should be readily visible on subsequent roentgenograms. The safest and easiest position for the initial thoracentesis, and for placement of the tube, is the second or third intercostal space on the mid-clavicular line. This level is easily identified by locating the angle of Louis, which represents the junction of the second rib with the sternum.

TECHNIQUE:

Although this book does not emphasize the techniques or procedures used in emergency departments, this is one emergency technique that is given, since it is life-saving and can be done without delay.

After all instruments are made ready and the anterior thorax is shaved, the entire area is prepared with suitable antiseptic and draped with sterile towels. A skin wheal is made with any suitable local anesthetic at the site of tube insertion, and infiltration extended down to the pleural surface. If the tube selected is large, say a 32F to 38F, the local anesthetic must be infiltrated widely throughout the intercostal muscles. If the small needle used for this infiltration is long enough, it may be passed through the anesthetized pleura into the pleural air pocket and aspirated for confirmation of the presence of air. Or, alternatively, a larger and longer needle, preferably with a short bevel, may be used for this purpose.

When the anesthetic has taken effect, a skin incision is made parallel to the ribs, the length of the incision depending upon the diameter of the tube, but usually being 1 to 2 cm long. Exactly how the tube is inserted is a matter of personal preference, but the emergency department physician should be familiar with all of the standard techniques. Probably the safest way is to widen the dissection below the skin incision with the gloved finger or large curved clamp, penetrating the pleura with the finger and palpating to be sure that the lung is not adherent to the parietal pleura. This step is even more important when the procedure is being done without benefit of preliminary roentgenograms, which is the case when there is extreme urgency or when a roentgenographic study is not readily available. The distal end of the tube is clamped. A curved clamp may be used to guide and push the proximal end of the tube into the pleural space. After the tube penetrates the pleura, it should be inserted several more centimeters to make sure that all side holes on the catheter are inside the pleura.

The distal end of the tube should then be connected to a suitable underwater seal and the clamp released. If the tube has been correctly placed, there should be an immediate rush of air bubbles through the escape hole of the first bottle or other unit. The patient should then be encouraged to breathe deeply and to cough slightly, the resulting air bubbles further confirming that the end of the tube is in the pleural cavity. If blood is present and if the tube is large enough, blood should escape along with the air as soon as the lung re-expansion is nearly complete. Suction should be added to the tube as soon as the tube is in place, or from the beginning of the procedure, depending upon the type of equipment being used. Suction is not always required for establishing and maintaining re-expansion of a collapsed lung where trauma is not involved. However, application of suction after tube insertion gives added assurance of early, complete lung re-expansion and avoidance of residual pockets of pleural air. Such pockets are frequently difficult to manage, if hours or days are allowed to pass during which time the pleura becomes adherent, which allows such pockets to form.

The diagnostic and therapeutic approach is the same for children, although smaller tubes are used. For some reason, blebs may be present in children but do not rupture until adolescence or the early twenties in most patients.

COURSE:

This patient had relief of her tension pneumothorax by needle insertion, followed immediately by insertion of a #28F silastic tube. Suction was applied, using an underwater seal technique, and the lung expanded fully within one hour, the expansion being confirmed by repeat roentgenography. Approximately 250 ml of serosanguinous fluid were recovered from the pleural cavity within the first few minutes after suction was applied. This is an unusually large amount of blood for a patient with spontaneous pneumothorax, even with tension. Since the mediastinum did not shift during the tension phase, it is probable that adhesions were present in the pleural cavity, and that one or more of these ruptured and bled as the lung collapsed. Such adhesions on the mediastinal side could have prevented a mediastinal shift.

The tube was removed on the third hospital day, but recurrence of pneumothorax required temporary reinsertion of the tube. A smaller tube may have been equally satisfactory in some patients, but in this patient, the presence of fluid in the pleural cavity was an indication for this size tube or a larger tube. The patient was discharged after five days. No blebs were visualized on her chest roentgenograms, but this is not unusual. When open thoracotomy is required for definitive therapy, small blebs have been found that were not detectable roentgenologically.

::

CASE 12: FEVER, SEVERE HYPOTENSION, HISTORY OF SCALP MALIGNANCY AND ULCER

HISTORY:

A 17-year-old girl arrived in the emergency department with a blood pressure of 60/0 mm Hg and temperature of 106°F (41.1^{o}C). Two years earlier, an epithelioid sarcoma of the scalp had been removed; the follow-up radiation therapy and chemotherapy had not prevented recurrence, and she had developed a large, chronic, ulcerative lesion of the scalp. She had had a similar episode of hypotension and fever three months earlier, at which time blood cultures and cultures of the wound had grown Pseudomonas aeruginosa. Pulmonary metastases were noted at that time. She was hospitalized for six weeks, gradually recovered, and had been home for several weeks before the present episode. However, for the two weeks preceding the present episode, her family had noted that she had progressive loss of interest, listlessness, anorexia and weight loss. For the two days preceding the present episode, she had had fever and chills.

On examination, her pulse was 140/minute and regular; respirations 28/minute. The ulcer was fairly clean because of the regular use of saline soaks at home. Her skin was warm and dry, and there was no evidence of cyanosis. Otherwise, the general examination was unremarkable.

QUESTIONS:

1. Which of the following is the most likely diagnosis in this patient?
   A. Occult hemorrhage
   B. Meningitis
   C. Septic shock
   D. Dehydration and malnutrition
   E. Widespread metastases

2. Common signs of septic shock include which of the following?
   A. Disorientation, confusion, mental obtundation
   B. Hyperventilation
   C. Fever
   D. Tachycardia
   E. Hypotension
   F. Leukocytosis

G. Cold, clammy extremities
H. Oliguria
I. All of the above

3. For early diagnosis, which of the following laboratory tests and special procedures are the most informative?
   A. Complete blood count
   B. Urinalysis
   C. Measurement of arterial blood gases and pH
   D. Determination of blood electrolytes, glucose, lactate, urea nitrogen, creatinine, enzymes
   E. Coagulation profile
   F. Culture of blood, sputum, urine and any wounds present
   G. Gram staining
   H. Measurement of central venous pressure or Swan-Ganz catheter measurements
   I. Electrocardiography
   J. Roentgenological examination of chest and abdomen
   K. Lumbar puncture
   L. All of the above

TRUE OR FALSE (Questions 4-7):

4. Septic shock can be caused by gram-negative or gram-positive bacteremia.

5. Septic shock frequently follows manipulative procedures, such as endoscopy, placement of indwelling catheters, and tracheostomy.

6. The mortality from septic shock is high despite vigorous therapy.

7. Septic shock occurs in approximately 25% of all bacteremias.

8. The pathophysiological mechanisms of gram-negative bacteremic shock involve which of the following?
   A. Activation, in turn, of complement, kallikrein and bradykinin
   B. Early arterial vasodilatation, with pooling of blood in peripheral tissues, and an increase in pulse pressure and cardiac output
   C. Increased capillary permeability, with loss of intravascular fluid
   D. Later decrease in blood volume and reduction in cardiac output
   E. All of the above

9. Immediate treatment includes which four of the following; secondary treatment includes which three of the following?
   A. Opening of at least two intravenous lines
   B. Maintenance of the airway
   C. Oxygen administration
   D. Intravenous administration of electrolytes and colloid solutions
   E. Antibiotics
   F. Vasoactive drugs
   G. Surgical intervention

10. Which of the following are complications of septic shock?
    A. Disseminated intravascular coagulation
    B. Respiratory failure
    C. Cardiac failure
    D. Renal failure
    E. Death
    F. All of the above

ANSWERS AND COMMENTS:

1. (C, D) Septic shock, complicated by dehydration and malnutrition, is the most likely diagnosis, although the other conditions may very well be present and should be searched for. While the patient did have pulmonary metastases, they were not thought to be contributory in this episode. Meningitis was ruled out by lumbar puncture yielding sterile, nonbloody spinal fluid under normal pressure. There was no evidence of a source of occult bleeding, such as a gastroduodenal stress ulcer, although such an ulcer might be expected in such a patient.

In this patient, the diagnosis was relatively easy to make because of the history of previous gram-negative bacteremia and the persistence of the scalp ulcer. The dehydration and malnutrition probably contributed to the shock syndrome by causing hypovolemia.

2. (I) All of these signs are rather nonspecific. Thus, diagnosis of septic shock is often a diagnosis of exclusion, that is, of considering the possibility of septic shock when the signs and symptoms do not fit into any other clinical picture. However, since a diagnosis of exclusion is usually made only after an exhaustive search for other diseases, such a prolonged search in most patients in septic shock will mean death, since irreversible changes occur early in this condition.

In the emergency department setting, there is often little or no history available. Frequently, elderly patients are brought from nursing homes by persons who know nothing about the patient's recent health. While disorientation and other symptoms of mental obtundation are common chronic symptoms in patients who have dementia of the presenile or senile type, they are often the earliest signs of septic shock in many nonsenile patients, occurring hours before other more definitive changes. Thus, mental confusion alone should always cause one to suspect septic shock and to make an effort to rule it out.

Acute hyperventilation syndrome (hyperventilation without obvious cause) is often based on emotional factors, such as stress or anxiety. Patients most susceptible to septic shock are not likely to suffer from this condition. Rather, the reason for their hyperventilation is an attempt to compensate for early metabolic acidosis, due to lactic acidemia; however, this cause of hyperventilation may not be suspected. The postoperative patient, whether still in the hospital or returning to the emergency department, may be thought to have atelectasis, pneumonitis, myocardial infarction, or pulmonary embolus; or may even be thought to be in the early phase of salicylate overdose, the latter being a common cause of hyperventilation in children.

Fever, tachycardia, hypotension and leukocytosis are not unusual in many malnourished patients who have underlying diseases that could cause such signs. However nonspecific these signs and symptoms are, they should suggest septic shock in any patient when they occur together, especially if mental confusion and hyperventilation are also present. On the other hand, the patient with septic shock may have no fever early on or may actually be hypothermic. Fever may not occur in the presence of severe infection in an elderly patient. Patients with atrioventricular block (and some elderly patients for unknown reason) may fail to develop tachycardia in response to obvious infection.

At least early in septic shock, the hypotension is due to a decrease in peripheral vascular resistance, probably produced by circulating vasoactive substances, such as kinins. By the time there is evidence of inadequate tissue perfusion, including oliguria and cool, clammy extremities, it is often too late to reverse the small vessel damage that has been done.

Further confusing the immediate diagnosis is the fact that, early in septic shock in some patients (this patient, for example), the skin may be warm and flushed, representing a hyperdynamic syndrome - so-called "warm shock." Most of us are conditioned to think of shock only if the blood pressure is low for that patient and if the skin, especially of the extremities, is cool and clammy. Thus, the patient with "warm shock" may not be diagnosed as having a serious illness or complication, unless certain other features, such as fever and hypotension, are also present.

If a good history is available and reveals the recent occurrence of chills, malaise, nausea with or without vomiting, jaundice and cardiac dysrhythmias without an obvious cause, especially if the patient is elderly, one should also suspect septic shock when the patient presents with the signs and symptoms just discussed.

3. (A, B, C, D, E, G, I, J, K) (A) With septic shock, there is usually marked leukocytosis and a shift to the left in the differential count. However, in the early stages of septic shock, the white blood cell count may be normal or low, suggesting severe endotoxemia, as well as adding to the difficulty of correct diagnosis. In many elderly patients, whether endotoxemia is present or not, there is little or no leukocytic response, even in the presence of severe infection. This fact must be remembered in interpreting the white blood cell count in any elderly patient. Severe leukopenia has been found in the late stages of septic shock, so the total white blood cell count, while it must be done, cannot always be used as a guide in diagnosis or prognosis.

(B) Urinalysis may be definitive for the diagnosis if it indicates severe infection. A Gram's stain of the sediment will often reveal the organism responsible, although other portals of entry into the blood stream must still be ruled out.

(C) Immediate measurement of arterial blood gases and pH is useful in diagnosis; serial measurements are useful in the management of the patient. Severe initial metabolic acidosis usually indicates a poor prognosis, since it usually means that the hyperventilation, with resultant respiratory alkalosis seen early, has already given way to metabolic (lactic) acidosis. A drop in PaO_2 suggests that arteriovenous shunting has already occurred. Elevated $PaCO_2$ frequently occurs in late stages of septic shock with respiratory insufficiency. The blood gases (PaO_2 in particular) and pH are a necessary guide to oxygen therapy.

(D) Severe hyperkalemia suggests a late stage of shock. An elevation of blood glucose may only indicate that catecholamines have been released, not that diabetes mellitus is present. Blood urea nitrogen and creatinine give early indication of the status of the renal parenchyma. Enzyme studies, especially SGOT, SGPT and LDH, are often elevated in cellular injury due to anoxia, and in all patients in severe shock. An elevated blood lactate level usually means advanced anaerobic metabolism.

(E) The coagulation profile should be done and should include bleeding and clotting times, platelet count, prothrombin time, partial thromboplastin time, fibrinogen titer, and fibrin split products. This is largely for a baseline, in the event the patient develops changes suggestive of disseminated intravascular coagulation.

(F) Positive cultures will not be obtained quickly enough to aid in establishing a working diagnosis. However, they are often essential to confirm that diagnosis and are, of course, along with sensitivity testing, important guides in therapy. (G) On the other hand, gram staining of smears of any abnormal tissue fluid is often helpful in early diagnosis.

(H) Every patient in shock should have either a central venous pressure (CVP) line or Swan-Ganz catheter in place. Since CVP monitoring can be started in any emergency department, this should be accomplished without delay, although serial readings are much more informative than the initial reading.

(I) An initial twelve-lead electrocardiogram is necessary to help rule out acute myocardial infarction and dysrhythmias. Oscilloscopic cardiac monitoring should be continued. In shock, nonspecific S-T segment changes and T-wave changes are often seen, but abnormal Q waves should not be present unless the patient has a new or old myocardial infarction. The serial electrocardiograms are helpful guides to low or high serum potassium levels, and it is usually quicker in most hospitals to get another electrocardiogram done than to get a potassium concentration report from the laboratory.

(J) Roentgenological examination (portable) of the chest is a must, and one of the abdomen is highly desirable. Both are helpful in pin-pointing the portal of entry of bacteria into the blood stream, and are also useful for differential diagnosis.

(K) Lumbar puncture is necessary if no other cause for the patient's obtundation and fever is found; it may also help determine the portal of entry of infection.

4. (True) Gram-positive bacteremic shock is caused by exotoxins, gram-negative shock by endotoxins. The organisms responsible for gram-positive bacteremic shock are staphylococcus, streptococcus, pneumococcus, Clostridium perfringens

(especially in septic abortion), Clostridium tetani, and Corynebacterium diphtheriae. This type of septic shock is rare, compared to gram-negative bacteremic shock.

Gram-negative bacteremic shock is caused by Escherichia coli, Klebsiella pneumoniae, Enterobacter species, proteus, pseudomonas (as was true in this patient), Serratia marcescens, and, less frequently, bacteroides, mima, herellea, and salmonella. It occurs in patients of all ages but is more common in neonates, in women with complications related to pregnancy, and in the elderly. Predisposing factors are diabetes mellitus; cirrhosis and blood dyscrasias; the presence of severe burns; other open wounds; and almost any type of malignancy, the last two of which are present in this patient.

5. (True) Septic shock (primarily gram-negative) may follow a manipulative procedure, including surgery, especially on the genitourinary tract or gastrointestinal tract. Treatment with corticosteroids, immunosuppressive drugs, and antimetabolites, as in this patient, may predispose to septic shock.

6. (True) Despite vigorous treatment, mortality from gram-negative septic shock ranges from 30 to 80%, depending upon the duration of shock before treatment is started and the predisposing and associated conditions, including advanced age. For all ages, organisms, and precipitating causes combined, mortality is approximately 50%.

7. (True) Forty per cent of all instances of bacteremia caused by gram-negative organisms are accompanied by shock, truly a problem of staggering proportions, considering the high mortality. This contrasts sharply with the 5 to 10% of cases of gram-positive bacteremia that result in shock.

8. (E) All. (A) The endotoxin produced by the wall of the bacterium activates the vasoactive amines listed, causing vasodilatation and direct injury to the endothelial cells. (B) This vasodilatation causes "warm shock," which was seen in this patient. Although "warm shock" occurs in some elderly patients, it is more common in young patients. Its presence must not lead to delay in the diagnosis, as this stage presents the golden opportunity for definitive treatment. The vasodilatation also causes relative hypovolemia.

(C) Damage to endothelial cells leads to leakage of intravascular fluid into the interstitial space. Hypovolemia results, aggravating the relative hypovolemia caused by early vasodilatation.

(D) The decrease in blood volume then leads to reduction in venous return and cardiac output. Cold extremities appear at this stage, because of increased peripheral arterial resistance.

9. (Immediate: A, B, C, D; Secondary: E, F, G) Immediate treatment is aimed at stabilizing the patient's precarious condition. (A) All medications must be given intravenously, hence the importance of having at least two intravenous lines established within one or two minutes of the arrival of the patient.

(B) In any patient in shock, the airway may become obstructed by sudden loss of consciousness, accumulation of mucus or blood, or aspiration of vomitus. Insertion of a cuffed orotracheal or nasotracheal tube assures maintenance of the airway during the remainder of the initial therapy.

(C) Oxygen therapy is absolutely essential for any patient in shock. It should be started immediately at maximum concentration, with adjustments made according to the PaO_2 levels. The PaO_2 should be maintained at a minimum of 75 to 80 torr, with an additional 7 to 8 torr for each degree of fever Farenheit, or 15 to 18 torr for each degree of fever Celsius. Respiratory failure is a common accompaniment or complication of septic shock. Respiratory support, including endotracheal intubation and mechanical ventilation, is usually necessary, unless the patient shows prompt improvement.

(D) As soon as the patient arrives and while the diagnosis is being made, intravenous fluids should be started and infused rapidly. At first, this fluid can be Ringer's lactate solution or 5% dextrose in water (safer in an elderly patient), but it should be changed to an electrolyte solution as soon as evidence of relative or absolute hypovolemia is found. Fluid challenge is appropriate at this stage. Either central venous pressure or pressures obtained by means of a pulmonary artery catheter are useful for this purpose, the latter being far superior. Colloid, in the form of albumin or plasma protein fraction, may be indicated if the initial response to fluid challenge is inadequate.

As soon as the previously mentioned steps have stabilized the patient's condition sufficiently, the following should be considered:

(E) Antibiotics, properly selected, will greatly improve the chances of survival. Their selection is based upon the clinician's assessment of the most likely infecting organism. When there is no indication of the causative organism, gentamicin may be used empirically, until culture reports are available. This patient received gentamicin plus carbenicillin, since this combination seems to work best for pseudomonas bacteremia, which is what she had had during the previous episode of septic shock. The important principle is to administer enough of the correct antibiotic or antibiotics to eliminate the infecting organism as rapidly as possible. Unless this can be done, the prognosis is extremely poor.

(F) Vasoactive drugs may not be necessary, but if necessary, are properly used only after adequate volume replacement and adequate oxygenation. The latter steps are often all that are required to reverse the shock state. However, if the patient fails to improve with these initial measures, dopamine is the vasoactive drug of choice, the dosage beginning with 2 to 5 micrograms/kg/minute. In severe shock, this may be increased to 20 micrograms/kg/minute, with due regard paid to the different pharmacological actions at different rates (see Case 19). Isoproterenol has potent myocardial stimulating effects, but it also causes tachycardia and cardiac dysrhythmias and must be used with caution. In general, levarterenol, metaraminol and the other vasoactive drugs should not be used.

(G) If a portal of entry can be found, such as ruptured appendix or septic abortion, surgical intervention is mandatory regardless of the condition of the patient.

10. (F) All. (A) Disseminated intravascular coagulation (DIC) is an intermediary mechanism of this disease, rather than a complication in the strictest sense of the word. As septic shock advances, microthrombi form in the capillaries, setting off a chain reaction leading to massive consumptive coagulopathy and irreversible shock.

(B) Almost from onset of the hypotension, the lungs bear the brunt of the pathological changes of septic shock. However, the effects on circulation and respiration cannot be separated in this syndrome, as they cannot in most others. There is a considerable increase in metabolic rate with fever (each degree Celsius elevation above normal increases the metabolic rate 12 to 13%), shivering and restlessness, as well as the increased work of breathing. The muscles of respiration, being relatively weak, become exhausted under the increased load, and ventilation and oxygenation fail at a time when they are needed more than normally. Long before this point is reached, such patients should be given assisted ventilation and usually require controlled ventilation if the shock is severe. Respiratory insufficiency may persist even after correction of the hemodynamic abnormalities. This frequently leads to delayed death by the mechanism outlined in E.

(C) Both the heart and the brain seem to be spared early in the shock, but not for long, if the inadequate tissue perfusion persists or becomes worse. Cardiac output is increased in gram-negative bacteremic shock, and even this is not enough to overcome the effects of the peripheral vasodilatation and relative or functional hypovolemia. The increased load, especially in patients who are elderly, is too much for a heart with little or no reserve. In later stages of the shock syndrome, myocardial depression occurs with diminished cardiac output and normal or elevated vascular resistance.

(D) In septic shock, the kidneys may be the earliest organs to fail if there is pre-existing renal disease. Otherwise, renal failure occurs only after prolonged and severe hypotension.

(E) Death is usually caused by single vital organ failure or multiple organ failure. The terminal event is usually pulmonary edema, with generalized hypoxia and secondary cardiac dysrhythmias, from which the patient cannot be resuscitated. The patient usually becomes comatose due to cerebral hypoxia, and the blood pressure can no longer be kept in a range compatible with life, primarily due to inadequate coronary perfusion.

The mortality rate is high in the emergency department, because so many patients arrive only after the shock syndrome is well established. In hospitalized patients, the syndrome may not be recognized until the pathophysiological processes are so far advanced that they cannot be reversed.

COURSE:

This patient again recovered from her pseudomonas bacteremic shock. However, she still had her malignant tumor and its metastases; and her prognosis is extremely poor.

::

CASE 13: FAINTING ATTACK PRECEDED BY NAUSEA

HISTORY:

A 27-year-old woman was brought to the emergency department because she had fainted. For one hour before she fainted, she had been nauseated with some retching but had not vomited. She had had no abdominal pain and had noted no melena. Nine months earlier, she had had an episode of massive upper gastrointestinal bleeding after taking aspirin. At that time, endoscopy had revealed esophagitis and gastritis but no bleeding site; barium studies had revealed a cloverleaf deformity of the duodenal bulb. She had progressed satisfactorily in the interim, taking antacids and avoiding aspirin. She denied alcohol usage.

Examination revealed a pale, sweaty woman whose pulse was 130 beats/minute and weak but regular and whose blood pressure was palpable at 80 mm Hg systolic. She had no epigastric tenderness, and the liver and spleen were not enlarged. Bowel sounds were hyperactive. The findings on the remainder of the examination were within normal limits.

QUESTIONS:

1. As you examine this patient, you suspect upper gastrointestinal bleeding with secondary shock. In the absence of hematemesis and melena, what evidence is there for this diagnosis?
   A. History of syncope
   B. Physical evidence of shock
   C. History of previous gastrointestinal bleeding
   D. History of taking antacids regularly
   E. Presence of nausea and retching
   F. Hyperactive bowel sounds
   G. All of the above

2. From this history and physical examination, which is the most likely diagnosis?
   A. Peptic ulcer with hemorrhage
   B. Esophageal varices with hemorrhage
   C. Acute gastritis with hemorrhage
   D. Mallory-Weiss syndrome

3. Initial laboratory determinations should include which of the following?
   A. Type and cross-match blood

B. Complete blood count
C. Arterial blood gases and pH
D. Blood urea nitrogen, creatinine, glucose and electrolytes
E. Liver function studies
F. Analysis of stomach contents
G. Stool examination for blood
H. Coagulation profile
I. Twelve-lead electrocardiogram
J. All of the above

4. The initial management of suspected massive upper gastrointestinal bleeding should consist of which of the following?
   A. Begin at least two intravenous infusions with Ringer's lactate or 5% dextrose in saline.
   B. Start whole blood intravenously.
   C. Administer oxygen by nasal prongs or mask.
   D. Insert a central venous line.
   E. Insert a large orogastric tube.
   F. Do gastric lavage with ice water or cold saline.
   G. Administer sympathomimetic amines, such as norepinephrine or metaraminol.
   H. Start antacid therapy.
   I. All of the above

5. Which of the following are useful for determining the site of bleeding in the early phase of the work-up for massive gastrointestinal bleeding?
   A. Esophagogastroduodenoscopy
   B. Selective arteriography
   C. Barium meal studies
   D. Laparoscopy
   E. Abdominal ultrasonography
   F. Computerized axial tomography
   G. Abdominal x-rays
   H. All of the above

6. Monitoring procedures should be instituted as soon as possible for which of the following?
   A. Urinary output
   B. Central venous pressure
   C. Vital signs
   D. Hematocrit
   E. Gastric contents
   F. Intake and output
   G. Arterial blood gases and pH
   H. Electrocardiographic changes
   I. All of the above

7. TRUE OR FALSE: Operation is never advisable for a patient with massive upper gastrointestinal bleeding, because it carries a prohibitive mortality.

ANSWERS AND COMMENTS:

1. (G) All. (A) Although it is possible that she only had vasovagal syncope or simple fainting, this is highly unlikely. One reason is that with simple fainting, the blood pressure promptly returns to normal as soon as the person lies or falls down. Although simple fainting may be preceded or followed by weakness and nausea, these symptoms should not persist for as long as an hour. Although not invariably the case, syncope, in the setting described here, usually means considerable, even massive, blood loss.

(B) Gastrointestinal bleeding should be suspected in any patient in shock, until such bleeding has been ruled out or some other cause is found. Evidence for bleeding is the finding of hypotension, tachycardia, thready pulse, and cool, clammy skin. A rectal examination is always indicated, unless it could be harmful, as it might be in cardiogenic shock (because of noxious reflexes). A chemical test of the stool for occult blood should be done if gross bleeding is not obvious. In a number of instances, patients have developed hypovolemic shock and died before there was any external evidence of bleeding. Therefore, gastrointestinal bleeding as a cause of undiagnosed shock should be strongly suspected.

It should be noted that the blood pressure reading is not a dependable indication of shock or impending shock because of reflex peripheral vasoconstriction, which temporarily masks the effect of decreased cardiac output. This reaction is likely to be more marked in younger patients.

(C) It is highly probable that this patient's upper gastrointestinal hemorrhage nine months earlier was from her chronic peptic ulcer, although the actual bleeding site was never identified. (D) If a patient with a history of acute peptic ulcer continues or resumes antacid therapy, it is likely that he or she still has a peptic ulcer or has recently had recurrence of an acute peptic ulcer. However, since many patients who take the antacid preparations have dyspeptic symptoms without actual pain, this historical point must be accepted with some reservations.

(E) Blood in the upper gastrointestinal tract causes nausea and vomiting in most patients. However, if the bleeding originates distal to the pylorus, blood may not be present in the stomach early on, and hematemesis will not be present. Retching, if severe, may result in tearing of the esophagogastric mucosa (Mallory-Weiss syndrome), a cause of upper gastrointestinal hemorrhage. However, this condition is typically preceded by vomiting of gastric contents, such as food material, severe retching, and then hematemesis.

(F) Hyperactive bowel sounds, along with the nausea, could mean early acute gastroenteritis. However, blood in the intestine is a more likely cause in the presence of syncope and shock. This patient did, in fact, have a large dark red stool shortly after arrival. The absence of black color could mean an origin of bleeding lower than the esophagus, stomach or duodenum, but is also compatible with a rapid intestinal transit time, the stool appearing less than two hours after onset of symptoms.

2. (A) The patient probably has bleeding from a chronic peptic ulcer of the duodenal bulb, the probable source of the bleeding nine months before. B, C, and D are all possibilities, but are much less likely in this patient, especially since she has no history to suggest any of the three.

These four entities are the cause of at least 95% of all upper gastrointestinal bleeding of severe degree. The only one of the entities that is manifested by positive physical findings (evidence of collateral circulation, spider angiomata, liver enlargement, palmar erythema, possible jaundice) in the presence of bleeding is esophageal varices, a manifestation of portal hypertension.

The epigastric pain and tenderness usually found in acute and chronic peptic ulcer disease decreases or disappears with the onset of bleeding, probably due to the buffering effect of the blood. If severe pain persists after bleeding begins, one should suspect perforation of an ulcer, usually of the confined type, that is, not into the general peritoneal cavity.

3. (J) All. (A) Blood typing and cross-matching are urgent, since the availability of adequate blood supplies may determine the type of treatment chosen (surgical or medical), as well as the patient's ultimate fate. At least eight units should be available, all typed and cross-matched. At least four of those eight will be needed immediately for a patient, such as this one, already in hypovolemic shock.

(B) A complete blood count, including measurement of hemoglobin and hematocrit, is useful, both for initial diagnosis and for a baseline for future care of the patient. However, it is unwise to decide early about the extent of bleeding on the basis of hemoglobin and hematocrit alone. A period of up to 24 hours may be required for re-equilibration of body fluids following hemorrhage. This patient's hemoglobin and hematocrit were both low (10 gm/dl and 24%, respectively).

(C) Arterial gases and pH should be determined for any patient in shock. The degree of metabolic acidosis must be determined, so that corrective measures can be taken if required.

(D) Blood urea nitrogen almost always rises when upper gastrointestinal bleeding occurs; this never happens when the blood originates in the colon. In fact, the first indication of upper gastrointestinal hemorrhage may be a rise in blood urea nitrogen, this rise occurring even in the absence of hematemesis and before melena occurs. The usual abnormal level is 30 to 35 mg/dl and is due to absorption of the products of digested blood protein. A level higher than this is probably due to other factors, as well. Decreased renal blood flow, as from the shock state itself, may contribute to the azotemia. Obviously, acute or chronic intrinsic renal disease must be considered if no gastrointestinal bleeding is confirmed. It must be remembered, too, that both conditions may be present in the same patient. The creatinine level does not rise with upper or lower gastrointestinal bleeding, so this measurement is helpful in diagnosis.

(E) Bilirubin, transaminases, and alkaline phosphatase should be measured and serum protein electrophoresis done. The presence of gross abnormalities would point strongly toward hepatic disease, portal hypertension and esophageal varices. However, here, too, it must be remembered that at least 35% of patients with liver disease, whether or not they have esophageal varices, also have peptic ulcer disease.

(F) In any patient such as this one, insertion of a nasogastric tube should be immediate and routine, even when there is vomitus available for visual or chemical identification of blood. Caution is required during insertion to avoid producing bleeding from esophageal varices or increasing it, if already present. Gentle aspiration at about 35 cm may yield blood if bleeding is coming from the distal esophagus. Blood found in the stomach indicates a bleeding site proximal to the ligament of Treitz, but that site could be as proximal as the nasopharynx, especially in children.

As a #18F nasogastric tube was being inserted in this patient, she vomited 400 ml of dark red blood. An additional 400 ml was recovered through the tube over the next 10 minutes (see Course).

(G) Stool examination for blood should be done in all patients who have gastrointestinal bleeding. However, the absence of melena does not rule out acute upper gastrointestinal bleeding, as was the case in this patient. Red blood is converted to black blood by the oxidation of heme by intestinal and bacterial enzymes. Thus, the color of the blood depends more upon how long the blood has been in the intestine than on the site of bleeding or even on the amount of bleeding, since only 50 to 100 ml of blood can cause melena.

(H) A coagulation profile should be done routinely, in order to screen for patients with systemic diseases that can cause bleeding. This profile should include bleeding and clotting times, prothrombin time, partial thromboplastin time and platelet count.

(I) A twelve-lead electrocardiogram should always be done to rule out, or determine the extent of, heart disease. Due to the frequency with which serious dysrhythmias develop in the presence of shock, regardless of the etiology, the patient should be kept on electrocardiographic monitoring until his or her condition stabilizes.

The results of all other laboratory tests on this patient were negative.

4. (A, B, C, D, E, F) Diagnostic, monitoring and treatment procedures should be carried out simultaneously. If there is a shortage of personnel, treatment of a patient in shock must take precedence over diagnosis, except for the brief initial evaluation. The objective in the first 30 to 60 minutes is to restore an effective blood volume, then to establish the diagnosis on which definitive therapy is to be based.

(A) Intravenous fluid should be run in rapidly through at least two large catheters. Both Ringer's lactate and saline solutions can substitute for whole blood to some extent, but the amount given has to be two to two and one-half times greater. In many patients, especially older ones, giving this much fluid may precipitate pulmonary edema, which can be difficult to control, even with diuretics and digitalis. Plasma can be given as a substitute for blood, but the risk of hepatitis is considerable.

This risk must be weighed against the risk of further delay while blood is being cross-matched.

(B) Whole blood transfusions should be started as soon as typing and cross-matching are completed. The blood should be given rapidly in an amount sufficient to raise the systolic blood pressure to 90-100 mm Hg and the central venous pressure by several cm H_2O, if it was low at the beginning. A common and serious error is to give too little blood to replace that which was lost. In the patient whose systolic blood pressure is 70-90 mm Hg, whose heart rate is 100-130 beats/minute, and who has other clinical signs of hypovolemia, the amount of blood required can be estimated as 25% of normal blood volume, or 18 to 20 ml/kg. However, if shock is severe, the initial resuscitation effort may require 40 to 50% of normal blood volume, or 30 to 35 ml/kg. There is no set formula - the clinical status of the patient is the best guide, and any continued bleeding during the time of transfusion will have to be taken into consideration. Cold blood from a blood bank, to be given rapidly, should always be warmed first. Fresh blood may be better than bank blood after the first few units have been given, if there is hyperkalemia, dilutional thrombocytopenia, or dilution of factor VIII with resulting generalized oozing. So-called "universal donor" blood (type O, Rh-negative) should be used only for the direct emergency situation, since there is a possibility of reactions, even fatal ones. This possibility must be weighed against the risk of delay.

(C) Every patient in shock needs supplemental oxygen to help combat the metabolic acidosis that invariably develops in hypoxic tissue metabolism, as well as to help prevent pulmonary insufficiency, one of the most serious complications of shock.

(D) A central venous catheter is useful for the rapid administration of fluid and blood, although these can ordinarily be given through peripheral lines. The central venous line is more important as a means of monitoring central venous pressure (CVP), since the amount of fluid to be given can be based on the CVP, and, as mentioned earlier, it is important to give not too little and not too much. If shock is severe or prolonged, a Swan-Ganz catheter must be used as a better guide to fluid management.

(E) The usual nasogastric tube is not large enough to allow removal of large blood clots. Thus, an Ewald tube, which requires oral intubation, is usually necessary in patients with massive upper gastrointestinal bleeding.

(F) Lavage of the stomach with ice water is well worth trying if bleeding is brisk. It should slow down the bleeding, if not actually stop it, and it is excellent preparation for endoscopy. Once the blood is removed by lavage, continued or recurrent bleeding can be determined by careful monitoring.

(G) There is no convincing evidence that vasopressors are useful in the treatment of hypovolemic shock. In fact, they may be harmful, in that they increase the degree of peripheral vasoconstriction and further decrease the flow of blood to the vital organs.

(H) Antacid therapy, started immediately, will compromise the ability of the endoscopist to visualize an ulcer. If endoscopy is available and contemplated in the management of the patient, antacid therapy should be withheld, at least initially. However, as soon as possible, it should be started for ulcer bleeding and continued hourly.

5. (A, B, C) (A) Endoscopic examination is an important tool in the diagnosis of the site and extent of upper gastrointestinal bleeding. Where available, it has largely replaced barium meal studies for this purpose. In spite of the difficulties of working with a restless or uncooperative patient, the endoscopist is usually able to do an examination that is thorough enough to contribute importantly to the patient's management. This is true even if the information gleaned is mainly negative, for example, that varices are not present.

Endoscopy is the only way to diagnose erosive gastritis.

(B) Selective arteriography is an excellent method of demonstrating the bleeding site if endoscopy cannot do so, and provided hemorrhage is still occurring at a minimum rate of 0.5 to 1.0 ml/minute. It is most useful in demonstrating bleeding from gastroduodenal stress ulcers or vascular lesions of the small intestine.

(C) Barium meal studies should be postponed if there is the possibility that either esophagogastroduodenoscopy or selective arteriography can be done. However, if neither of these special procedures is available, barium meal studies should be considered, since they can usually differentiate between esophageal varices and peptic ulcer disease. This is the distinction that is so important to make in planning therapy. However, it must be remembered that, even if esophageal varices are identified by this method, there is no assurance that they represent the source (or the only source) of the bleeding.

(D, E, F) These are not usually indicated in a patient with frank upper gastrointestinal bleeding, unless primary or metastatic malignancy is suspected. In that case, one or more palpable abdominal masses would suggest the diagnosis.

(G) Flat and upright (or lateral decubitus) roentgenological studies of the abdomen are not likely to reveal the source of the hemorrhage. However, they may be useful screening devices to rule out malignancy, hepatomegaly, splenomegaly, and gallstones (which can erode mucosa and cause bleeding), as well as free air from a perforated viscus. Occasionally, both bleeding and perforation complicate a peptic ulcer at the same time. Metallic and certain non-metallic foreign bodies would be revealed by such films, also giving guidance in the proper definitive therapy.

6. (I) All. (A) Monitoring the output of urine every 30-60 minutes until the patient's condition is stabilized is one of the best indices of tissue perfusion. However, in the presence of renal disease, urinary output may be misleading, and too much fluid may be given under the erroneous impression that hypovolemia is still present. (B) Frequent CVP readings can help one avoid this pitfall, since CVP is the most precise, generally available measurement of fluid or blood loss and the best method for determining the adequacy of fluid and blood replacement.

(C) Initially - and for monitoring possible further bleeding - the vital signs associated with postural changes are the ones most helpful in determining whether stabilization of blood volume has been obtained. The tilt test is easily and safely done (if the patient is not actually in shock at the time) by recording the blood pressure with the patient supine, and then raising the head of the bed at least 45 degrees and recording the blood pressure again after 10 minutes. Alternatively, the patient can be asked to sit up with his feet dangling over the side of the bed, but this could be dangerous if his hemodynamic status is severely compromised (in which case, the test would probably not be necessary). The tilt test is most useful when the blood pressure and pulse are not clearly diagnostic of shock but are suggestive of borderline hemodynamic compensation.

(D) Hematocrit determinations made every two hours, until the patient's condition is stabilized, are useful for monitoring blood loss, as well as for following the response to therapy. Each unit of blood is expected to raise the hematocrit by 1.5 to 3.0%

when it is below 30% and if there is no further bleeding. The precautions outlined in answer 3B should be noted in interpreting hematocrit readings.

(E) Repeated or continuous aspiration of the gastric contents, using irrigation as needed, is very helpful in determining the presence of persistent or recurrent bleeding.

(F) Measurement and recording of the intake and output are essential, at least until the patient's condition has stabilized.

(G) Serial measurements of arterial blood gases and pH allow for a precise adjustment of oxygenation and ventilation, as well as for the regulation of acid-base balance related to metabolic processes and electrolyte losses.

(H) Electrocardiographic monitoring is a must for reasons previously outlined (answer 3I).

7. (False) Immediate operation for control of bleeding should be done whenever it is obvious that persistent massive bleeding and resulting shock cannot be counteracted by the rapid administration of large amounts of blood or blood substitutes. If the patient is in severe shock on arrival and fails to respond to rapid initial electrolyte fluid replacement and to 1000 ml of blood replacement given in 10-15 minutes, he should be prepared for immediate operation.

Early operation should always be considered in elderly patients, since they seem to tolerate the surgical procedure better than they tolerate persistent or recurrent bleeding and multiple blood transfusions. Regardless of his age, the patient with massive rebleeding, after initial stabilization by blood transfusions, is a candidate for operation.

On the other hand, in the patient with jaundice or ascites, tamponade of the varices with a Sengstaken-Blakemore tube should be attempted, since the risk of immediate operation is probably prohibitive.

COURSE:

Endoscopy was performed within one hour of the patient's arrival. No bleeding site could be found in the esophagus and stomach following removal of another 500 ml of bright red and dark red blood. However, active bleeding was seen from an ulcer of the duodenal bulb.

Blood was administered in the amount of 2000 ml over a 12-hour period, 1500 ml in the first two hours. The patient had no further bleeding and her condition remained stable.

Upper gastrointestinal barium studies done a few days later showed a clover-leaf deformity of the duodenal bulb, with no significant obstruction. Medical treatment was continued during and after her two-week hospital stay.

::

CASE 14: ANAPHYLACTIC SHOCK

HISTORY:

A 37-year-old woman had a severe cough of one week's duration, aggravated by her two-pack-per-day cigarette habit. She saw her local physician, who, on the basis of clinical and roentgenological findings, diagnosed bilateral pneumonia of the lower lobes. After eliciting a negative history of penicillin sensitivity, he injected 600, 000 units of aqueous procaine penicillin intramuscularly. Almost immediately, she became apneic and cyanotic and collapsed to the floor. Her heart was still beating strongly at 74 beats/min. The physician administered epinephrine, 0. 3 ml subcutaneously and started mouth-to-mouth ventilation, the latter being changed within 30 seconds to bag-valve-mask ventilation, via an oropharyngeal airway with 6 liters/min flow of oxygen. Her cyanosis disappeared promptly, but her pulse became rapid and weak, and her blood pressure dropped from 124/74 to 80/50 mm Hg. No skin rash developed.

The patient was taken to the emergency department one block away, via ambulance. En route, she was given a rapid intravenous administration of 1000 ml of lactated Ringer's solution through a large-bore catheter in one arm, 5% dextrose in water and the following medications in the other arm: diphenhydramine, 50 mg; and hydrocortisone sodium succinate, 250 mg.

When she arrived at the emergency department, her blood pressure was 90/60 mm Hg; her respirations were 24/min; and her pulse was 140/min. She was conscious but drowsy. History revealed that only a few months earlier, she had received penicillin by intramuscular injection for acute tonsillitis thought to be due to Group A hemolytic streptococcus. She had had no allergic reaction then, and had no personal or family history of drug allergy or sensitivity.

QUESTIONS:

1. Which of the following statements about systemic anaphylaxis are true?
   - A. Systemic anaphylaxis, anaphylactic reaction, anaphylactoid reaction and immediate hypersensitivity reaction are all terms used interchangeably.
   - B. There are many predisposing factors to anaphylaxis.
   - C. Anaphylaxis is always quite severe.

D. It affects several body systems.
E. Sensitivity reactions may become progressively worse.
F. The most common drug cause is penicillin.
G. The most common non-drug cause is Hymenoptera sting.
H. All of the above

2. The etiology and pathogenesis of systemic anaphylaxis are along which of the following lines?
   A. Precipitation by certain known substances
   B. Release or formation of chemical mediators which act primarily on smooth muscle and vascular tissue
   C. A and B

3. The diagnosis of penicillin anaphylaxis is based on which of the following?
   A. The history of a very recent (seconds to hours) injection of penicillin
   B. Respiratory difficulty
   C. Transient hemiplegia
   D. Skin symptoms and signs
   E. Cardiovascular collapse
   F. All of the above

4. TRUE OR FALSE: Urticaria and angioedema are almost always ominous signs of anaphylaxis.

5. Initial therapy for anaphylaxis is which of the following?
   A. Administer epinephrine.
   B. Place the patient in the supine position and elevate the lower extremities.
   C. Obtain and maintain a patent airway.
   D. Administer oxygen.
   E. Open an intravenous line and administer saline or lactated Ringer's solution.
   F. Administer diphenhydramine.
   G. Apply a tourniquet proximal to the injection (or sting) if on an extremity.
   H. All of the above

6. Supplemental therapy should be tailored to the type of reaction the patient is having and to the response to initial or primary therapy. Which of the following should be considered for a patient with a severe anaphylactic reaction who has responded only slightly to initial treatment?
   A. Aminophylline intravenously for bronchospasm
   B. Vasopressor therapy for hypotension
   C. Corticosteroid therapy

D. Isoproterenol
E. Calcium
F. Monitoring of vital signs, electrocardiogram, urinary output, plus serial chest roentgenograms, arterial blood gases and pH
G. Hospitalization
H. All of the above

7. In addition to the treatment outlined in questions 5 and 6, the correct management of systemic anaphylaxis, due to hymenoptera sting, includes which of the following?
   A. Remove the stinger with the venom sac, if present.
   B. Institute measures to prevent stings in the future.
   C. Institute measures to decrease the severity of stings in the future.
   D. Arrange for the patient to have an insect sting kit with him at all times.
   E. Arrange for him to have identification as being hypersensitive to insect sting.
   F. All of the above

ANSWERS AND COMMENTS:

1. (A, D, E, F, G) (A) In practice, no distinction is made in the meaning and use of these various terms. In actual fact, there is more than one mechanism involved, which accounts for the earlier distinction between anaphylaxis (the preferred term) and anaphylactoid reaction.

A good definition of anaphylaxis is a life-threatening response appearing within minutes after exposure of a sensitive person to a specific antigen.

Anaphylactic reactions were at one time considered those that had been clearly shown to be immunological, IgE-mediated, whereas anaphylactoid reactions were those in which an immunological basis had not been demonstrated. However, this distinction was somewhat artificial and has been largely abandoned.

(B) In essence, there are no predisposing factors, except exposure to some immunogen in the past. However, such exposure is usually not evident in the patient's history, and must be based on clues in both the patient's history and those of the family members. The following are suggestive of predisposition to allergic response. A history of an atopic background (personal or familial tendency to asthma, rhinitis, urticaria or eczematous dermatitis) predisposes to anaphylaxis, especially, it seems to penicillin allergy, although not as clearly to other types. Special precautions must be taken in patients with this history. However, anaphylaxis may develop in patients with no such history. Additional evidence of predisposition to anaphylaxis is the fact that IgE levels are elevated in most patients who have a history of atopic allergy.

The history of previous reaction to certain drugs, especially penicillin and related preparations, must be sought but it is often difficult to evaluate. Even by careful and time-consuming questioning, it is often impossible to be certain whether or not the symptoms described represent true hypersensitivity. If there is any doubt about this, it is better to avoid administering the drug in question, since the reactions tend to become more severe with each exposure to the sensitizing agent (see E). As illustrated by this patient, absence of a history of previous reaction is no assurance that a serious reaction will not occur.

(C) Anaphylactic reactions vary from mild to severe. They may begin with mild symptoms and signs which rapidly become severe; they may remain mild and soon disappear; or they may be immediately severe, as in this patient. The quicker the symptoms appear and the more rapidly they progress, the severer the reaction and the greater the likelihood that the outcome will be fatal. This fact emphasizes the importance of immediate diagnosis and treatment. To repeat, not all mild reactions will progress to life-threatening proportions, but it is safest to assume that they will, especially when the patient is acutely exposed to an allergen or substance known to cause anaphylaxis.

(D) The systems in which major manifestations of anaphylaxis occur in man are cutaneous, respiratory, gastrointestinal, ophthalmological, and cardiovascular. The most common symptoms are cutaneous and respiratory, with the respiratory symptoms, chiefly laryngeal edema or bronchospasm, usually occurring after the appearance of erythema, pruritus, and urticaria. The patient described here was exceptional in that (1) her apnea occurred first, presumably due to laryngospasm or laryngeal edema; and (2) she never did develop cutaneous manifestations or bronchospasm. Prompt treatment with epinephrine may have prevented these symptoms.

(E) Sensitivity reactions due to antigen-IgE interaction tend to become progressively worse. This fact makes screening of patients, on the basis of history, especially difficult and uncertain. If a former reaction had been mild, it may have gone unnoticed, and there is no warning that the next one may be severe, even fatal. Even more baffling is the fact that a patient may have received a dozen or more courses of penicillin without incidence and then experience anaphylaxis the next time he receives it.

(F, G) Allergic reactions to penicillin and to Hymenoptera sting make up most of those treated in emergency departments. These reactions are due to interaction of antigen with IgE. There are from 100 to 300 fatal anaphylactic reactions to penicillin annually in the United States. Many others are mild to severe but without a fatal outcome, usually due to prompt and adequate treatment, as in this patient. The incidence of hypersensitivity to penicillin is estimated to be 1 to 5% among adults in the United States but is much less frequent in children. Whether this is due to less vigorous antibody response in children, less previous drug therapy, differences in drug metabolism, or lower allergic reactivity, is not known. Fortunately, acute life-threatening anaphylactic reactions are very rare (0.05%).

There were 400 deaths reported from Hymenoptera stings (bees, wasps, yellow jackets and hornets) in the United States from 1963 to 1973. Although this is only 40 deaths per year, all were preventable. The recent invasion by fire ants of the southern states will increase the number of anaphylactic reactions to insect stings seen in emergency departments.

2. (C) (A) The substances capable of causing anaphylaxis are, by group or type, proteins, such as heterologous serum; antibiotics, local anesthetics, and hormones; prophylactic vaccines; insect venom; diagnostic agents; pollen extract and other hyposensitizing agents; and foods. The most common of these are drugs, diagnostic agents, foods, and insect stings.

Most of the points made about hypersensitivity to penicillin apply to other drug reactions and Hymenoptera reactions. Therefore, only penicillin anaphylaxis, which this patient had, will be discussed in detail. Question and answer 6 will present some information about hypersensitivity reactions to Hymenoptera stings.

(B) The mediators that are released or produced are histamine, slow-reacting substances of anaphylaxis (SRS-A), and kinins, as well as several other substances that have recently been identified and are now being characterized. Histamine is apparently the most important substance, being released from its storage site (the mast cell granules) when the allergen combines with IgE antibodies on the surface of the mast cells. This same degranulation of mast cells can be precipitated by way of the complement system, in which case, kinins are also released or produced. Kinins presumably cause the vasodilatation and shock that occur without any other symptoms. The precursor sites of SRS-A are unknown.

3. (A, B, D, E) (A) There is no difficulty with diagnosis in the patient who has an immediate reaction after receiving an injection of penicillin. However, onset varies from a few seconds, as in this patient, to several hours, with well over 90% of reactions beginning within the first 30 minutes. Immediate reactions are more likely to be severe, and fatal reactions begin almost invariably within a few seconds to a few minutes following injection.

The particular pattern of the immediate hypersensitivity reaction in man probably depends upon genetic factors, the immunogen that originally causes the hypersusceptible state, and the relative proportions of the different antibodies involved. The most frequently seen pattern is (1) pruritus with urticaria formation; (2) either upper respiratory obstructive symptoms or bronchospasm; and (3) then vascular collapse. However, one or more of these types or phases (which can serve as warning signals) may be bypassed, and the more life-threatening ones appear without any warning.

The most common steps in fatal anaphylaxis are severe respiratory distress with asphyxia, vascular collapse, and death within 15 minutes. The first two steps were exhibited by this patient; she was treated successfully before the third step could occur. The other variant is profound vascular collapse without antecedent respiratory symptoms. With this variant, the blood pressure drops precipitously, and the patient suffers cardiac arrest, for which immediate treatment is required if the patient's life is to be saved. Since there is no time for capillary leakage to account for the hypotension, it probably is due to widespread, severe vasodilatation, as well as severe myocardial depression.

The most important point about diagnosis is that it must be made promptly, by suspicion and careful observation of any high-risk patient, and by attention to any clues, however slight, to a beginning reaction. One such clue, although unusual, is cramping abdominal pain of sudden onset, due to spasm of the intestinal smooth muscle. If the patient says he must go to the rest room, he must be accompanied by a professional who can recognize the progression of symptoms and signs indicating impending anaphylaxis.

For the patient who is receiving penicillin and several other drugs orally and parenterally at home and who has a reaction while eating, the specific cause is very difficult to determine. The same applies to Hymenoptera reactions if there is no clear-cut history of one or more stings.

(B) The respiratory symptoms are usually diagnostic if they are straight-forward and if the clinician has a high index of suspicion. Hoarseness or choking may be the earliest symptom, and it must not be disregarded. On the other hand, fulminant bronchospasm, unresponsive to treatment, may be the only respiratory symptom. Both laryngeal edema and bronchospasm may appear simultaneously or only one may be present throughout the attack. This variability in anaphylaxis is a pitfall for the unexperienced or unwary clinician.

(C) Although some central nervous system symptoms may appear, it is not likely that hemiplegia, either transient or permanent, will be one of them. Rather, the symptoms are apprehension, with a feeling of impending doom; weakness; vertigo; dilatation of the pupils; blurred vision; syncope; or, as in this patient, sudden unconsciousness. Some, or all of these, are due to developing hypotension and hypoxia.

(D) See answer 4 for a discussion of the cutaneous signs and symptoms.

(E) Shock following cutaneous and respiratory signs and symptoms is due to hypoxia and hypovolemia, the latter caused by a rapid increase in capillary permeability and leakage of fluid from the vascular compartment. Pooling of blood, especially in the splanchnic area is also a factor. If the shock occurs without antecedent cutaneous or respiratory signs or symptoms, the patient may not have time to call for help or may not know to do so if he thinks that his weakness, faintness, vertigo, pallor or nausea are to be expected following his injection. If he has been left alone, he may be in cardiac arrest by the time the nurse or other professional returns to his room. This emphasizes the importance of constant observation of the patient by a responsible member of the staff or the family, until it is obvious that an early allergic reaction will not occur. In a patient with a history suggestive of the risk of anaphylaxis, that constant observation is necessary for several hours.

4. (False) Although urticaria and angioedema are the cutaneous

forms of the clinical syndromes of both immediate and delayed hypersensitivity, they must be viewed in context if their significance is to be determined. Urticaria involves only the superficial portion of the dermis, with elevated, well-demarcated, non-pitting, serpiginous lesions called wheals, whelps, or hives. They are almost always pruritic and can be quite extensive, coalescing into giant wheals or giant hives.

Angioedema (formerly called angioneurotic edema) is well-demarcated, localized swelling that involves the deeper portion of the dermis, as well as the subcutaneous tissue. It is frequently pruritic but not as often as, or to the extent of, urticaria. It can become quite extensive, especially when it involves the face and neck.

Both urticaria and angioedema are caused by increased capillary permeability in the areas of swelling. Both can occur simultaneously in the same patient. Both represent a localized cutaneous form of anaphylaxis, although they are not only caused by allergy. Other causes, especially of chronic or recurrent forms, are infections, physical factors, such as exposure to cold, certain systemic diseases, and emotional stress. Any food or drug is capable of causing urticaria or angioedema, and ingested allergens are much more frequent causes than inhalants.

The important point here is that not every patient with urticaria or angioedema is having the prodrome of anaphylaxis; most are not, and urticaria is a very common isolated problem seen in emergency departments.

Determination of the offending agent(s) is often difficult or impossible, and recurrence or chronicity is common despite what would seem to be adequate treatment. The relation, if there is any, between these conditions and immediate hypersensitivity reactions is unclear.

5. (H) All. As usual in a true emergency, the therapeutic procedures are carried out <u>while</u> the diagnosis is being made, and all therapeutic steps are carried out simultaneously, if possible, not one at a time, as implied in the listing of them. Nor, if they must be carried out one at a time, are they in the exact order of priority in this list, except that epinephrine is <u>always</u> the first drug given, not diphenhydramine, not corticosteroid, not any other drug.

(A) A therapeutic dose of epinephrine should be given at the earliest symptom or sign, if there is any suggestion that the patient might be at high-risk for anaphylaxis. The interval from the beginning of pruritus, in even a small area, with no visible wheal or swelling, to the occurrence of bronchospasm, laryngeal spasm or edema, can be only a few seconds or minutes. Thus, it is important to treat the patient on the suspicion that a reaction is occurring. Patients should be observed and warned to report even the slightest symptom not present before the injection was made. It is not safe to wait for the full-blown clinical picture to develop, or to quibble about whether the patient is just tense about the treatment, whether his choking sensation may merely represent globus hystericus, or whether his cardiac condition or blood pressure is such that he may not be able to tolerate epinephrine. There is too much at stake to allow any delay. For the high-risk patient, the epinephrine should be loaded in the syringe and almost literally in the hand of the physician or other person present who is authorized to administer it.

Epinephrine probably functions in at least two ways: (1) it increases cAMP, and (2) it decreases or prevents the release of histamine and SRS-A. It also reverses end-organ responses, such as smooth muscle contraction, vasodilatation, and increased capillary permeability.

Epinephrine 1:1000 should be given to an adult in a 0.3 - to 0.5 - ml dose in the undersurface of the tongue, which is highly vascular and where absorption is rapid. The dose may be repeated every 3 minutes in a severe reaction, every 10 to 20 minutes otherwise. If the patient will not, or is unable to, open his mouth, the intramuscular (deltoid) or subcutaneous route should be used.

The first dose of epinephrine may be given intravenously, if the clinical situation warrants the risk of producing ventricular fibrillation, although this risk is slight in most patients. If given intravenously, the epinephrine should be diluted in at least 10 ml of saline. The dose for children should be 0.01 ml/kg (a maximum of 0.3 ml) of 1:1000 epinephrine, diluted at least 30 to 50 times. Epinephrine should not be administered directly into the chambers of the heart unless the situation is desperate. Again, the reason is the risk of causing ventricular fibrillation, which is likely to be refractory if the epinephrine is inadvertently placed into the myocardium. Epinephrine may also be given as a 0.2 - ml dose into the site if the antigenic material was injected into an extremity, in the hope that the reduced absorption will prevent further progression of the symptoms.

In this patient, four doses of epinephrine were given 15 minutes apart. The first dose was given subcutaneously, the second one intramuscularly, the last two subcutaneously. Her blood pressure returned to normal over one hour from the start of symptoms, presumably helped by the beta effect of the epinephrine on the heart and its alpha effect on the peripheral arteries.

(B) The patient must always be placed in the recumbent (supine) position at the first indication of a reaction. Although this seems self-evident, it must be done even when the patient protests and prefers to "walk around" because he is suddenly restless. If his reaction progresses to shock and unconsciousness, he may hurt himself if he falls. Also, elevation of the lower extremities may help prevent or alleviate the hypotension that frequently develops (see pathophysiological mechanisms in answer 2).

(C, D) Frequently, the mechanism of respiratory-tract involvement is edema of the glottis, which can cause total obstruction within a few seconds, as in this patient. There may have been an element of laryngospasm contributing to her obstruction, since positive-pressure ventilation with mouth-to-mouth ventilation, and then administration of a high concentration of oxygen, allowed adequate oxygenation until the epinephrine took effect and the glottic obstruction began to subside. In a setting such as this, one should always try mouth-to-mouth (or mouth-to-mask) ventilation, since the rescuer's lungs are an excellent bellows system. Use of bag-valve-mask ventilation may be totally inadequate if done by inexperienced personnel. Ideally, suction should always be available, so that no time will be lost in removing excessive saliva or vomitus from an obtunded patient.

If assisted ventilation is needed, and if the ventilation and oxygenation are inadequate, endotracheal intubation must be done if the extent of laryngeal edema does not make it impossible. This is one of the situations where cricothyreotomy done immediately and rapidly is life-saving.

The other way in which the respiratory system may be involved is by bronchospasm, which may also appear within seconds or minutes and be life-threatening. Diagnosis is by auscultation of the chest; treatment is by aminophylline, administered intravenously, discussed in answer 6 (A).

As soon as possible, the administration of high concentrations of oxygen should be substituted for mouth-to-mouth ventilation.

This should relieve the hypoxia that develops due to upper airway obstruction or bronchospasm. It also assists in preventing or abolishing the anaerobic metabolism caused by both the respiratory impairment and the hypotension with decreased tissue perfusion.

(E) It is extremely important that an intravenous catheter be inserted as quickly as possible, and intravenous fluids started, usually 5% dextrose in saline or lactated Ringer's solution. This catheter also gives a route of access to the cardiovascular system for the fluids and medications that are the mainstay of treatment of this condition.

Either solution should be infused rapidly, at first, in order to replace the intravascular fluid lost to the extravascular fluid compartment, due to increased capillary permeability. Regardless of the patient's age or cardiac status, if he is hypotensive or if he becomes hypotensive during the reaction, it is wiser to administer lactated Ringer's solution or saline, rather than 5% dextrose in water.

Although pulmonary edema is a possibility in any patient who receives fluid or colloid by rapid intravenous administration, it is highly unlikely in most patients with anaphylaxis. However, central venous pressure, as well as urinary output, may be used as guides to the amount and rapidity of such infusions, especially after the first 30 to 60 minutes.

(F) Diphenhydramine hydrochloride, administered intravenously in aqueous solution, should be given early, especially if epinephrine fails to improve the patient's condition. In adults, it is usually given in an initial dose of 50 to 100 mg, the dose repeated in 15 to 30 minutes, if necessary. In less urgent situations, 50 mg may be given intramuscularly and repeated in 30 to 60 minutes, if necessary. The dose of diphenhydramine for children is 10 to 50 mg, given intramuscularly or intravenously. The mechanism of action is to further diminish the effect of the histamine by competing at the cellular histamine-binding sites.

If the patient fails to improve with one or more injections of epinephrine and one or more injections of an antihistamine, such as diphenhydramine, some other antihistaminic drug, such as cyproheptadine or hydroxyzine, should be administered. There is frequently more response to one antihistamine than to others.

The antihistamines are useful in many types of allergic disorders, including anaphylactic reactions. However, they must never be used as a substitute for epinephrine, only as an adjunct to it. One reason for this is that mediators other than histamine are usually involved in anaphylaxis, in which case the patient may die despite adequate antihistamine therapy, if epinephrine is not used primarily.

Topically applied antihistamines are not recommended both because of their limited benefit, and because they produce sensitization, which at times results in dermatitis.

(G) Although there is some question about the efficacy of a tourniquet applied proximal to the site of injection or sting on an extremity, it should be tried. It may prevent further antigen from getting into the general circulation at a time when the adverse reaction <u>may</u> be partly dose-related. The tourniquet should be tight enough to impede lymphatic and venous drainage, but not so tight that it impedes arterial flow. To prevent edema and possible ischemia, it should be removed for at least one to two minutes every 10 to 15 minutes. The only effect of the tourniquet is to allow time for the treatment drugs to take effect, so it is usually useful for only 15 to 30 minutes.

6. (H) All. (A) Of the four clases of drugs that are useful in anaphylaxis, namely, adrenergic agents, antihistamines, methylxanthines and corticosteroids, the first two have already been discussed. The prototype of the methylxanthine group is aminophylline, which, if it is used at all, is always administered intravenously. Its only indication in the treatment of anaphylaxis is the appearance of bronchospasm that cannot be controlled with epinephrine and antihistamines. Aminophylline should not be given in the presence of shock unless it is absolutely necessary. The reason is that it tends to cause hypotension or make it worse, even when given over a period of 10 minutes in the recommended dose of 250 mg diluted in 10 to 20 ml of saline. This dose can be followed by 500 mg in 500 ml of 5% dextrose in water titrated at a rate no faster than 5 mg/minute, for the first few hours. The dose of aminophylline for children with bronchospasm is 4 mg/kg, given intravenously over about 30 minutes.

The mechanism of action of aminophylline is inhibition of the degradation of cAMP by phosphodiesterase. This increases the level of cAMP, which, in turn, decreases the release of histamine and SRS-A.

(B) As soon as it is obvious that the patient's hypotension is not responding to adequate amounts of electrolyte-containing fluid, it is time to add a vasopressor. Either metaraminol or levarterenol may be used. The dose of metaraminol is 2 to 10 mg given intravenously, followed by a titrated infusion of 100 mg in 500 ml of 5% dextrose in water. The dose for children is 0.3 to 2.0 mg/kg in 500 ml of 5% dextrose in water, titrated for the desired effect.

The dose of levarterenol is 8 mg diluted in 5% dextrose in water. Care must be taken to prevent extravasation into the tissues around the site of the centrally placed indwelling venous catheter, because of the risk of necrosis. The dose for children is 0.1 microgram/kg/min.

(C) Hydrocortisone sodium succinate is useful in alleviating prolonged reactions or in preventing the recurrence of symptoms. The dose in adults is 100 to 200 mg, given intravenously and repeated every 4 to 6 hours; the dose in children is 10 mg/kg, given intravenously.

However, hydrocortisone has little or no place in the initial management of anaphylactic shock, largely because the time required for its beneficial effect is measured in hours rather than minutes. Since it is difficult to predict how long the reaction, especially bronchospasm, will last, it is probably wise to give hydrocortisone, in the dose mentioned, to patients with severe reactions. It must be stressed, however, that the use of a steroid must never divert the clinician from the primary therapy, namely, epinephrine administered early and repeated as necessary.

(D) In the patient without hypotension, who has bronchospasm unresponsive to epinephrine and aminophylline, a dose of isoproterenol should be tried, concomitant with careful electrocardiographic monitoring. It may be given as an intravenous infusion, 1 mg in 250 ml of saline, or as an aerosol with intermittent positive pressure ventilation, 0.5 mg diluted 1:200 in saline.

(E) In the event that the patient has little or no response to epinephrine and vasopressors administered in adequate doses by appropriate routes, the clinician should consider the possibility of epinephrine-fastness. This can be the case in patients who take propranolol regularly, of which there is an increasing number each year. In such patients, the dose of epinephrine should be kept at the therapeutic level, since the alpha effect of epinephrine on the peripheral arterioles would still be of value in preventing hypotension or in correcting it.

Whereas much of the beta effect of epinephrine on the heart is prevented by propranolol or other beta blockers, the effect of some other drugs is not. One such drug, if the beta-blockade is not complete, is calcium, which releases endogenous catecholamines. It may be administered intravenously as calcium chloride, calcium gluconate, or calcium gluceptate. In this setting, calcium is not likely to cause cardiac dysrhythmias, because these should be controlled by the propranolol. Also, cardiac rate and force should increase, unless the patient already exhibits tachycardia, which is unlikely in the presence of propranolol.

Other preparations should be used for other complications, but the ones previously outlined are the main ones required. If therapy is begun early, they are almost invariably adequate for a successful outcome.

(F) Knowledge of vital signs, as well as arterial blood gases and pH, is necessary in order to monitor the patient's progress. The urinary output should help the clinican determine the adequacy of total fluid intake. It is not unusual for electrocardiographic changes to occur during or after an episode such as this patient had. In an older, less vigorous patient, such an episode of hypovolemic shock might very well have precipitated cardiopulmonary decompensation, including decreased cardiac output and pulmonary edema.

(G) For minor reactions, or for those that respond promptly to treatment, it may not be necessary to admit the patient to the hospital for observation and further treatment. However, there is no doubt that a patient having as severe a reaction as this patient had should be admitted. As a general rule, such patients should be observed in the hospital setting for at least 12 to 24 hours, since recurrence of symptoms may follow discontinuation of therapy or changing from parenteral to oral therapy.

7. (F) All, most of which are self-explanatory. Local reactions do not usually require such intensive care, although they can be prolonged and very uncomfortable for the patient. There is some evidence that patients have more severe reactions with subsequent stings or with multiple stings, especially about the head, face and neck. There are serious medicolegal implications in failing to prescribe an insect sting kit and failing to refer the patient for allergy consultation following a severe reaction. The identification, such as a bracelet, necklace, or wallet card, is also very important for the patient to have. Although the whole-body extract presently available for hyposensitization

is not entirely satisfactory, it should be strongly recommended for any patient who has had anaphylaxis following a sting. It is hoped that venoms, in addition to pure bee venom, will be available for treatment within a few years. In the meantime, emphasis should be placed on avoidance of stings.

COURSE:

Following emergency treatment, as mentioned in answers 5 and 6, this patient was admitted to the hospital for observation. Her electrocardiogram showed no abnormality except sinus tachycardia, and her chest roentgenogram showed no change in the infiltrate known to be present in both lung bases. Her only symptom was slight hoarseness, which disappeared over a period of three days. No attempt was made to intubate her trachea, so the hoarseness was presumably due to laryngeal edema, producing complete obstruction of her glottis. Had she not responded so promptly to positive pressure ventilation and oxygenation, cricothyreotomy or tracheostomy may well have been indicated, assuming that endotracheal intubation was not possible. Erythromycin was started before she left the hospital and was well tolerated. She made a complete recovery within 48 hours.

She was cautioned to never again take penicillin or related products by any route. She was given an identification card, as well as a bracelet, for Medic Alert.

::

CASE 15: SYNCOPE

HISTORY:

An 18-year-old man was standing in line at a restaurant at 7:00 a.m., waiting to be seated for breakfast. He suddenly felt weak and dizzy, "things got black," and he fell to the floor. He regained consciousness promptly and felt much stronger after drinking some milk and coffee. Two weeks earlier, he had had a viral syndrome, thought to be influenza, from which he had gradually recovered. His only similar fainting episode had occurred one year earlier under similar circumstances. His medical history and that of his family were noninformative.

Forty-five minutes after the incident, the results of general and neurological examinations were entirely normal. His blood pressure was 114/94 mm Hg; pulse, 70/min; temperature, 97.2°F (36.2°C) orally. Since he had not had a physical examination for several years, blood was obtained for a complete blood cell count, fluid and electrolyte levels, glucose, and blood urea nitrogen. All were normal.

QUESTIONS:

TRUE OR FALSE:

1. The most likely diagnosis in this patient is vasovagal or vasodepressor syncope.

2. When the patient is in the upright position, syncope occurs only after 10 to 15 seconds of total cessation of blood flow to the brain.

3. Diagnosis of syncope is made almost solely by the history, unless the attack occurs in the presence of the physician. Which of the following statements about the historical, physical or laboratory diagnostic clues are true?
   A. Hysterical syncopal attacks are suggested by normal skin color, pulse, and blood pressure, occurrence of the attack in the recumbent patient, or the patient's graceful fall from the upright position.
   B. If the history indicates that the patient stood up and fainted, it probably indicates postural (orthostatic) hypotension.
   C. Simple or vasovagal (vasodepressor) syncope is sug-

gested in a young person who has weakness and pallor while upright and under emotional stress.

D. A cardiac cause is likely if the patient is elderly or has heart disease, especially if the attack occurs in the recumbent position.

E. If the patient had tonic or clonic movements, epilepsy is the most likely diagnosis.

F. The twelve-lead electrocardiogram and rhythm strip may be diagnostic.

G. Holter monitoring for 24 hours may reveal a temporal relationship between syncope and the cardiac rhythm or rate.

4. Syncope occurring with exertion is likely to be due to which of the following conditions?
   A. Aortic stenosis
   B. Idiopathic hypertrophic subaortic stenosis (IHSS)
   C. Cardiac tumor, producing a ball-valve effect
   D. Ball-valve thrombus
   E. All of the above

5. In addition to the fact that it often occurs with the patient recumbent, which of the following are true about syncope due to cardiac causes?
   A. It occurs in older patients.
   B. It is usually due to acute subendocardial myocardial infarction.
   C. The syncope of Adams-Stokes syndrome is caused by supraventricular tachycardia.
   D. Syncope due to aortic stenosis only occurs with effort.
   E. Syncope due to idiopathic hypertrophic subaortic stenosis (IHSS) usually occurs immediately after exertion.

6. Which of the following are true regarding treatment?
   A. Simple fainting usually requires no treatment.
   B. Associated injuries, as from a fall, should be searched for and treated.
   C. Postural hypotension, as a cause of syncopal attacks, can be frequently treated by adjustment of drugs and dosages.
   D. Cardiac syncope frequently requires an artificial pacemaker.
   E. Valve replacement is usually necessary for aortic stenosis with syncopal attacks.
   F. All of the above

ANSWERS AND COMMENTS:

1. (True) By far, the most common cause of fainting in a young person with this history is vasovagal syncope.

Syncope is the sudden transient loss of consciousness, due to a reduction in cerebral blood flow. The precise mechanism of vasovagal syncope is not well understood.

The cause of the reduction in cerebral blood flow and underperfusion of the brain is loss of the systemic arterial vasoconstriction, that normally prevents excessive pooling of blood in the venous and arterial systems. In the patient who faints because of psychic disturbance, this change in vascular tone is reflexly mediated from the cerebrum through the vagus nerve, with bradycardia as one result. Normally, three-fourths of the blood of the body is located in the venous system. Any pooling of additional blood in the venous system interferes with venous return to the heart. The decreased venous return and the bradycardia combine to decrease the blood pressure below a critical level. When cerebral perfusion is reduced by approximately 50%, syncope results.

Vasovagal syncope is rare during physical exercise, since the exercise helps prevent the bradycardia; the muscular activity, especially of the lower extremities, promotes venous return to the heart.

The onset of syncope is usually sudden, although most patients experience a premonitory, brief period of weakness or nausea immediately prior to losing consciousness.

Syncope must be differentiated from dizziness, vertigo, hysteria, head trauma, convulsive states and epileptic equivalents (including petit mal with "absences"), shock, cardiac arrest, and coma. The latter is due to extreme depression of cerebral function from various causes, whereas syncope is restricted to loss of consciousness due to cerebral ischemia. Syncope has the following essential criteria: a rapid or sudden loss of consciousness due to generalized lack of cerebral blood flow, with loss of postural tone; upright position, with the victim falling if unsupported; and short duration of the attack.

The circumstances are usually similar to those of this patient: a recent illness, standing position (often waiting in line before a meal), and no food intake for several hours. However, this is not to suggest that the sudden development of hypoglycemia is the cause of the fainting. It usually is not, and the blood sugar in most such patients is normal.

Syncope is frequently precipitated by a stressful situation, such as the prospect of, or the actual experiencing of, pain (receiving an injection or having blood drawn), or discussion about injury to or operation upon someone else, especially a close friend or relative.

Multiple causes of syncopal attacks in an individual patient are not infrequent. An example is postural hypotension, hypoglycemia and hyperventilation, or any combination of these conditions. Patients with diabetes mellitus are subject to such multiple causes. Hypoglycemia, alone, may cause syncope, but it is usually preceded by profound weakness and bizarre behavior and merges with coma; and the patient is unlikely to recover without receiving sugar or other carbohydrates.

The examination and any routine laboratory tests done prove to be almost always negative for any precipitating cause. The clinician is usually torn between not doing any special tests and performing certain screening tests, especially if the patient has had one or more similar episodes previously, or if he has not had a physical check-up in a long time. Usually, in young, healthy patients, these tests turn up nothing except possibly equivocal or incidental findings, which should then be followed up. Since disease detection is one of the proper functions of an emergency department, there is no harm in obtaining selected screening tests, although most emergency departments are not set up for carrying out comprehensive examinations with continuity of care. The exception to this is the physician in practice in a community where he covers the emergency department in a local hospital, and can, therefore, follow such patients in his office or clinic. Otherwise, selective referral for follow-up or consultation is obviously indicated for any significant clinical or laboratory abnormalities.

There is renewed emphasis upon the differential diagnosis of the causes of syncope. One reason is the availability of the artificial electronic cardiac pacemaker, which makes it possible to prevent many of these attacks when due to cardiac disease. This is a worthwhile effort, since cardiac-induced syncope is often fatal.

2. (False) After only 1.5 to 2 seconds, an upright patient feels dizzy, and in 3 to 4 seconds, he loses consciousness. Thus, there is only a very brief period during which the patient may

take protective action, such as lying down or asking for assistance. The recumbent patient who has cessation of cerebral blood flow becomes unconscious in only 7 to 12 seconds; again, this is usually too short a time for the patient to obtain help.

It should be pointed out that the amount of warning, which is measured in seconds, it not helpful in the differential diagnosis in most patients.

3. (A, B, C, D, F, G) (A) Hysterical syncope can easily be differentiated if a good history can be obtained from the patient (difficult at times), usually a young woman, or from one of the many witnesses usually present. They relate that there was no pallor or sweating and the pulse and blood pressure were normal, if these were checked. The patient's description of the incident will be very unemotional, with no outward display of anxiety. The attack is likely to have happened in such a way that the patient is unlikely to have harmed herself. It frequently occurs, or can recur, when the patient is recumbent. The patient is not truly unconscious in this condition. The only other condition likely to have the same history is cardiac syncope, which may require differentiation, although there is usually no difficulty in this.

(B) The patient who suddenly stands up from a sitting or recumbent position, and has syncope, almost certainly has postural or orthostatic hypotension due to pooling of blood in the lower extremities and failure of the baroreceptor reflexes. These reflexes usually respond promptly to a sudden drop in blood pressure - such as occurs when a person stands up - by elevating the blood pressure and increasing the heart rate. When these protective mechanisms fail, the patient faints.

Once the diagnosis is made from the history, the problem is to determine the cause. Certain drugs may interfere with normal postural reflexes, such as nitrates used in treatment of angina, ganglionic blocking agents, such as guanethidine, phenothiazine (particularly following parenteral use), and levodopa. Drugs that reduce blood volume are also a common cause of postural hypotension, especially thiazide diuretics or the potent diuretics, such as furosemide or ethacrynic acid.

Another possible cause is decreased circulating blood volume from occult bleeding, for example. The tilt test for detecting occult bleeding is described in Case 13.

Blood volume depletion and syncope can occur with dehydration from any cause, especially severe or prolonged vomiting or diarrhea, or both.

Excessive venous pooling can cause syncope in patients with normal blood volume. These include patients who have extensive varicose veins of the lower extremities; normal persons who have stood for a long time in hot weather; and any patients who have recently had a febrile illness, as had this patient. Pregnant patients are subject to syncopal attacks for a variety of reasons, including pressure on the inferior vena cava by the gravid uterus, most often in the last trimester.

(C) Simple syncope is by far the most common type, especially in adolescents and young adults. The diagnosis is not made by exclusion, although an effort must be made to eliminate any other serious causes (see question and answer 1).

(E) The presence of a few clonic movements of the face or limbs during a vasovagal syncopal attack does not mean epilepsy, and one must be careful not to label it as such, especially from a history that may not be reliable. Differentiation of that type of syncope from a convulsion is usually not difficult. In syncope, the loss of consciousness precedes the clonic movements; it is the reverse in a convulsion. Syncope is characterized by almost immediate recovery of consciousness once the patient is recumbent, and no residual headache, drowsiness or mental confusion, as are characteristic of the postictal state. A grand mal seizure is characterized by tonic-clonic movements that would be hard to miss by reliable witnesses. It must be remembered that a patient with an Adams-Stokes attack may have a grand mal seizure if his cardiac output is interrupted for 10 to 15 seconds (see question and answer 5). If there is any doubt about the significance of clonic movements as described by witnesses, further investigation, including neurological consultation, must be considered.

(F) An electrocardiogram is frequently, although not always, indicated in the investigation of the cause of fainting. One was not done in this patient, because the diagnosis was fairly certain and it did not seem necessary. Within a short time (less than one hour), the electrocardiogram and monitor strip may show an obvious cause of the attack, although this is most likely in older patients. Prolongation of the Q-T interval may be associated with syncope. Large U waves, as well, are also present in a heterogenous group of patients who have taken phenothiazine, who have hypokalemia of any cause, or who have Jervell and Lange-Nielsen syndrome. In the latter, congenital deafness is usually, but not invariably, present, and sudden death is common.

(G) If attacks are frequent, Holter monitoring should be done in the hope of finding an association between syncope and a tachy- or bradydysrhythmia. The monitoring may have to be repeated several times for patients who have infrequent attacks and normal electrocardiographic findings between attacks.

4. (E) All. If the history reliably indicates that syncope occurred during physical exertion, these are some of the conditions that must be considered, depending somewhat upon the patient's age.

5. (A, E) Not every patient with a significant cardiac lesion who faints does so because of his heart problem. Such patients can have all of the other causes of fainting as well. For that reason, the emergency department physician should not overreact and request a lot of laboratory studies for every cardiac patient with syncope.

On the other hand, the most important group of patients whose syncope is checked in emergency departments comprises those with heart disease. The reason for that importance is that these patients may, at any time, require an artificial pacemaker, without which the next attack may be fatal. All cardiac syncope results from a significant, usually sudden, drop in cardiac output. It is caused by transient asystole, transient ventricular tachycardia or fibrillation, a change from sinus rhythm or partial block to complete atrioventricular block, or slowing of the idioventricular pacemaker secondary to drug action or electrolyte imbalance.

As a rule, older patients are the ones who have cardiac syncope. The cause is usually complete heart block or dysrhythmia, either bradycardia or tachycardia.

(B) Subendocardial infarction does not cause syncope, but anteroseptal transmural infarction infrequently does. Syncope is rare with inferior infarction.

(C) The Adams-Stokes syndrome is not due to any type of tachycardia, but is syncope associated with the bradycardia of complete heart block. However, not every patient with bradycardia, even at the rate of 30 to 40 beats/min, will have syncope, especially when recumbent.

(D) Syncope due to aortic stenosis usually occurs with exercise or some type of effort, but it can occur in the patient at rest. In either case, it is always an ominous sign, whether or not it is associated with angina. Warning symptoms are often absent; when they occur, the symptoms are weakness or lightheadedness with pallor. Sudden death is due to either ventricular fibrillation or ventricular asystole.

(E) It is true that the exercise period, itself, is not as dangerous for the IHSS patient as the period immediately following the exertion. The reason is that while the exercise is going on, the heart has increased venous return. As soon as the exertion ceases, the venous return reverts to normal. However, the hypertrophied ventricular septum may obstruct the flow of blood from the heart, since the force of the cardiac contractions is still increased. If syncope does not occur from this obstruction of the outflow tract, it may occur secondary to the transient tachycardia that accompanies or immediately follows exertion in these patients.

6. (F) All. The syncopal attack, itself, rarely needs treatment, because it is corrected by the patient's becoming recumbent. Treatment for the cause of syncope is sometimes necessary. Only a few illustrative points are made here, related to the most common causes of syncope.

(A) Simple fainting usually requires no treatment, except that the patient should be reassured and cautioned about the circumstances that caused it. If attacks persist, further investigation should be arranged. Prevention of future attacks is often possible by advising the patient to avoid the precipitating factors or by "deconditioning" the patient. In any case, the patient should lie down while under the type of stress that may cause fainting.

(B) It is unusual for a person who has experienced vasovagal syncope to be injured in the fall, primarily because the few seconds of premonitory symptoms allow him to slump, rather than "crash", to the ground. A faint in a dangerous location, as at a height, can cause serious injury. A general examination should always be done to rule out associated injuries, as is done in cases of convulsion.

There is little or no warning before the syncope that is due to cardiac cause or postural (orthostatic) hypotension. Such patients do sustain injuries from falls, frequently falling forward on the face and sustaining lacerations and fractures. These may take precedence over the syncopal attack for both diagnosis and therapy.

(C) If postural hypotension is due to drugs, adjustments in the amount or the schedule can frequently be made. Adverse interactions between drugs may be involved, and underlying cardiac or other disease is present in many patients. In the emergency department, it is not unusual to find that an elderly patient being investigated for syncope has been taking six to twelve drugs prescribed by as many as three to five physicians.

(D) An artificial pacemaker is almost always required in a patient who has an Adams-Stokes attack. The sooner it is placed, the better, since the next attack may be fatal.

(E) A patient with aortic stenosis may have syncope from some other cause, as can any patient with heart trouble. If it is determined that his syncopal attacks are caused by the aortic stenosis, valve replacement is indicated as soon as possible.

CASE 16: COMA IN AN ALCOHOLIC PATIENT

HISTORY:

A 51-year-old man was found on the street, nonresponsive and hyperventilating. EMT-As, summoned to the scene, transported him promptly to the emergency department by ambulance, administering oxygen at 12 liters/min by face mask en route. No history was available, and no warning about diabetes mellitus, allergies, or other special conditions could be found among his belongings.

EXAMINATION:

The patient was unconscious and made no response to painful stimuli. He was unkempt and there was the odor of alcohol on his breath. Blood pressure was 90/50 mm Hg; pulse, 110 beats/min; respirations 40/min; rectal temperature, 100°F (38°C). There were no reflex nor motor abnormalities, and there was no evidence of injury.

QUESTIONS:

TRUE OR FALSE (Questions 1 and 2):

1. The patient probably has alcohol intoxication and should be allowed to "sleep it off" without being disturbed.

2. The patient may be having a disulfiram (antabuse) - alcohol reaction.

3. Which of the following <u>initial</u> steps should be taken to establish a diagnosis?
   A. Do rapid-method semi-quantitative blood glucose determination, such as with Dextrostix®.
   B. Administer 50 ml of 50% glucose intravenously.
   C. Administer naloxone (Narcan®) intravenously.
   D. Intubate the trachea with a cuffed tube, and administer a high concentration of oxygen.
   E. Draw arterial blood for pH and gas determinations.
   F. Administer thiamine hydrochloride, 100 mg intravenously or intramuscularly.

4. Which of the following additional measures for diagnosis and treatment should be carried out?

A. Start an intravenous infusion of dextrose.
B. Insert a Foley catheter into the bladder, and send a urine specimen for routine analysis and drug screening.
C. Draw blood for drug screening (if facilities for this test are available) and measurement of electrolytes, true glucose level, and alcohol level.
D. Start cardiac monitoring with a 12-lead ECG as soon as possible.
E. Do a complete blood cell count, serum amylase measurement, and urine culture; obtain skull and chest roentgenograms; examine stool for occult blood.
F. Do a lumbar puncture.

5. TRUE OR FALSE: Alcoholic patients almost never need gastric lavage.

6. The mechanism of hypoglycemia in acute and chronic alcoholism is:
   A. Direct effect of the alcohol on cerebral glucose regulating centers
   B. Acute and chronic pancreatitis
   C. Inadequate food intake
   D. Depletion of glycogen stores in the liver
   E. All of the above
   F. None of the above

7. TRUE OR FALSE: After his recovery from coma, the patient should be screened for diabetes mellitus.

8. What other complications are commonly found in alcoholic patients?
   A. Pneumonia
   B. Urinary tract infection
   C. Upper gastrointestinal hemorrhage
   D. Pancreatitis
   E. Polyneuropathy
   F. All of the above

ANSWERS AND COMMENTS:

1. (False) It is a serious mistake to assume anything about a comatose patient who smells of alcohol, especially in the absence of any history. Even if the patient is a known alcoholic and has been treated repeatedly for this problem in the same facility, he may, this time, be in coma from another cause. Coma of this degree from ethanol is uncommon, unless the alcohol has been consumed rapidly in large amounts or has been

combined with other drugs, such as the sedative-hypnotic-tranquilizer type, or with methyl alcohol (methanol) or other poisons.

The danger is that alcohol may not be the sole problem or may not be the problem at all. Assuming alcoholism in such patients, without work-up, can cause misdiagnosis of a serious, even fatal, condition. The problem is compounded in a busy emergency department when the care of other patients seems more urgent. However, at the very minimum, such patients require a fairly complete examination and screening laboratory tests, plus recording of whatever history can be obtained from relatives and friends, EMT-As, old records, and any other possible sources. While a period of observation is essential after the definitive diagnosis has been made and definitive, or at least supportive, treatment has been started, this observation is different, by far, from letting the patient "sleep it off" on the off-handed assumption that he is in a drunken stupor.

2. (False) The signs and symptoms of a disulfiram-alcohol reaction are flushing of the face, sweating, hypotension, drowsiness, hyperventilation, headache, dyspnea and apprehension. If the intake of alcohol is great, coma and even death may ensue. Since this patient was comatose, the headache and apprehension could not be determined. He was indeed comatose, hyperventilating and hypotensive. However, the almost pathognomonic signs of sweating and flushed face were absent, and a diagnosis of disulfiram-alcohol reaction was not entertained. (Note: Due to the low blood pressure, evaluation and treatment should be done with these patients lying down when such a reaction is suspected. Treatment is with antihistamines.)

3. (A, B, D, E, F) (A) The Dextrostix® in this patient measured "near zero" and his true blood glucose was 20 mg%. (B) He responded promptly to intravenously administered 50% glucose (50 ml initially, then another 75 ml for a total of 125 ml, because his Dextrostix® finding was so low). Within a minute or two, he awoke and asked, "Where am I?" His speech was slurred, but he was no longer comatose. His blood glucose after 4 hours was 114 mg/dl. (D) Any comatose patient should be intubated, if for no other reason than to protect his airway and to allow controlled ventilation. Also, it is very likely that some degree of acidosis, as in this patient, will require treatment. Initially, high concentrations of oxygen are in order until a preliminary diagnosis is made. (E) Arterial blood for pH and gas determinations should always be done as soon as possible, whether the patient has already received oxygen or not. These tests are indispensable in determining whether the patient has electrolyte

and acid-base imbalance, and, if so, which type of disturbance and the degree of each type. This patient's blood gases were: PaO_2, 120 torr; $PaCO_2$, 31 torr. Blood pH was 7.26; HCO_3^- was 13.4 mEq/l. Since he was able to take fluids and food orally so promptly, he was not given sodium bicarbonate intravenously for his moderate metabolic acidosis. His hyperventilation was probably secondary to metabolic acidosis. Six hours later, arterial pH was 7.48; PaO_2 was 139 torr; $PaCO_2$ was 31 torr; HCO_3^- was 22 mEq/l. These changes no longer indicate metabolic acidosis. (F) Thiamine hydrochloride should be administered to any alcoholic or suspected alcoholic in a 100-mg dose, which may require repeating every 12 hours for 2 to 4 doses. The first dose should be given intramuscularly or intravenously, even in a patient who is alert, and it should be given before glucose is given, to prevent sudden and irreversible Wernicke-Korsakoff syndrome[2] (see Case 17). The mechanism causing the Wernicke-Korsakoff syndrome appears to be blockage of oxidative decarboxylation of pyruvate to acetyl coenzyme A, with the accumulation of pyruvate in the absence of thiamine. Such depletion of thiamine is more likely to be present when prolonged heavy alcohol intake is combined with severe starvation and profound hypoglycemia, as in this patient.

If he had failed to respond promptly to the glucose infusion, then C would have been a logical additional step to take. Naloxone is not an antidote for alcoholic coma, and there is, as yet, no specific drug for this purpose. In fact, there is not even a drug available that will speed up the metabolism of alcohol in the body. The value of naloxone is that it is a specific antagonist for overdosage of opiates, and thus is of both diagnostic and of therapeutic value. No serious problems have developed from its use in this manner. It is not necessary that the patient have a slow respiratory rate for the diagnosis of opiate toxicity to be entertained, since the respirations may be normal or rapid on the basis of some other cause. Thus, naloxone for this patient, in the absence of a response to the glucose, would have been wise. The dose is 0.4 mg (1 ml) for adults and 0.01 mg/kg for neonates and children, initially administered intravenously, intramuscularly, or subcutaneously. It may be repeated intravenously at 2- to 3-minute intervals, but the absence of significant improvement suggests that the coma may be partly or completely due to non-opioid drugs or to other causes.

4. (A, B, C, D, E initially; F if the patient still fails to respond) (A) It is always important to have one or more large-bore intravenous lines open and running in any comatose patient. Intravenous medications can be given through such lines, the fluids

speeded up as desired, and the type of fluid changed as needed. Usually, these are established at the scene where the patient is found. In this particular instance, the patient was found close to an emergency department, and immediate transportation there seemed advisable. Dextrose 5% in 0.9% saline was an arbitrary choice in this patient, but it served the purpose until more diagnostic information could be obtained.

(B) Every comatose patient should probably have an indwelling catheter for obtaining a clean specimen of urine and for determining urinary output. In this patient, urinalysis was within normal limits except for moderate ketones. Urinary screening for drugs should be done even though the report may not be available immediately. It was negative in this patient.

(C) Blood screening for drugs was not available for this patient. Serum electrolytes were normal, except for bicarbonate level of 17 mEq/l and potassium level of 6.9 mEq/l (see answer D). Measurement of alcohol level should be done more often than it is. The results are not always available immediately, and most physicians think there is a legal problem about doing this test. The only problem that arises is if the test result is shared with some unauthorized person (such as a police officer), without the patient's informed written permission. If the test is needed for clinical care of the patient, there should be no hesitation about performing it. It was not done in this patient, because he became conscious so quickly, and it appeared that his problem could be controlled without the data the test would have provided.

(D) Cardiac monitoring is vital in any adult patient who is obtunded or acidotic, because of the possibility of dysrhythmia developing. Also, the 12-lead ECG is very helpful in ruling out myocardial ischemia, infarction, bradyarrhythmias that could indicate heart block, digitalis toxicity, and the presence of hypo- or hyperkalemia. This patient's serum potassium was later reported as 6.9 mEq/l, with no reference to hemolysis of the specimen, a frequent cause of elevated levels of potassium in patients seen in an emergency department. However, there was no evidence of hyperkalemia on his electrocardiogram. The elevated potassium level was probably due to a shift of potassium from the intracellular space in the presence of metabolic acidosis.

(E) This patient's blood cell count showed no abnormality. His serum amylase test (to rule out acute pancreatitis) was reported as less than 100 Somogyi units (within normal limits). A chest roentgenogram and urine culture, routine procedures in a febrile or obtunded patient because of the possible role of infection, showed no abnormalities. In men, the prostate should be palpated rectally for possible evidence of infection, and this, and some other parts of the physical examination, will need to be rechecked when the patient is alert and able to indicate areas of tenderness. The stool should always be checked for occult blood, since both alcohol ingestion and aspirin ingestion (frequently associated) cause acute and chronic upper gastrointestinal bleeding. The test was negative in this patient. Skull roentgenograms should be obtained in any obtunded alcoholic patient who may have fallen or sustained a blow over the head. Head injury is frequent in alcoholic patients, and the emergency department physician should maintain a high index of suspicion in this regard. A careful neurologic examination should always be done and repeated later after the patient improves (that is, after a few hours of observation). Each examination should be documented on the emergency department record. Cervical spine films are also required if the blow to the head could have caused cervical trauma. If a history is not obtainable or is not considered accurate, these screening films may be justified in any alcoholic patient, especially if he is, or has been, unconscious. The yield of such examinations is very low, however.

(F) Lumbar puncture should be done in any obtunded or febrile alcoholic patient who does not respond promptly to initial treatment measures. In most patients, this will rule out meningitis and subarachnoid hemorrhage, but not subdural or epidural hemorrhage. However, lumbar puncture is never the first diagnostic test done. It is a test done only if lower-risk tests are noninformative, and, as mentioned, there is no response to initial treatment measures.

5. (False) Many patients with an overdose of alcohol (ethyl or other types) should have gastric lavage, with the airway protected by a cuffed endotracheal tube. The lavage is usually followed by instillation of sodium bicarbonate into the stomach. Unfortunately, the alcohol is usually absorbed (30 to 120 minutes) into the system before lavage can be done, but it should be tried in the hope of removing any residual alcohol, as well as any other drugs that may have been taken and that may be contributing to the patient's cerebral and respiratory depression. Since alcohol is not adsorbed by charcoal, charcoal followed by emesis would not be feasible. Gastric lavage was not necessary in this patient because of his prompt response to intravenously administered glucose. This indicated that his coma was due to alcoholic hypoglycemia, rather than to an overdose of ethyl alcohol.

6. (C, D) (C) It was learned later that this patient had been on a drinking binge for at least a week and had eaten poorly during that time. As is so often the case, this history was not available at the time he was brought in, comatose. It is usually safe to presume that any alcoholic patient is malnourished and deficient in multivitamins. This patient was also ketotic, presumably due to his starvation syndrome, though alcohol itself apparently can contribute to the development of ketosis. (D) Alcohol has a deleterious effect on several body functions, one of which is carbohydrate metabolism. This effect is, at least in part, an inhibition of hepatic gluconeogenesis with depletion of hepatic glycogen stores. In the presence of starvation, this effect is enough to produce profound hypoglycemia, as was found in this patient. This risk is increased by the simultaneous ingestion of oral hypoglycemic agents and alcohol. All patients taking these drugs should be advised not to drink alcoholic beverages, especially when there is limited caloric intake from other sources. The risk is also increased in the presence of alcoholic liver disease.

Although this form of hypoglycemia is not common in alcoholics, all binge drinkers should be warned of its possibility, as well as the possible irreversible brain damage that frequently results from profound and repeated hypoglycemic episodes.

7. (True) The point here is that if the patient has diabetes mellitus, he may have hypoglycemia secondary to an overdose of insulin (or oral hypoglycemic drugs) or to his usual dose of insulin followed by inadequate food intake. The history, when obtainable, is the best clue to pre-existing diabetes mellitus. Previous hospital records should always be consulted, if available, and calls to other physicians or hospitals may be very fruitful, although time-consuming. A maximum effort should be made to contact the patient's relatives, not only for a history, but because he will need to be released under their care if he is not admitted to the hospital.

There was nothing to suggest diabetes mellitus in this patient.

8. (F) All. Pneumonia (A) and urinary tract infection (B) are the two most common secondary findings. The former may be due to aspiration while the patient vomits during alcoholic stupor. Urinary tract infection, as well as other infections, can occur as a result of the lowered resistance to infection associated with malnutrition, and probably other factors. Gastric irritation (C) is usual with alcoholic intake, and bleeding can occur from the esophagus, stomach or duodenum, especially if peptic ulcer

is present. Gastritis is far more likely if the patient has taken aspirin concomitantly. Pancreatitis (D) is a frequent accompaniment of acute and chronic alcoholism, although the exact mechanism is not well understood (see Case 1). It is always difficult to determine the cause of upper abdominal pain and tenderness in such patients. The most frequent causes are acute alcoholic gastritis, peptic ulcer disease exacerbated by alcoholic intake, pancreatitis and alcoholic hepatitis. Appropriate screening studies must be undertaken in all such patients, with arrangements made for repeating some of the tests later if there is still doubt about the diagnosis.

The mechanism of peripheral neuropathy (E) is not clear, but the disorder is very common in patients with acute or chronic alcoholism who have a poor dietary intake.

COURSE:

This patient was observed for six hours following his dramatic response to intravenous glucose. He was able to be up walking around, with assistance; he was allowed to go home, with an appointment for clinical evaluation within a few days. He was warned of the seriousness and the danger of these episodes. He failed to keep his appointment and has not been treated again in this facility.

REFERENCES

1. Becker, C.E., et al.: Alcohol as a Drug: A Curriculum on Pharmacology, Neurology and Toxicology. New York: Medcom Press, 1974.

2. Victor, M., et al.: The Wernicke-Korsakoff Syndrome. Philadelphia: F.A. Davis Co., 1971.

::

CASE 17: ALCOHOL WITHDRAWAL SYNDROME

HISTORY:

A 63-year-old man was transferred from another general hospital, because that hospital's rules would not allow admission of alcoholic patients. The record transferred with him included the following information: He had had a generalized seizure, during which he had severely lacerated his tongue; a sublingual hematoma developed over the next two hours. He had been drinking alcoholic beverages daily for three months (mostly "moonshine" whiskey, according to his wife), with a history of binge drinking for 20 to 30 years. When drinking, he would almost quit eating. There was no history of head injury or of seizure disorder, except possibly one or two seizures during alcohol withdrawal in the preceding five years. His liver had been enlarged "for some time." He had hypertension of many years' duration, for which he had taken some kind of medication; however, at the time of admission, he was taking no medications and no vitamins. Prior to transfer, he had been given chlordiazepoxide, 25 mg intramuscularly, and this was repeated in 20 minutes with some improvement in his restlessness. He was also given diphenhydramine, 25 mg intramuscularly; the reason for this was not stated in the transfer note. Nasal oxygen was also started at six liters per minute.

EXAMINATION:

Examination revealed a postictal state - the patient could state his name and nothing else. There was no tremor, pallor, or jaundice. The undersurface of his tongue was lacerated, and there was a hematoma beneath his tongue, which posed no immediate threat to his airway. His rectal temperature was 102°F (38.8°C); pulse, 130 per minute and regular; blood pressure, 200/100 mm Hg. Diffuse rales and rhonchi were noted over both mid and lower lung fields. His liver was smooth and enlarged to 3 cm below the costal margin at the midclavicular line, but was only slightly tender. His reflexes were hyperactive throughout; there was an equivocal Babinski sign on the left. Otherwise, the neurologic examination was negative. There was no lead line on his gums.

LABORATORY DATA:

Hemoglobin: 13.7 gm/dl

Hematocrit: 41%
Red blood cells: unstippled
White blood cell count: 15,200 with 66% segmented neutrophils, 6% bands, 19% lymphocytes, 9% monocytes
Urinalysis: negative
Blood studies:
Sodium: 138 mEq/l
Potassium: 3.1 mEq/l
Chloride: 97 mEq/l
CO_2 combining power: 23 mEq/l
Blood urea nitrogen (BUN): 17 mg/dl
Creatinine: 0.8 mg/dl
Glucose: 129 mg/dl
Calcium: 8.2 mg/dl
Magnesium: 1.1 mg/dl
Uric acid: 6.3 mg/dl
Total protein: 6.9 gm/dl
Albumin: 3.4 gm/dl
Total bilirubin: 1.6 mg/dl
Lead concentration: 83.3 micrograms%
LDH: 424 I.U./l
SGOT: 135 I.U./l
Alkaline phosphatase: 80 I.U./l
Amylase: less than 100 Somogyi units
Ammonia: 89 micrograms%

Arterial blood gases: (while patient was receiving oxygen by nasal prongs at six liters per minute)
PO_2: 60 torr
PCO_2: 31 torr
pH: 7.52
Australian antigen: negative
Coagulation profile: normal prothrombin time, partial thromboplastin time - 36.4 seconds; platelet count - 165,000/mm^3
Creatinine clearance: 100 ml/min (normal range - 90-130 ml/min)
Stool: black, strongly positive for blood (guaiac)

Gross blood was obtained from the nasogastric tube. This stopped spontaneously after three hours, which suggests that it may have originated from the tongue laceration.

X-rays: No definite infiltration was seen on chest x-rays, but there was moderate diffuse pulmonary emphysema, calcific sclerosis of the aortic arch, pleural thickening on the right side and healed rib fractures. Skull x-rays were within normal limits. No lead line was noted in the long bones.

Electrocardiogram: sinus tachycardia (110/min) with no other definite abnormality. Brain scan was within normal limits.

Lumbar puncture yielded clear fluid under normal pressure; cell count, protein and glucose were normal; no organisms were grown from the fluid. Blood culture was also negative. Sputum cultures revealed Staphylococcus aureus, Hemophilus influenzae, and Klebsiella pneumoniae.

QUESTIONS:

1. In addition to chronic alcoholism, hypertension, postictal state from alcohol withdrawl and secondary laceration of the tongue with sublingual hematoma, this patient had:
   A. Laennec's cirrhosis
   B. Upper gastrointestinal bleeding
   C. Lead intoxication, mild
   D. Aspiration pneumonitis with emphysema
   E. All of the above

2. Which of the following symptoms and signs characterize the minor, or prodromal, state of withdrawal syndrome?
   A. Agitation and anxiety
   B. Tremulousness
   C. Anorexia, nausea and vomiting, diarrhea
   D. Tachycardia, sweating and fever
   E. All of the above

3. In addition to worsening of the symptoms and signs of the previous question, which of the following are characteristic of severe withdrawal from alcohol?
   A. Hallucinations
   B. Delirium
   C. Seizure activity
   D. All of the above

4. Which of the following are complications of the full-blown alcohol withdrawal syndrome?
   A. Hyperthermia
   B. Circulatory collapse
   C. Infection
   D. Dehydration and electrolyte imbalance
   E. Cardiac arrhythmias
   F. Hematological disorders
   G. Trauma
   H. All of the above

5. TRUE OR FALSE: Withdrawal from alcohol and withdrawal from sedative-hypnotic drugs are easily distinguishable clinically.

6. Treatment for moderate to severe alcohol withdrawal syndrome consists of which of the following?
   A. Adequate tranquilizers to control symptoms
   B. Hospitalization and careful observation for several days
   C. Thiamine and other vitamins
   D. Proper diet
   E. All of the above

7. Another nutritional complication is called the Wernicke-Korsakoff syndrome. Which of the following are typical of this syndrome?
   A. Ataxia
   B. Nystagmus
   C. Paralysis of the extraocular muscles
   D. Disturbances of consciousness, memory, intellect
   E. Confabulation
   F. Polyneuropathy
   G. All of the above

ANSWERS AND COMMENTS:

1. (E) All, although B and C are questionable, as indicated below. (A) The patient's enzyme studies confirmed serious liver disease, presumably Laënnec's cirrhosis. On this admission, there was no evidence of encephalopathy due to liver disease, although he was given lactolase to prevent such symptoms. All of his mental changes were thought to be due to postictal state and alcohol withdrawal syndrome. (B) It was not certain whether he had acute upper gastrointestinal hemorrhage or whether all of the blood recovered from the nasogastric tube had been swallowed. Since his initial stool guaiac test was strongly positive and his stool was black, it is probable that he had some acute gastrointestinal bleeding. The bleeding cleared overnight and was presumed to be due to alcoholic gastritis. (C) The history of drinking "moonshine" whiskey for at least three months, and his elevated blood lead concentration (above 80 micrograms %), confirmed the diagnosis of lead intoxication. Although this condition can cause seizures, even coma, it was not thought that lead poisoning was the basis of this patient's neurologic problems. (D) The initial chest x-ray failed to show evidence of any type of pneumonitis. This is common, the diagnosis in the early post-aspiration period usually being made on the basis of history of seizure or other predisposing or precipitating factor and the

physical examination. His initial PaO_2 of 60 torr while he was receiving oxygen, as well as his subsequent course, confirmed this diagnosis.

2. (E) All. Psychomotor agitation (A) and tremor ("the shakes") (B) are characteristic of both early and late withdrawal. Characteristically, the tremor occurs early in the morning and is relieved by alcohol, at least at first. If something prevents further drinking, such as gastritis, nausea or vomiting, the tremor becomes worse. Accompanying it are irritability, hostility, restlessness, exaggerated startle response, inability to concentrate, easy distractability, and impairment of memory and judgment. Tremulousness is a sign of both physical dependence on alcohol and of withdrawal, and there is no difference in the tremor of the two conditions. Usually, the total clinical picture allows one to make the distinction. The history makes it easy, but a history is not always available, or if available, is not always reliable. Agitation can be a sign of hypoxia, since many alcoholic patients smoke heavily, have chronic obstructive pulmonary disease, and have aspirated during or following a seizure, all of which this patient had, or had done. Arterial blood gases and pH should always be measured, as they will help rule out ketoacidosis and other causes of metabolic acidosis, including lactic acid accumulation in the blood following a seizure. These tests help determine the degree of the respiratory alkalosis that occurs with the hyperventilation of alcohol withdrawal, as seen in this patient. They also define the extent of the respiratory acidosis that is present in many patients with chronic obstructive pulmonary disease.

Gastrointestinal disturbances (C) progress to severe vomiting and diarrhea in some patients, who then very quickly become dehydrated and develop electrolyte imbalance. Autonomic hyperactivity (D) is reflected by tachycardia, sweating and slight fever, as well as an increase in tremulousness. This stage of withdrawal is sometimes called "impending DTs," but frequently it does not progress to full-blown delirium tremens, even without treatment.

3. (D) All. (A) Hallucinations are of two types in alcohol withdrawal. Alcoholic hallucinosis, as it is called, occurs early after cessation of alcohol and represents the less severe form. The hallucinations are usually auditory, and the patient's sensorium remains clear. This type of withdrawal syndrome can be treated with a phenothiazine, haloperidol, although such drugs are no longer recommended in the treatment of the more severe types of withdrawal, since they may precipitate seizures. The

dose is 2.5 to 5 mg intramuscularly, and this dose may be repeated every hour up to two to three times, if necessary. The exact relationship of this subtype of withdrawal to the more severe types described later is not clear, but it is important to differentiate between them, a differentiation that can usually be made on clinical grounds in a cooperative patient. If there is a history of previous seizure disorder - idiopathic, post-traumatic or withdrawal type - diazepam would probably be safer and just as effective, since it has anticonvulsant properties.

The other type of hallucinations in the withdrawal syndrome is that associated with delirium (B), frequently called delirium tremens. This is a more advanced stage of withdrawal than alcoholic hallucinosis and is much more serious. It has a mortality rate of 10 to 15%. By definition, the patient is disoriented and the hallucinations are very vivid and usually visual in type, although they may be of almost any type. Delusions, if present, are paranoid in nature and frequently merge with the hallucinations, adding to the patient's agitation and restlessness. It should be determined whether these aberrations occur at times other than during withdrawal before a diagnosis of functional psychosis can be entertained.

The blood sugar level should be determined in any alcoholic patient whose mental status is abnormal. On suspicion of hypoglycemia or on the finding of low blood sugar on Dextrostix® testing, the patient should be given 50 ml of 50% glucose intravenously, immediately. In fact, this should be done if there is any question about whether all of the mental changes are due to alcohol or alcohol withdrawal.

A seizure (C) or a series of two or three seizures may occur 24 to 48 hours after total cessation of drinking, although they tend to occur earlier than that. In the reported series, seizures have occurred in 8 to 10% of patients presenting at emergency departments with alcohol withdrawal syndrome. These "rum fits" may be the only seizures the patient has ever had; many patients admit to having had them before, when they attempted to quit drinking. Usually the seizure episode (one or more seizures) has occurred before the patient arrives at the emergency department and is the reason he is brought there. Status epilepticus occurs in some patients during alcohol withdrawal.

Although abstinence from alcohol is a frequent cause of seizures, it must not be assumed to be the cause until studies have ruled out other causes, such as head injury. Subdural hematoma does not usually cause seizures but is such a common injury in alcoholics that it must always be thought of and ruled out by appropriate studies. The seizures of abstinence syndrome are almost always generalized; but focal or generalized seizures can occur with the hypoglycemia that sometimes accompanies withdrawal, as it accompanies alcohol intoxication.

Long-term seizure treatment should not be considered at this time and should never be instituted if alcohol withdrawal appears to have been the sole cause of a seizure.

There is some overlap between minor or prodromal stages and the major or severe withdrawal syndrome. The severity of the syndrome usually depends upon how long the patient had been drinking and how much he had drunk. However, the spectrum of behavior during withdrawal is wide; and it is difficult to determine exactly where the patient is on that spectrum at any one time. It is even more difficult to predict whether the patient will improve or suddenly get worse. A period of observation is an absolute necessity for such patients; and most, if not all of them, should be treated in the hospital. In most instances, the entire spectrum of alcohol withdrawal syndrome, including delirium tremens, is over in 72 to 96 hours. For patients with only the mild, or early or prodromal, phase, it may all be over in 24 to 30 hours, although 7 to 10 days are usually required for all signs and symptoms to return to normal.

4. (H) All. Just as the alcohol intoxicated patient is subject to complications, so is the withdrawing patient, some of the complications in the latter being even more serious than in the former. (A) Hyperthermia of uncertain cause can occur and may be difficult or impossible to control. The proper treatment is cooling blankets or ice bags, plus aspirin or acetaminophen, started as soon as a rising temperature is recognized.

Circulatory collapse (B) is a serious threat and must be guarded against by every possible means, including monitoring of various parameters on an hour-to-hour basis. Treatment consists of administration of intravenous fluid, usually a balanced salt solution, in quantities sufficient to replace fluid lost through excessive perspiration and hyperventilation, as well as that lost by vomiting and diarrhea. Whole blood or blood components may be necessary. Either of these dangerous complications (hyperthermia and circulatory collapse) can occur rapidly. They account for most of the deaths directly attributable to withdrawal.

Infection (C) is one of the most frequent complications, and it should always be searched for if the patient has fever, as this patient did, although slight fever can occur from the autonomic hyperactivity of moderate to severe withdrawal, as discussed in answer 2. Lumbar puncture is usually necessary to rule out cerebrospinal infection, meningitis in particular, although a spinal tap is not likely to reveal evidence of epidural or subdural hematoma, except indirectly by showing an increased pressure. Pulmonary infections are common and must be treated vigorously when present. Urinary tract infection is next in frequency. Blood cultures should be performed early and repeatedly if the initial examination shows the patient to be febrile. Additional causes of infection are alcoholic hepatitis and acute pancreatitis.

Fever, per se, is a symptom, not an illness, but it is frequently associated with dehydration (D), and such patients may require 6000 to 8000 ml of intravenous fluid daily. Special precautions, such as careful intake and output recordings, must be taken to avoid overhydration with resulting cerebral edema, pulmonary edema and other complications.

Electrolytes must be monitored carefully. Withdrawing patients are subject to cardiac arrhythmias (E), so continuous electrocardiographic monitoring is also mandatory. Potassium levels should be carefully adjusted, in order to decrease the chances of fatal arrhythmia due either to high or low serum potassium concentrations. Cardiac arrhythmias are more likely to occur in alcohol withdrawal than in intoxication, and are more likely to recur if they have occurred in the past, with or without the withdrawal syndrome.

Hematologic disorders (F) are also common and require diagnosis and prompt treatment, especially hypoprothrombinemia and anemia. The former is usually secondary to severe liver disease and vitamin K deficiency. The latter is frequently due to both iron deficiency and folic acid deficiency. Replacement therapy is vital in these patients. Gastrointestinal bleeding is a common complication and is more frequently due to alcoholic gastritis than to esophageal varices or peptic ulcer.

Trauma (G) is found in withdrawing patients as frequently as in intoxicated patients, and screening studies must be made at the time of admission. Also, special precautions should be taken to prevent further trauma, such as from seizures or falls, after the patient arrives at the hospital. Usually, mechanical, as well as pharmacologic, restraints are required, along with constant attendance, preferably in an intensive care unit for the first few days.

Other complications that can occur are those that this patient had as outlined in the case presentation and in answer 1.

5. (False) It is impossible to distinguish alcohol withdrawal symptoms from those of, for example, phenobarbital withdrawal. Also, simultaneous withdrawal from both agents, or several agents, is not uncommon. Such multiple withdrawals increase the agitation and tremor, as well as the susceptibility to seizures, including status epilepticus.

Another point to remember is that if barbiturates are involved along with alcohol, the onset of withdrawal is delayed by several days and the duration of the syndrome is prolonged. A urinary drug screening should always be done (and a blood drug screening should also be done if this test is available) in the hope of finding residual levels of such drugs, since the patient may have continued them parenterally, after onset of vomiting prevented further oral intake.

6. (E) All. It has never been proved that medications will stop the progress of withdrawal syndrome, but they do help alleviate the severe agitation and calm the patient, helping him to conserve his strength. (A) Chlordiazepoxide, 50 to 100 mg orally, intramuscularly or intravenously, or diazepam, 10 to 20 mg orally, intramuscularly or intravenously (preferred if extreme agitation is present), is useful initially, and the dose may be repeated in 2 to 4 hours, if necessary. The unusually large doses are required because of cross-tolerance between alcohol and most sedative-hypnotic-tranquilizer drugs. However, intravenous administration of diazepam has been reported to cause respiratory arrest and should be given cautiously in the lowest dose that will control the symptoms. The long half-life of chlordiazepoxide (30 hours) makes it useful for patients who are being treated on an out-patient basis. This use may tide a patient overnight or over a weekend, until his admission to an alcohol facility can be arranged. Hydroxyzine should not be used to treat alcohol withdrawal because of its antihistaminic and anticholinergic properties, which could precipitate seizures. The improper use of stronger (major) tranquilizers and the problem of hospitalization (B) are discussed in answer 3.

(C) Most, if not all, alcoholics have clinical or subclinical vitamin deficiencies. Alcohol is the only common drug that is also a food. Seven calories are produced from each gram of alcohol (2 ml of 100-proof liquor), and there is a tendency for binge drinkers to live off the alcohol and not consume food of other types. This creates a double problem from the nutritional standpoint: the alcohol, itself, must be metabolized, which requires certain vitamins, and it contains no vitamins. Therefore, it is not surprising that persons who drink regularly, instead of eating, develop nutritional deficiencies, especially vitamin deficiencies. Polyneuropathy is a manifestation of vitamin deficiency, although the exact mechanism of its development is still unclear. It is seen in alcohol intoxication, as well as in withdrawal, as an isolated complication, both the sensory and the motor type. Since administration of vitamin supplements carries no hazard, it should be routine during treatment of alcohol withdrawal. The especial value of thiamine is discussed in answer 7. Thiamine should be given to all alcoholics intravenously with glucose solution, or intramuscularly in a dose of 100 mg, or in a dose of 50 mg by each route. (D) Since the alcoholic withdrawing after a prolonged binge is apt to be in a clinical state of starvation, his diet during treatment should be nutritious, as high in calories as his weight dictates, and bland at first, since he probably has gastric irritation. Diet is usually the concern of the emergency physician for only the first 24 hours or so if the observation period is carried out in the emergency department or an adjoining facility.

7. (G) All. Wernicke's encephalopathy is characterized by ophthalmoplegia, ataxia and disturbances of consciousness. It has an acute onset in the patient who has been drinking alcohol heavily and who has severe nutritional deficiencies, especially thiamine deficiency. Korsakoff's psychosis refers to an abnormal mental state, in which memory and learning are affected out of all proportion to other cognitive functions. The encephalopathy and the psychosis are two facets of the same disease and may be called Wernicke's disease, with or without Korsakoff's psychosis, or the Wernicke-Korsakoff syndrome, in patients with both components of the disease.

This syndrome, although rare, represents a medical emergency. The eye signs are easy to check and should be given careful attention in every acutely intoxicated patient, although 15% of one series showed withdrawal symptoms, as this patient did. The eye signs progress from horizontal and vertical nystagmus to bilateral lateral rectus palsy, conjugate gaze paralysis, and, eventually, complete paralysis of all eye movements. The defect in recent memory must be differentiated from that in an intoxicated, noncooperative patient.

Thiamine is the specific treatment of the Wernicke-Korsakoff syndrome. It should be administered promptly if the syndrome is suspected, both as treatment and as prevention. The prompt use of thiamine reverses the lesions and is crucial in preventing the development of an irreversible and incapacitating amnesic psychosis. The prognosis for recovery of mental function is grave unless treatment is prompt; even so, recovery of mental function is slow and often incomplete. Thiamine should be administered in a divided dose, 50 mg intravenously and 50 mg intramuscularly, the latter dose being repeated each day until the patient resumes an adequate diet.

There is a special risk in giving alcoholics glucose without concomitant thiamine, since the glucose, alone, may precipitate Wernicke's disease or cause an early form of the disease to progress rapidly.

It is good practice to administer all of the B vitamins, in addition to thiamine, to all alcoholic patients requiring parenteral glucose, whether the patients are intoxicated or in withdrawal. The metabolic defect in the Wernicke-Korsakoff syndrome appears to be an excess of pyruvate, due to the blockage of oxidative decarboxylation of pyruvate to acetyl coenzyme A in the absence of thiamine. Adequate thiamine prevents that blockage.

COURSE:

After two hours of treatment and observation in the emergency department, this patient was admitted to the intensive care unit. He remained confused and disoriented for several days, although he had no more seizures.

The dose of thiamine (100 mg intramuscularly) that had been administered in the emergency department was repeated daily for three days, along with multivitamins orally. Chlordiazepoxide was continued as needed to control agitation, which was rather prominent after the postictal phase. Penicillin was started from the beginning, since aspiration pneumonia was suspected. This drug was replaced by cephalothin sodium and kanamycin after sputum culture and sensitivity reports were available.

On the fifth hospital day, patchy pneumonia and left lower lobe atelectasis were apparent on clinical and roentgenologic examination, and the patient required endotracheal intubation and intensive treatment for acute respiratory failure. The tongue laceration healed well and the hematoma resolved slowly. At no time was it a threat to his airway and there was no secondary bleeding or other evidence of a bleeding tendency. There was no further upper gastrointestinal bleeding, but arrangements were made for barium studies to be done on an out-patient basis. He was discharged afebrile and was doing quite well on the twenty-first hospital day.

No treatment was required for lead poisoning. He was strongly advised to stop drinking alcohol and to have repeat liver function studies in three months.

::

CASE 18: ABDOMINAL DISTRESS IN A 37-YEAR-OLD MAN WITH DIABETES MELLITUS

HISTORY:

A 37-year-old man with a history of hypertension, type IV hyperlipidemia, and mild diabetes mellitus, controlled by diet, was brought to the emergency department because of generalized abdominal pain of 24 hours' duration, malaise and anorexia of two weeks' duration. Recently, he had had balanitis, probably due to monilia, which was improving with treatment. Circumcision had been recommended, but the patient had still not decided to have it done. He had had an inferior myocardial infarction three years before; at that time, a diagnosis of three-vessel coronary artery disease was made. He was taking methyldopa, hydrochlorothiazide, nicotinic acid and propranolol. He had lost 20 pounds over the last four months.

The patient was a mildly obese black man with moderate abdominal distress. There were signs of mild dehydration. His respirations were deep at 20 per minute and his breath had a fruity odor. His temperature was 98.8°F (37°C); his pulse was 104/min on admission, 80/min 30 minutes later and regular. Blood pressure was 140/100 mm Hg. Examination of his heart and lungs revealed no abnormality. There was mild, diffuse abdominal tenderness but no masses or enlarged organs; peristalsis was normal.

LABORATORY DATA:

Hemoglobin: 14.1 gm/dl
White blood cell count: 7,700/mm^3, with normal differential
Urinalysis: negative, except for 3+ ketones and 3+ glucose
Serum levels:
- Sodium: 125 mEq/l
- Potassium: 5 mEq/l
- Chloride: 77 mEq/l
- Carbon dioxide combining power: 13.5 mEq/l
- Urea nitrogen: 33 mg/dl
- Glucose: 720 mg/dl
- Ketones: not recorded

Arterial blood:
- pH: 7.34
- HCO_3^-: 14 mEq/l
- PCO_2: 28 torr
- PO_2: 100 torr (patient breathing room air)

QUESTIONS:

1. The most likely diagnosis in this patient is:
   A. Mesenteric venous thrombosis
   B. Acute recurrent myocardial infarction
   C. Diabetes with ketoacidosis
   D. Compensated metabolic acidosis
   E. Hypertension
   F. Type IV hyperlipidemia
   G. Coronary atherosclerosis

2. TRUE OR FALSE: This patient should have been admitted to the hospital.

3. Which of the following general statements about diabetes mellitus are true?
   A. It is the third leading cause of death in the United States.
   B. There are two fairly distinct forms, "juvenile onset diabetes" and "maturity onset diabetes."
   C. The most important acute complications of diabetes mellitus are ketoacidosis, hypoglycemia, and hyperglycemia, hyperosmolar nonketotic coma.
   D. All of the above

4. Which of the following general statements about diabetic ketoacidosis are true?
   A. It is more common in men.
   B. It occurs only in adults.
   C. It results in a high mortality rate.
   D. It is a state of insulin deficiency, characterized by hyperglycemia, hyperketonemia and metabolic acidosis.

5. For a patient with diabetic ketoacidosis, which of the following treatments are used?
   A. Insulin
   B. Fluids
   C. Electrolytes
   D. Sodium bicarbonate routinely
   E. Potassium intravenously from the beginning
   F. Glucose in all intravenous fluids
   G. All of the above

6. Which of these statements about hyperosmolar nonketotic diabetic coma are true?
   A. Blood glucose levels usually range between 600 and 2000 mg/dl.
   B. Hypernatremia and severe dehydration are characteristic.

C. Initial treatment is rehydration, insulin therapy and evaluation of the precipitating disease process.
D. The mortality is approximately 50%.
E. All of the above

ANSWERS AND COMMENTS:

1. (C, D, E, F, G) (A) The abdominal pain and tenderness were probably secondary to the patient's ketoacidosis and not due to intra-abdominal disease, per se. At least no such disease was found. The mechanism of that abdominal pain and tenderness is not well understood.

(B) His electrocardiogram was compatible with an old inferior myocardial infarction, with no evidence of an acute process (see answer G).

(C) He had diabetes mellitus, complicated by moderate ketoacidosis. He is the type of patient who, had he waited another day or two, would probably have arrived at the emergency department comatose. Fortunately, ketoacidosis usually has a gradual onset over several days. The laboratory studies confirmed the presence of metabolic acidosis (acidemia), partially compensated by hyperventilation (D).

The most common metabolic abnormalities seen in an emergency department are those involving glucose metabolism. Although this patient illustrates the problem, most of the patients with ketoacidosis are much sicker than he was.

(E, F) Hypertension and type IV hyperlipidemia were diagnosed by history, as was coronary atherosclerosis (G), previously confirmed by coronary angiography. The extent of the changes in the vessels, and the presence of ventricular dyskinesia, ruled out operative intervention. The patient's decreased sodium level may have been secondary to his hyperlipidemia, but the concomitant decreased serum chloride suggested moderate loss of both ions through renal obligatory mechanisms, secondary to the hyperglycemia and glycosuria. However, it should be noted that his serum potassium level was not decreased, although his total body potassium was probably diminished, since that is usually the case in ketoacidosis.

Renal insufficiency is probably also present, aggravated by the dehydration. The patient also had starvation ketosis of uncertain extent.

2. (False) This patient represents the multiple-problem patient seen so often in emergency departments. The importance of reviewing such a patient's hospital record is clearly reflected in this case, since such review saved an unnecessary admission. It is likely that in-patient care would have been chosen by most physicians for a patient with a blood glucose concentration of over 700 mg/dl and several other serious acute and chronic medical problems, but no harm followed the decision not to admit him. In addition, the consultant who made the decision not to admit the patient was able to check him in the clinic within 48 hours and found him much improved. Many diabetic patients with ketoacidosis have such mild symptoms, signs, and metabolic and fluid derangements that they can be treated at home and followed up by their physician on a daily basis, if necessary.

COURSE:

The patient improved greatly during the eight hours he remained in the emergency department. He received oxygen by nasal prongs, electrolytes intravenously, potassium (40 mEq) in the third liter of fluid, and low-dose insulin therapy (see answer 5). There was a fall in his blood glucose concentration to 300 mg/dl, at which point he was allowed to go home.

After the episode described, he was started on insulin in small doses. After two months, the insulin was discontinued in favor of dietary control of his diabetes mellitus. That was only mildly effective, but the patient would not take insulin regularly. The use of alcoholic beverages contributed to his lack of compliance, but the extent of his alcohol use could never be determined. On subsequent hospitalizations, he was found to have mild renal failure, and he developed angina on exertion. He failed to comply with instructions about medication and had several bouts of mild congestive heart failure and pneumonitis. Treadmill electrocardiography, eight months after the episode reported here, could not be interpreted because of poor patient effort. However, he did develop trigeminy. His blood pressure was not well controlled. As is so frequently the case, he failed to return after 12 months of follow-up care, despite several efforts to have him do so. During that 12-month period, he had had no further episodes of ketoacidosis.

3. (D) All. (A) The cause of diabetes mellitus is poorly understood. This disease is characterized by widespread organ involvement and leads to serious acute and chronic complications, including early death. It is surpassed in causing death only by cardiovascular disease (of which it is a potent breeder, as

exemplified by this patient) and malignant tumors. (B) The two forms mentioned have differing clinical problems in diagnosis and management, but both have the complications listed in 3C. Hyperosmolar nonketotic coma with hyperglycemia is more likely to present in the elderly patient with maturity onset diabetes (MOD) (see question and answer 6). Patients with juvenile onset diabetes (JOD) tend to have an absolute insulin deficiency and are much more likely to develop ketoacidosis; patients with MOD are characterized by a relative insulin deficiency. (C) The care of patients with diabetes mellitus in an emergency department is usually for their complications: ketoacidosis, hypoglycemia, and hyperosmolar nonketotic coma. Occasionally, lactic acidosis occurs, but is usually not associated with these complications of diabetes mellitus. It does occur with the use of phenformin as an oral hypoglycemic agent. That drug has been withdrawn from the market by the FDA.

4. (D, which is a good definition of diabetic ketoacidosis) (A) Diabetic ketoacidosis is two and one-half times more common in women than in men. The reasons are not clear, although some believe that female sex hormonal factors have an effect, since many of the patients have their acidotic episode near the beginning of a menstrual period.

(B) Diabetic ketoacidosis occurs in children as well, since they tend to have the more severe form of diabetes.

(C) Fortunately, the mortality rate in diabetic ketoacidosis is not high in children who receive proper treatment. In adults, the mortality rate depends greatly upon associated and secondary medical problems. The slow onset in both children and adults allows most patients to obtain proper treatment.

5. (A, B, C) (A) Because ketoacidosis is the result of the effect of insulin deficiency on carbohydrate, protein and fat metabolism, it is clear that insulin administration is the most important aspect of therapy. Even if the patient is not comatose, oral hypoglycemic agents are not suitable. In all instances, regular (crystalline) insulin should be given. There are two generally accepted plans by which it may be given. The traditional plan is to give insulin in doses of 2 to 4 units/kg of body weight to patients with severe acidosis and coma; as little as 1 unit/kg to those less critically ill. In adults, that means 50 to to 100 units in the first hour of therapy but up to 200 units in the sickest patients. Half of the dose can be given intravenously, and half subcutaneously, provided the patient's blood pressure is adequate. If the blood pressure is low, all of the insulin should be given intravenously. After the blood glucose level

falls to 250 to 300 mg/dl, glucose should be added at a rate of approximately 10 grams (200 ml of 5% dextrose in saline) per hour. From that time on, the patient's hourly insulin dose should be regulated by the glucose levels in blood and urine, levels that should be measured at least every four hours.

Recently popularized is the other basic plan of treatment, low-dose intravenous insulin administration. It involves a priming injection of 0.1 units/kg of body weight followed by 0.1 units/kg/hour. The rate should be reduced to 1 to 5 units/hour when the blood glucose level drops below 250 mg/dl.

It is obvious that one must decide in advance which plan to use and to use it from the beginning. The choice is partly a matter of personal preference and partly a matter of experience, since both methods seem satisfactory for the management of ketoacidosis, at least in adults. The second plan is less well accepted for children. Occasionally, because of inadequate or delayed response, the low-dose intravenous method will have to be changed to a high-dose intravenous or subcutaneous method, but that is unusual. It should be remembered that an adequate response means correction of the ketoacidosis, not just a drop in the blood glucose level.

(B, C) Fluid administration is extremely important in the treatment of ketoacidosis. For at least the first 12 to 24 hours, all fluids must be given intravenously, even in the absence of vomiting. The rapidity with which fluids are given depends somewhat upon the magnitude of the dehydration and whether significant circulatory insufficiency is present. During the first hour, normal saline, approximately one liter or 20 ml/kg of body weight, should be administered if there is evidence of moderate to severe volume depletion, such as tachycardia in the absence of obvious infection, hypotension, or loss of skin turgor. During the first eight hours, a total of 3 to 5 liters should be given to a patient with a 10% fluid deficit, approximately half of that as half normal saline, the rest as normal saline.

(D) Sodium bicarbonate should not be given before the report on arterial blood gas and pH is available. That is because with vomiting of several days duration - not unusual in ketoacidosis - the patient may have ketoalkalosis, which, naturally, should not be treated with alkali. In general, alkaline solution is not indicated unless the blood pH is below 7.0, indicating a life-threatening situation.

(E) Potassium therapy is usually not required for the first two to four hours, thus usually beginning after the patient has been admitted to the hospital. However, the serum potassium level falls rapidly with correction of the acidosis. A good rule is to add 20 to 40 mEq of potassium chloride to the second or third liter of fluid and to aim at giving a total of 120 to 160 mEq during the first 24 hours. The amount needed can be monitored with the electrocardiogram, so that the results are available immediately. The serum concentration is what determines the cardiac effects of potassium. However, the serum level does not accurately reflect the deficit in total body potassium, which is usually 300 to 400 mEq.

Because diabetic ketoacidosis is clearly associated with decreased 2, 3-diphosphoglycerate (DPG) and increased affinity of hemoglobin for oxygen, it is important to replace phosphate, which plays an important role in the metabolism of DPG. The increased affinity for oxygen by hemoglobin prevents release of oxygen to the tissues, adding to the tissue hypoxia and compounding the acidosis by enhancing the formation of lactic acid. Therefore, potassium phosphate may be used for replacement of both potassium and phosphorus.

(F) Glucose should not be included in the initial replacement fluid, although it should, as mentioned earlier, be added after the blood glucose concentration reaches approximately 250 to 300 mg/dl. That means that electrolyte solution (i. e., containing no glucose) is used initially.

6. (E) All. (A) The degree of hyperglycemia is greater than that for ketoacidosis, levels of 1200 mg/dl being not uncommon. It would seem that the pancreas can secrete enough insulin to prevent the formation of ketone bodies, but not enough to prevent increasing levels of glucose in the blood. A vicious cycle is set up with the appearance of dehydration and azotemia. It is noteworthy that many of these patients have previously undiagnosed diabetes, although the disease is usually mild. Differentiation from ketoacidosis is made by determination of arterial blood gases and pH (see answer C), as well as the presence of normal or near-normal levels of blood and urinary ketones.

(B) The severe dehydration is secondary to decreased water intake and obligatory water excretion. The hypernatremia (150 mEq/l or more) is a manifestation of the dehydration. The high plasma osmolarity of 350 to 450 mOsm/l is due to the marked hyperglycemia and the hypernatremia.

(C) Rehydration should be accomplished cautiously with 0.45%

saline, not 0.9% saline, partly because the free-water deficit is great and partly because a high serum sodium concentration is usually present. In addition, many elderly patients with diabetes also have compromised cardiovascular systems. At least 6 to 12 liters are required in the first 24 hours. Potassium replacement should be started early, since potassium moves into the cells as the blood sugar is lowered and as acidosis, if present, is corrected.

Low-dose constant insulin infusion is ideal for these patients, provided their blood glucose levels are carefully monitored. These patients are probably more sensitive to insulin than ketoacidotic patients. If the high-dose method is used, 50 units may be given initially, subcutaneously, and may be repeated every two hours, until the blood glucose level is approximately 300 mg/dl.

The underlying or precipitating process is usually infection, which must be diagnosed and then treated vigorously.

(D) One reason the mortality is as high as 50% is that the patients tend to be elderly and have underlying cardiovascular and other serious diseases. The late diagnosis and a lack of aggressive treatment also contribute to that high mortality.

CASE 19: PARASTERNAL CHEST PAIN, MALAISE ON AWAKENING

HISTORY:

A 53-year-old man woke up in the morning with right parasternal chest pain, weakness, sweating, and nausea but no vomiting. The pain lasted above five minutes and did not radiate. It recurred a few minutes later, lasting about eight minutes. There was no dyspnea. The sweating and nausea persisted and he had diarrhea. He rode the bus to the hospital where he worked as a custodian, but, because he continued to feel weak and nauseated, he reported to the emergency department almost two hours after the attack had begun. He still had vague discomfort in his sternal region, with no radiation.

The patient had had hypertension for 12 years and gout for 6 years. He also had idiopathic hypertrophic subaortic stenosis (hypertrophic cardiomyopathy) of mild to moderate degree. Ten hours before onset of the present illness, he had taken 14 tablets of colchicine, 0. 5 mg each over a one-hour period, because of a flare-up of gouty arthritis of his right knee. He usually took colchicine in this amount over an 8- or 10-hour period. The pain was quickly relieved; the expected diarrhea and severe nausea and vomiting developed within one hour. Additional medications that he had been taking routinely for some time were triamterene, 100 mg daily; furosemide, 40 mg daily; allopurinol, 100 mg three times daily; methyldopa, 500 mg four times daily; and isosorbide dinitrate, 5 mg sublingually as needed for chest pain. Recently, he had started taking clonidine, 0. 1 mg twice daily, because blood pressure control had been inadequate, probably due, in part, to poor compliance. He had a 20-year history of alcohol abuse.

Examination revealed a moderately obese, alert, restless and anxious patient who was pale and diaphoretic; the skin of his extremities was cool. His blood pressure was 60/30 mm Hg; pulse, weak at 148/min; respirations, 20/minute; and temperature, 99°F (37. 2°C). There was a grade III/VI holosystolic murmur at the cardiac apex, radiating to the left sternal border and to the axilla. His lungs were clear. His liver was palpable two cm below the right costal margin and was tender. No other abnormalities were found on physical examination.

QUESTIONS:

1. On the basis of the clinical examination alone, which of the following are most important in this patient?
   A. History of chest pain
   B. History of vomiting and diarrhea
   C. History of hypertension and diuretic therapy, as well as methyldopa treatment
   D. History of idiopathic hypertrophic subaortic stenosis
   E. History of chronic alcoholism
   F. Negative history of diabetes mellitus, heart attack, peptic ulcers, or trauma
   G. Finding of hypotension and weak, rapid pulse
   H. Finding of restlessness, pallor, cool and sweaty skin
   I. Finding of loud systolic murmur
   J. Finding of liver enlargement and tenderness
   K. All of the above

2. For such a patient, which of the following tests can be done with almost immediate results available (5 to 15 minutes)?
   A. Determination of blood glucose
   B. Examination of the urine
   C. Identification of the cardiac rate and rhythm
   D. Determination of electrolytes
   E. Determination of central venous pressure
   F. Twelve-lead ECG
   G. Determination of arterial blood gases and pH
   H. Chest roentgenogram
   I. Blood typing and cross-matching
   J. Review of previous hospital records and electrocardiograms, if available
   K. A complete blood count
   L. All of the above

3. On the basis of information provided so far, what is the most likely diagnosis in this patient?
   A. Cardiogenic shock due to myocardial infarction
   B. Cardiogenic shock due to tachycardia
   C. Hypovolemic shock due to vomiting and diarrhea
   D. Cardiogenic shock due to obstruction of the left ventricular outflow tract
   E. All of the above

4. The initial therapeutic maneuvers are which of the following?
   A. Establish at least two intravenous lines and begin administration of 5% dextrose in water through one, and Ringer's lactate or 5% dextrose in saline in the other.

B. Administer a fluid challenge.
C. Begin oxygen by mask, in high concentrations.
D. Administer medication for severe pain.
E. Give lidocaine intravenously.
F. Elevate the head and trunk 10-15 degrees.
G. Insert a nasogastric tube.
H. All of the above

5. Which of the following statements about cardiogenic shock are true?
   A. It is defined as shock of cardiac origin, with decreased blood flow and evidence of peripheral circulatory abnormalities.
   B. It occurs in 10% to 20% to hospitalized patients who have acute myocardial infarction.
   C. It is the principal cause of death during the hospital care phase of acute myocardial infarction, accounting for around 50% of these deaths.
   D. It is usually found in patients who have a transmural infarction of 40% or greater of the left ventricle.
   E. It is caused only by acute myocardial infarction.
   F. Patients with hypertension, and the elderly, are probably predisposed to it when acute myocardial infarction develops.
   G. There is a frequent history of previous acute myocardial infarction.
   H. About half of the patients who develop cardiogenic shock as a complication of myocardial infarction do so within 24 hours.
   I. It usually appears abruptly and progresses rapidly.

COURSE:

Within 10 minutes of the patient's arrival at the emergency department, two intravenous catheters had been inserted, an infusion of dextrose 5% in water and one of Ringer's lactate were started; a urinary catheter was inserted; a central venous pressure (CVP) catheter was inserted; and bag-valve-mask ventilation, with 60% oxygen, was begun. Morphine, 2 mg, was given intravenously and relieved his discomfort without causing vomiting or respiratory depression. An intravenous drip of dopamine, 5 mcg/kg/min, was started and sodium bicarbonate, 44.6 mEq, was given after the arterial blood gases and pH had been measured. There was no evidence of pulmonary edema. His improvement was such that tracheal intubation was not necessary, nor was an additional dose of sodium bicarbonate. He was admitted to the coronary intensive care unit.

6. Which of the following statements are true about dopamine in the treatment of cardiogenic shock due to acute myocardial infarction?
   A. It should be started as soon as possible after onset of cardiogenic shock, regardless of whether hypovolemia is present.
   B. It increases myocardial contractility and cardiac output.
   C. It increases blood flow in the renal and mesenteric beds, with a secondary increase in urinary output.
   D. At different flow rates, it has different physiological effects.
   E. All of the above.

ANSWERS AND COMMENTS:

1. (K) All. (A) The chest pain was not typical of myocardial ischemia or infarction, but was severe enough to require treatment at home with isosorbide dinitrate and in the emergency department with morphine sulfate, 2 mg administered intravenously.

(B) Severe nausea, vomiting and diarrhea are usually well tolerated by a young adult with a normal cardiovascular system, but would not be well tolerated by a patient such as this.

(C) The patient's usual blood pressure was 160-180/100-120 mm Hg. This means that he would probably have inadequate myocardial, as well as peripheral, perfusion at blood pressure levels much lower than that. Certainly, a pressure of 60/30 mm Hg, as was initially recorded, would be dangerous. The long-term diuretic therapy would tend to contract his blood volume even before the loss, by vomiting and diarrhea, occurred, making the margin of safety even smaller. Taking large doses of methyldopa chronically - if indeed this patient did take it regularly - raises several other questions, including the possibility of orthostatic hypotension.

(D) Idiopathic hypertrophic subaortic stenosis (IHSS) is not usually accompanied by marked coronary atherosclerosis but may be associated with angina pectoris and exertional dyspnea.

(E) The history of chronic alcoholism and the finding of an enlarged tender liver (J) raise the question of hepatic failure, especially under physiological stress, as well as the possibility of bleeding from esophageal varices or other sites due to hypoprothrombinemia.

(F) All negative points in this history are important, including absence of diabetes mellitus, since the presence of diabetes would suggest hypoglycemia or ketoacidosis; absence of peptic ulcer disease, since ulcers, when present, can cause acute or chronic bleeding; and absence of trauma, since trauma, when present, can provide other sources and sites for occult bleeding. The absence of previous heart attacks is also significant, since such previous attacks make the patient more likely to have another attack.

(G, H) The physical findings in this patient are definitive for some form of shock. In shock, the blood pressure is usually, but not always, low and the pulse is fast and weak. The patient is usually restless and anxious, but may be somnolent and apathetic; he is usually pale, or even cyanotic, with cool, sweaty skin, especially over the hands and feet.

(I) The finding of a loud, systolic, apical heart murmur was unexpected, more so since the patient had no history of such a murmur.

2. (L) All. Obviously, accomplishment of these tests in the first 5 to 15 minutes requires a team approach with well-trained persons who have been pre-assigned their tasks. Also, it must be remembered that the time required for reporting tests varies widely among hospitals. The emphasis here, as in most of these case studies, is on the ancillary studies that are required for immediate management in the emergency department.

(A) For such a patient, blood glucose determination should be done routinely with Dextrostix®, regardless of the history. If it was done immediately on this patient, it was not recorded. The "true" glucose level reported later was 90 mg%, well within the normal range.

(B) It is a good rule to insert an indwelling urethral catheter in any comatose or hypotensive patient. The sooner it is in place, the better. The few exceptions to this rule, such as the presence of a drop of blood at the urethral meatus, which suggests urethral damage, do not apply to a patient with no history or evidence of trauma.

The amount of urine flow should be measured every 5 to 15 minutes at first, then every 30 to 60 minutes, until the patient's condition stabilizes. This patient's urinary output was only 5 ml in the first 20 minutes after catheter insertion, but was 20 ml at the end of the first hour. Immediate semi-quantitative bedside tests on the urine include determination of protein, glucose and ketone (acetoacetic acid and acetone) levels, all of which were normal. The usual nitroprusside tests (Acetest® or Ketostix®) will not identify beta-hydroxybutyric acid, which is not a ketone, per se.

(C) Electrocardiographic monitoring was instituted immediately by means of electrode-defibrillator paddles and continued with regular electrodes. On the rhythm strip, the heart rate was 145/min and regular, and P waves were identifiable. The diagnosis was sinus tachycardia. (F) The twelve-lead electrocardiogram confirmed this diagnosis and showed elevation of the S-T segment in leads V_1, V_2, and V_3, suggestive of anterolateral ischemia and acute anterior myocardial infarction. Voltage criteria for left ventricular hypertrophy were also present.

(D) Determination of electrolytes, including sodium, potassium, chloride, blood urea nitrogen, and bicarbonate, is a very important screening test for renal disease and endocrinological imbalance, and can also indicate acid-base imbalance. However, acid-base imbalance is best determined by arterial blood gas and pH measurements (G), which, in most hospitals, can be done more quickly than electrolyte measurements. None of the electrolytes were significantly altered; the arterial blood gases were PO_2, 60 torr; PCO_2, 34 torr; and HCO_3^-, 18 mEq/l; pH was 7.30, indicating moderate metabolic acidosis.

(E) In almost all patients in shock, a central venous pressure line should be inserted early and the baseline reading recorded. In this patient, the baseline reading was only 5 cm H_2O, which suggested, but did not confirm, the presence of hypovolemia (see answer 4B).

(H) The chest roentgenogram done with portable equipment is absolutely essential for ruling out obvious conditions, such as pneumonitis, pulmonary infarction, pneumothorax with or without tension, hemothorax (even in the absence of a history of trauma), and enlargement of the cardiac silhouette, the last suggesting cardiac tamponade. Widening of the thoracic aorta is suggestive of dissecting aneurysm, especially if there is progressive widening on serial films. This patient's chest roentgenogram showed no abnormalities.

(I) Blood must be typed (10 minutes required) and cross-matched (45-60 minutes required), because the patient may have occult bleeding. Although blood substitutes can be used at first with restoration and maintenance of adequate blood volume, whole blood must be administered in the presence of persistent blood loss or if the blood pressure drops secondarily.

(J) Unfortunately, this patient's previous hospital record with previous electrocardiograms could not be obtained immediately, so the physician attempting the clinical evaluation was severely handicapped.

(K) The complete blood count is useful in determining a baseline for hemoglobin and hematocrit. Even moderate hemorrhage does not cause a drop in hemoglobin or hematocrit in less than several hours. Therefore, it is possible for a patient to be in severe shock, including the hypovolemic type, and to have a normal hemoglobin and hematocrit. The white blood cell count is expected to be high because of the stress of the shock state.

Other tests required for hospital admission, or for clarification and refinement of the diagnoses, can be done for later reporting. These include blood lactate, not done on this patient, however.

3. (E) The patient probably had a combination of all of these pathophysiological mechanisms, except that there was little evidence of myocardial infarction. However, this could not be ruled out in the first hour or so, and the patient had to be managed cautiously as if he had had a massive acute myocardial infarction.

The initial clinical diagnoses were (1) acute anteroseptal myocardial infarction with possible papillary muscle dysfunction or ruptured interventricular septum; (2) cardiogenic shock; (3) idiopathic hypertrophic subaortic stenosis; and (4) hypertensive cardiovascular disease.

4. (A, B, C, D, E, F) (A) The reason for having at least two intravenous lines is that the patient must be given all medications intravenously, and some of them are not compatible with certain intravenous fluids. This is especially true in the treatment of cardiac arrest, a constant threat to any patient in shock. Also, the patient may need rapid infusion of fluid if he is found to be hypovolemic. In that case, both intravenous lines should be used for an electrolyte solution and a plasma substitute. In this patient, caution was indicated as to the amount and type of fluid, because of the presence of IHSS and the possibility of acute myocardial infarction with secondary cardiogenic shock.

The risk of precipitating pulmonary edema was considerable in this patient. However, that risk was matched by the risk of not giving enough fluid fast enough and having his cardiovascular status deteriorate even further, probably causing his death. This dilemma is one of the reasons a central venous pressure line is needed (see answer 2E).

On the basis of an initial low-normal CVP reading in this patient, a fluid challenge (B) of 200 ml of Ringer's lactate injection was given. The result was a rise in CVP of only 2 cm H_2O at 10 minutes. His blood pressure rose to 80/50 mm Hg over 20 minutes and to 100/70 mm Hg over 50 minutes; he became less restless and his skin began to warm up. Approximately 400 ml of 5% dextrose in water were given within the first hour.

For the patient who remains in shock for some time, that is, the patient who is unresponsive to treatment, it is essential to measure other variables, including left ventricular performance through a Swan-Ganz catheter. This approach is always indicated for optimal management of patients whose main problem is left ventricular failure of moderate to severe degree, as in many patients with myocardial infarction. This patient had such a catheter inserted in the second hour after his arrival, and, on the basis of its evidence, a larger fluid challenge was given safely and effectively, with a gradual rise in blood pressure to 120/80 mm Hg and an increase in urinary output.

(C) Every patient in shock needs oxygen in as high a concentration as possible, at least at first. In general, oxygen by nasal prongs or face mask is not adequate, and endotracheal or nasotracheal intubation should be considered. One need not fear oxygen toxicity, even with administration of 100% oxygen, until several (6 or more) hours have elapsed. However, as soon as possible, the concentration should be reduced. The decision to reduce the concentration of oxygen is based on several factors, chiefly, the arterial blood gases and pH. If the PaO_2 remains low after administration of a high concentration of oxygen, the airway should be rechecked and pulmonary embolus ruled out.

(D) The pain of severe myocardial infarction must be relieved, since it, in itself, sets up noxious reflexes. A small dose (2 to 4 mg) of morphine given slowly (over 2 minutes), intravenously, seems to work best. It can be repeated in 10 minutes if neither nausea nor respiratory depression occurs. For a patient with a history of nausea following morphine administration, dimenhydrinate, 50 mg, may be given intravenously to decrease the likelihood of nausea and vomiting.

(E) Although lidocaine administration may aggravate rather than alleviate cardiogenic shock, it probably should be used early in any adult patient with severe chest pain thought to be due to acute myocardial infarction. The risk of developing ventricular tachycardia or ventricular fibrillation is too great to wait for the appearance of premature ventricular contractions (PVCs).

(F) The patient's head and trunk may be elevated 10-15 degrees for cardiogenic shock, higher than this if pulmonary edema is present. There is no evidence that the traditional Trendelenberg position helps, so its use has largely been abandoned in such patients.

(G) A nasogastric tube should be inserted if upper gastrointestinal hemorrhage is suspected, but usually not if myocardial infarction is probable. Unless it is urgently needed to empty a stomach distended sufficiently to interfere with ventilation, the procedure may have to be delayed until the diagnosis becomes clearer. In this patient, it was not necessary.

If the patient's shock state is prolonged, an intra-arterial catheter should be inserted for more accurate and continuous measurement of arterial pressure, as well as for an accessible means of obtaining arterial blood for gases and pH.

5. (A, B, C, D, F, G, H, I) (A) Cardiogenic shock is characterized by failure of the pump itself, whereas hypovolemic shock represents inadequate fluid in the vascular system, and vasomotor shock represents pooling of the blood in some part of the system.

Some authorities[1] limit the use of the term cardiogenic shock to that type due to massive acute myocardial infarction, and such a cause should be assumed if no other cause is known. The point is that in the prehospital and emergency department phases of care, it is often difficult or impossible to be certain of the etiology. Therefore, the patient should be treated as if he has myocardial infarction complicated by shock, provided the clinical evaluation and preliminary ancillary studies all point in that direction. If a hypovolemic cause alone, or in association, is suspected, this should be carefully tested and, if present, corrected with appropriate monitoring and repeated fluid challenges. Since as many as 20% of patients with acute myocardial infarction have some degree of hypovolemia, this approach seems sound and may be curative of the shock problem in a patient similar to the one presented here.

(B) As many as one out of every five patients admitted to the hospital for acute myocardial infarction will develop cardiogenic shock. Death occurs in over 80% of patients, usually the result of massive transmural damage to the left ventricle (D). As more dysrhythmias are being brought under control by the care given in cardiac intensive care units, cardiogenic shock is claiming a higher proportion (now around 50%) of patients who die in the hospital of myocardial infarction (C).

(E) There are other causes of cardiogenic shock, although acute myocardial infarction is the principal cause. Some of these other causes are major dysrhythmias, rupture of a papillary muscle, rupture of the interventricular septum or the heart itself, and filling problems, such as pericardial tamponade or pulmonary embolism. Since some of these are amenable to surgical correction, they should be looked for and, when found, treated aggressively. Another cause is obstruction of the left ventricular outflow tract as by end-stage valvular disease or IHSS, the latter present in this patient. Apparently, the obstruction became more severe as his blood volume, already reduced by various mechanisms, was acutely reduced even further.

(F, G) Predisposition to cardiogenic shock, due to myocardial infarction, occurs in patients with hypertension, as in this patient, and the elderly, as well as in those who have had one or more previous myocardial infarctions. The mechanism of this predisposition is not clear.

(H, I) Cardiogenic shock, due to myocardial infarction, usually appears suddenly and progresses rapidly, patients often dying within a few hours. About half of the patients who develop cardiogenic shock do so within 24 hours, although about one-sixth do not develop it until a week or more later. In the latter instance, the shock often appears when an extension of the infarct occurs.

6. (B, C, D) (A) Dopamine should be administered only after any hypovolemia has been corrected. If normovolemia is present, dopamine should be started as soon as possible after onset of cardiogenic shock.

(B) At low doses, dopamine increases cardiac output by increasing myocardial contractility, the latter brought about by its stimulation of the beta-adrenergic receptors of the heart. (C) Also at low doses, dopamine dilates mesenteric and renal vessels through stimulation of dopaminergic receptors. This increases urine output in most patients.

(D) The infusion rate of dopamine must be individually titrated for the desired effect. A beginning rate of 2-4 micrograms/kg/ minute is recommended for patients who are likely to respond to low doses. However, in more seriously ill patients, the initial infusion rate should be 5 micrograms/kg/minute, gradually increased up to 20 micrograms/kg/minute, if necessary. To obtain this control, dopamine should be prepared by diluting 200 mg (the contents of one 5-ml container) in 500 ml of 5% dextrose in water, making a concentration of 400 micrograms/ml.

COURSE:

After the first day in the intensive care unit, the patient's convalescence was uneventful. Serial electrocardiograms and serial enzyme studies failed to confirm acute myocardial infarction. There was no evidence of ruptured interventricular septum, and the loud systolic murmur diminished in intensity. Its cause was never determined. Renal function returned to normal, with gradual increase in urinary output to 50 ml/hour.

Since there was no evidence of acute pancreatitis, gastrointestinal bleeding or other acute process to account for the hypotensive episode, it was presumed to be due to volume depletion by vomiting and diarrhea, with inadequate fluid intake. These apparently caused an increase in the functional and mechanical obstruction of the outflow tract of the left ventricle (IHSS). Thus, this patient had a combination of hypovolemic and cardiogenic shock, without evidence of acute myocardial infarction. He was discharged on the fifth hospital day.

REFERENCE

Rackley, C. E., et al.: Cardiogenic Shock: Recognition and Management. In: A. N. Brest (Ed.), Cardiovascular Clinics: Innovations in the Diagnosis and Management of Acute Myocardial Infarction. Philadelphia: F. A. Davis Co., 1975.

::

CASE 20: EPIGASTRIC DISCOMFORT AND PAIN

HISTORY:

A 47-year-old man was in good health until eight days before admission, when he experienced a substernal burning sensation while hiking. The pain did not radiate, it lasted only 15 minutes, and it did not recur when he resumed hiking at a slower pace. Over the next several days, he had burning epigastric discomfort, not related to meals or to exertion. On the day before admission, he experienced the same epigastric discomfort while climbing stairs. He became worried about his heart and reported to the emergency department in a very casual manner for a "check-up." He had had glaucoma for eight years, but had no history of other disease. He had smoked two packs of cigarettes daily for 30 years. His father had died of myocardial infarction, and one sister had had triple bypass surgery for coronary artery disease.

Examination showed him to be in no obvious distress and to have no diaphoresis. His blood pressure was 110/72 mm Hg; pulse, strong and regular at 76 per minute; respirations, 18 per minute and regular; temperature, 98.6°F (37°C). The lungs were clear to auscultation; there was no cardiac enlargement, irregularity, or murmurs. Examination of the abdomen and extremities showed no abnormalities. ECG monitor showed normal sinus rhythm with no premature ventricular contractions.

QUESTIONS:

1. TRUE OR FALSE: On the basis of these findings, this patient should be suspected of having a serious cardiac problem.

2. Which of the following are the most life-threatening to this patient?
   A. Reflux esophagitis
   B. Abdominal diseases
   C. Acute myocardial infarction
   D. Dissecting aortic aneurysm
   E. Unstable angina
   F. Pulmonary embolism
   G. Acute pericarditis
   H. Musculoskeletal (chest wall) origin
   I. All of the above

3. Initially, which of the following laboratory tests are most important in making the diagnosis in this patient?
   A. Electrocardiographic monitoring
   B. Twelve-lead electrocardiography
   C. Portable chest x-ray
   D. Measurement of cardiac enzymes
   E. Status of liver function
   F. Measurement of serum and urine amylase
   G. Flat plate and upright x-ray studies of the abdomen
   H. Rectal examination with examination of stool for blood
   I. Measurement of arterial blood gases and pH
   J. All of the above

4. A twelve-lead ECG was being run when this patient suddenly became unresponsive and stopped breathing, and ventricular fibrillation appeared on the ECG. In such an instance, what are the proper steps to take?
   A. Open the airway.
   B. Deliver a precordial thump.
   C. Defibrillate immediately.
   D. Begin mouth-to-mouth ventilation or bag-valve-mask ventilation with supplemental oxygen.
   E. Begin external cardiac compression if spontaneous heartbeat fails to resume promptly.
   F. Intubate the trachea as soon as possible and administer 100% oxygen.
   G. All of the above

5. Which of the following are true about this patient? (Read answer 4 first)
   A. He was clinically and biologically dead when he developed ventricular fibrillation.
   B. He responded in the usual way to defibrillation, administered early after onset of ventricular fibrillation.
   C. He should have been given sodium bicarbonate and epinephrine intravenously before being defibrillated.
   D. If this patient had not been attached to the monitor at the time of his cardiac arrest, he could have had what is called "blind" defibrillation.
   E. All of the above

6. If this patient had not been attached to the monitor at the time of sudden unconsciousness, how would you have checked to see if he had developed cardiopulmonary arrest?
   A. Try to arouse him by shouting and shaking his shoulders.
   B. Palpate the carotid or femoral pulse.
   C. Look at his eyegrounds to determine if blood is moving through the arterioles.
   D. Take his blood pressure.

E. Check his pupils.
F. Check his reflexes.
G. Check his breathing.

7. Which of the following are true about chest pain due to acute myocardial infarction.
   A. Such pain can usually be distinguished from that arising in other structures in the chest on the basis of the history alone.
   B. The cardiac origin must usually be confirmed by electrocardiography and other laboratory studies.
   C. The pain almost never occurs in the back or epigastrium.
   D. It is usually substernal.
   E. It is usually sharp.
   F. It frequently radiates to the left upper extremity.
   G. It can usually be localized by the patient with one finger.
   H. All of the above

8. Which of the following are true about unstable angina?
   A. Synonyms are accelerated angina, crescendo angina, decubitus angina, nocturnal angina, preinfarction angina, impending myocardial infarction, and the intermediate syndrome.
   B. All patients with this syndrome should be admitted to a coronary intensive care unit for at least 48 hours of continuous electrocardiographic monitoring.
   C. It is characterized by a change in the pattern of pain and in the usual favorable response to rest or nitroglycerin.
   D. Its course is unpredictable.
   E. Serial (at least daily) electrocardiograms and cardiac enzyme determinations are helpful in making the diagnosis and in differentiating this disease from myocardial infarction.
   F. Coronary arteriography is frequently indicated.
   G. All of the above

9. Besides oxygen and lidocaine, what other drugs may be helpful in cardiopulmonary resuscitation if the patient fails to respond as promptly as this patient did?
   A. Sodium bicarbonate
   B. Epinephrine
   C. Atropine sulfate
   D. Calcium chloride
   E. Isoproterenol
   F. Propranolol
   G. Dopamine
   H. Procainamide

I. Vasoactive drugs
J. Potent diuretics
K. All of the above

ANSWERS AND COMMENTS:

1. (True) Despite the absence of any clinical signs in this preliminary examination, this patient has a history of chest pain, and any patient with chest pain should be suspected of having a serious cardiac problem. Also, epigastric pain on exertion is known to be a substitute symptom of myocardial disease.

The differential diagnosis for a patient who has chest pain is often surprisingly simple, and at other times, surprisingly complex. Initially, the most important asset is a high index of suspicion. The most life-threatening of the probable diseases must be suspected first.

2. (C, D, E, F) When a patient, especially an adult, arrives in the emergency department with chest pain, a three-pronged approach is used: (1) diagnosis is made as rapidly as possible; (2) treatment is started promptly; and (3) complications are prevented, if possible. This patient illustrates the importance of this approach.

While items C-F were selected on the basis of their threat to life if undetected and unprepared for, the others certainly should be considered in the differential diagnosis. However, the worst possible causes must be ruled out before the more common, but less serious, conditions can safely be considered. All relevant factors must be taken into account, such as age, associated medical conditions, and whether the patient is thought to be exaggerating or understating his symptoms. Family members can frequently confirm or refute how correct the history is, how frequently the attacks of chest pain occur, and how severe they are. This is especially helpful in diagnosing chest pain, since most patients will try to deny that they are having a heart attack and will try to minimize their symptoms as much as possible, as did this patient.

While the best approach for the emergency department physician is to consider all of the listed possibilities as the patient gives his history, there is often insufficient time for a complete history. Careful monitoring and, if possible, treatment must frequently take precedence over definite diagnosis. For these life-threatening diseases, treatment should begin as soon as the working diagnosis points toward a particular condition.

(C) Acute myocardial infarction is a definite possibility in this patient. The usual history is of crushing substernal chest pain, but the symptoms are not always so dramatic. A few patients have no symptoms, although, in these, a careful questioning of both the patient and his family will usually reveal discomfort in the past. As many as 15% of patients with proved myocardial infarction deny having experienced any discomfort. The most difficult diagnostic problems arise when the patient has few, if any, symptoms, a negative physical examination, then a negative ECG. It is this type of patient whose problem taxes the physician's diagnostic skill and frequently requires consultation and observation with careful monitoring and serial diagnostic studies before the correct diagnosis and management can be arranged. As the public becomes more and more sophisticated in matters of health, there will be many more such patients presenting themselves to emergency departments with such vague symptoms, patients who will tax even further our diagnostic acumen and our facilities for screening and monitoring.

(D) Dissecting aortic aneurysm is another lethal disease that must be diagnosed rapidly. Diagnosis can frequently be made on the basis of a history of excruciating pain in the anterior and posterior chest, which is usually most severe at onset and radiates into the epigastrium, lumbar regions, or lower extremities. Wide differences in blood pressures and pulses between the upper and lower extremities are frequently noted. Progressive widening of the aorta on serial roentgenograms, with definitive aortography, often leads to the correct diagnosis.

(E) Unstable angina pectoris would be a very likely diagnosis in this patient, even though his pain did not consistently reappear with exertion. The symptoms of this disease vary greatly, and one should strongly suspect it in any middle-aged person, especially a man, with these or similar symptoms (see answer 8).

(F) Pulmonary embolism with pulmonary infarction has more subtle symptoms, and may be forgotten when diagnoses are being considered. The initial portable chest x-ray may be helpful, but is frequently negative, at times even after pulmonary infarction has begun. Measurement of arterial blood gases and pH should be routine, since a PO_2 lower than normal for the patient's age would suggest the presence of pulmonary embolism in the absence of other obvious causes, such as pneumonia. The finding of peripheral thromboembolic disease is also helpful, but the most likely source of a pulmonary embolus is phlebothrombosis of the lower extremities; this condition is often asymptomatic and cannot be detected by physical examination.

If indicated, pulmonary radionuclide scan and pulmonary arteriography can be done and are diagnostic.

If none of these appear to be the cause of the chest pain, or while tests are being done to confirm them or rule them out, consideration can be given to the remaining diseases on the list.

(A) Acute esophagitis is a common diagnosis in emergency departments, but it should be based largely on exclusion of other conditions that cause similar symptoms. It is usually of the reflux type and may or may not be associated with esophageal hiatal hernia. Even when a patient has a history of such a hernia, with reflux symptoms, the physician should not ascribe the chest pain to this condition until he has made every effort to rule out brief or prolonged myocardial ischemic attacks. This can usually be done by the history of a change in the character of the pain from that which the patient usually has (see answer 8). Patients with reflux esophagitis usually obtain dramatic relief when given antacids, but it must be remembered that an occasional patient with myocardial ischemia does so, also.

(B) It can be very difficult to differentiate abdominal diseases from the syndrome of myocardial ischemia or infarction, since the pain of both may be referred to the upper abdomen. The abdominal diseases most likely to cause confusion are acute pancreatitis, acute cholecystitis with or without cholelithiasis (biliary colic), and peptic ulcer disease, especially with penetration or perforation. Physical examination is usually helpful; x-ray examination is sometimes definitive; electrocardiography is rarely positive in the patient with abdominal disease alone. However, in a patient who has angina pectoris also, or if there are S-T depressions associated with shock, the situation may be very hard to resolve, and hospital admission for observation is required.

(G) Acute pericarditis may be part of the pattern of acute myocardial infarction, but, when due to that cause, is usually associated with a friction rub. The rub may be evanescent and should always be listened for repeatedly in any patient with chest pain. In acute idiopathic pericarditis, widespread S-T elevation may be present on the ECG, and abnormal Q waves are usually absent.

(H) Chest pain of musculoskeletal origin is largely a diagnosis of exclusion, although a few entities are clear enough to make a definitive diagnosis possible without further studies. For example, a hematoma in the chest wall muscle is easy to diagnose if the history indicates an injury or strain. Costochondritis (costosternal syndrome, or Tietze's syndrome), etiology unknown, affects the upper two or three chondrosternal or costochondral junctions and responds gradually to conservative symptomatic treatment.

3. (A, B, C, I) In light of the difficulties in differential diagnosis outlined in question and answer 1, it is obvious that these four are the tests that should be done first. The others can be started, but either they will not be reported in time (a common problem in emergency departments), or they are not necessary for the initial evaluation. (A) Any adult coming to the emergency department with chest pain should be connected immediately to the ECG monitor or checked immediately with combination electrode-defibrillator paddles. These give immediate, definitive information on the electrical function of the heart. Such monitoring should be continued without interruption, until it is decided that the patient has a condition unlikely to cause myocardial instability.

(B) A twelve-lead ECG is very helpful in adults with chest pain, both for what it may show and what it may not show. It cannot be emphasized too often that a negative resting ECG in a patient with chest pain does not rule out myocardial ischemia or infarction. Serial ECGs, repeated several times over a period of 12 to 48 hours, preferably with the patient in the hospital, are needed to rule in or rule out myocardial ischemia or infarction. Exercise recordings are hardly feasible or safe to obtain in most emergency departments, but information of a positive exercise test in the past is very helpful.

(C) A portable chest x-ray is very helpful and can usually be obtained quickly, without disturbing the patient. All obvious pulmonary lesions can be detected in this manner, although some of the most lethal conditions, such as pulmonary embolization with pulmonary infarction, do not show up on a plain film, especially a single portable view. Additional views, at least posteroanterior and lateral views, should be taken as soon as possible, whenever a pulmonary lesion is found or is strongly suspected.

(D) Measurement of cardiac enzymes is useful if the results are immediately available, but this is not usually the case. If the first results are normal, serial enzyme studies, along with serial ECGs, may be needed for definitive diagnosis. (E) Liver function studies are not usually helpful initially, and the reports are usually delayed for hours or even overnight. (F) Serum amylase and a timed urinary amylase are useful findings in the diagnosis of acute pancreatitis, but here, too, these tests are not usually reported early enough to be of help in the initial management of the patient. (G) Roentgenographic studies of the abdomen may be diagnostic of ruptured viscus, calcific deposits or intestinal obstruction. (H) Rectal examination with a guaiac test for blood in the stool may be very helpful if gastrointestinal bleeding is suspected, such as from an esophageal lesion, a gastric or duodenal ulcer, or other lesion.

(I) Arterial blood gases and pH are very valuable in screening patients with possible pulmonary embolization and certain other pulmonary lesions, such as pneumothorax, pneumonitis, and chronic obstructive pulmonary disease with acute exacerbation. Such a test is useful in helping one decide whether radionuclide pulmonary scanning should be done. It is also wise to obtain arterial blood gases and pH if oxygen therapy is contemplated, since a baseline reading, with the patient breathing room air, is a helpful guide to such therapy.

4. (A, C, D, E, F, and in that order, if they cannot be done almost simultaneously) (A) As soon as the patient becomes unconscious, his tongue falls against the posterior pharyngeal wall, obstructing the airway. The easiest, quickest, and safest way to open the airway (in the absence of neck injury) is to extend the head and elevate the neck. If possible, one member of the resuscitation team should be given the responsibility of maintaining the airway and ventilating the patient. (D) Mouth-to-mouth ventilation delivers only 16% oxygen, but the bellows action of the rescuer's lungs is excellent for delivering the 800 to 2000 ml tidal volume of air that is needed. However, a stronger concentration of oxygen (21%) can be obtained by the use of one of the usual non-rebreathing bags of the AMBU type, in which case an oropharyngeal airway should be used along with extension of the head. Supplemental oxygen should be added as soon as possible. As soon as it can be done thereafter (usually after rapid oxygenation), a cuffed endotracheal tube should be inserted and 100% oxygen given (F). This tube assures an open airway and prevents aspiration if the patient regurgitates.

The defibrillator was charged to the maximum setting and defibrillation was done (C). All of this was accomplished in 10 to 15 seconds, as it should be in a well-organized emergency department, using the team approach. The proper setting on the unit was for defibrillation, not synchronized cardioversion. With the latter, the unit will not fire in the absence of an R wave and there are no R waves in ventricular fibrillation.

Within 5 seconds, sinus rhythm resumed at 108 beats/minute; an occasional premature ventricular contraction (PVC) was present, easily controlled with a bolus of lidocaine followed by a continuous intravenous infusion of lidocaine at 2 mg/minute.

Unless the patient responds immediately to defibrillation, as this patient did, external cardiac compression should be started (E). The rule is that the patient should not be left without cardic compression for more than 5 seconds, before or after defibrillation. This patient's carotid pulse was strong as soon as the normal sinus rhythm reappeared on the monitor, so no cardiac compression was required.

A precordial thump (B) is now recommended only in a monitored situation such as this. However, it is not recommended for ventricular fibrillation, since defibrillation is the specific treatment for this dysrhythmia. On the other hand, for asystole, the other major cause of cardiac arrest, a single precordial thump is indicated. While drug therapy and other treatment modalities are being prepared or administered, it is sometimes possible to pace a patient's heart by delivering repeated precordial thumps, using the monitor and pulse as guides. However, if a spontaneous beat is not resumed, it is probably better to substitute cardiac compression without further delay.

COURSE:

This patient's blood pressure one minute after defibrillation was 100/60 mm Hg. He was then admitted to the CCU, where further studies and the subsequent course confirmed acute inferior myocardial infarction. He had no further episodes of ventricular irritability, but was continued on prophylactic lidocaine infusion intravenously for the first 48 hours after admission. From the initial and subsequent electrocardiograms, it appeared that his infarction had occurred at about the time he arrived at the emergency department. The discomfort he experienced over the preceding eight days probably represented pre-infarction or unstable angina. In his case, it was probably on the basis of near-total occlusion of at least his right coronary artery.

He was doing well when discharged on the nineteenth hospital day. Coronary angiography was scheduled for three months after discharge.

5. (B, D) (A) Clinical death is present when the patient's heart and respirations stop, which were once the criteria for pronouncing a patient dead. Biological death does not occur until

irreversible changes occur in the brain. The brain is the organ most vulnerable to anoxic changes in the body and the one in which the changes become irreversible earlier than all others. The interval between these two forms of death is only 4 to 6 minutes; and it is only during this interval that life-restoring measures can be carried out without it being almost certain that permanent brain damage will remain if the patient is resuscitated.

(B) This patient showed the usual response to defibrillation when it is administered within the first few seconds of cardiac arrest, due to ventricular fibrillation. The earlier the defibrillation is delivered, the more likely it is to be successful. After total cessation of blood flow, for as briefly as 30 to 60 seconds, the patient may not respond as promptly as this patient did. Nevertheless, defibrillation at full power should be tried immediately, without waiting for intravenous lines to be opened or medications to be administered (C). If there is no response, cardiac compression and artificial ventilation should be continued while the medications are quickly administered intravenously; then, as soon as possible thereafter, a second defibrillation (and more if needed) should be tried.

(D) An adult patient who suddenly becomes unconscious, pulseless, and breathless (apneic) should have defibrillation without waiting for ECG monitoring, unless the monitoring can be accomplished within a few seconds. This procedure is called "blind" defibrillation, since the dysrhythmia is not known. In an adult, the probability that ventricular fibrillation is the cause of cardiac arrest is great, being approximately 75%. The other predominant cause is ventricular standstill (asystole). Clinically, there is no way to differentiate between these two conditions, but defibrillation will not harm the patient with asystole. Neither will it help him, but it will help those patients with ventricular fibrillation. Such blind defibrillation is not recommended in children, since cardiac arrest in children is frequently of the hypoxic type and due to asystole, rather than to ventricular fibrillation. With the combination electrode-defibrillator paddles and machines now available in most emergency departments, the rhythm can be determined immediately in any patient of any age, provided the paddles can be applied and the monitoring done within seconds.

6. (A, B, G) (A) When a person seems to be unconscious, he may only have dozed off to sleep, in which case he will awaken when his name is shouted or when he is shaken vigorously. On rare occasions, simple fainting can confuse the issue, since

the patient may then be unable to respond momentarily. A postictal patient may be stuporous, but will usually respond to noise or painful stimuli.

(B) The most important test is palpation of a central type pulse, usually in the carotid or femoral arteries. The radial artery is too peripheral to be used. In small children, the precordium can be palpated in lieu of the carotid or femoral vessels. If the pulse cannot be felt after careful palpation, preferably at both the carotid and femoral locations and taking at least 5 to 10 seconds, it must be assumed that the patient has cardiac arrest. Whenever absent pulse, absent respirations (G), and unresponsiveness (A) concur, immediate cardiopulmonary resuscitation is indicated.

C, D, E, and F are a waste of time, since unresponsiveness, pulselessness and breathlessness are sufficient for the diagnosis of cardiac arrest. In particular, one should not worry about checking pupils to diagnose death (E), since death by this criterion is clinical death and may be reversible.

7. (B, D, F) (A) It is almost impossible to determine the source of the pain by this history alone. However, the history is probably the most helpful single aspect of the clinical evaluation for ruling in or ruling out cardiac origin of the pain. For confirmation, electrocardiography is always necessary, and certain other laboratory studies, including cardiac enzyme determinations, are often necessary (B). The roentgenographic examination of the chest and the total clinical picture must also be considered.

(D) The pain, when present, is usually substernal, but may occur in the interscapular area (C), in which case it suggests dissecting aneurysm. When the pain is only in the epigastrium, it is confused with that of esophageal disease, peptic ulcer disease, cholecystic or pancreatic disease or other abdominal conditions. While it is likely to be crushing, pressing, burning, vise-like or aching, the pain of acute myocardial infarction is almost never sharp (E).

Patients will frequently point with one finger to the cardiac apex as the site of pain. While it is possible for the pain of coronary disease, including acute myocardial infarction, to be limited to that area, this location usually means functional (nonorganic) pain (G). The more localized the pain, the more likely it is not to be due to acute myocardial infarction. An exception to this rule is the occasional patient whose pain of myocardial infarction is referred to a single area, such as the jaw or elbow.

(F) Typically, if it radiates at all, the pain radiates to the left upper extremity, usually along the medial aspect of the arm and, at times, the forearm as well. However, it may be felt only in the left side of the neck, the chin, or the right upper extremity.

8. (G) All. The term unstable angina is usually reserved for the patient with long-standing angina whose pattern of pain has changed. His attacks occur more frequently or with less provocation, there is usually a less reliable response to rest, and there may be minimal or no relief from pain from even repeated doses of nitroglycerin. Unstable angina, after a variable period of time, is followed by myocardial infarction, and the patient with such angina should be admitted to the hospital promptly for monitoring and further studies. Coronary arteriography will usually show marked narrowing of one or more of the coronary arteries, in which case, coronary artery surgery may be required. In brief, until the diagnosis is decided upon, the patient with unstable angina should be managed as if he has sustained an acute myocardial infarction. This is the important point for emergency department physicians to remember, since the patient with unstable angina sent home from the emergency department is very likely to have myocardial infarction when he returns.

9. (K) All. In the "Standards for Cardiopulmonary Resuscitation (CPR) and Emergency Cardiac Care (ECC)"[1] and in the Manual for Training in Advanced Cardiac Life Support,[2] these drugs are divided between "essential" (A - D, plus oxygen, lidocaine and morphine sulfate for pain) and "useful" (E - J) drugs. All providers of advanced CPR are strongly advised to take a course in the use of these drugs. In this discussion, only a brief explanation of the role of each drug will be given. Dosages are for adults except where otherwise noted, and all drug administration in the treatment of cardiac arrest is intravenous.

(A) Sodium bicarbonate is administered in a dose of 1 mEq/kg of estimated body weight as soon as possible after cardiac arrest (but not before defibrillation, if this can be done quickly). Its purpose is to correct the metabolic acidosis that appears almost immediately and progresses rapidly, because anaerobic metabolism allows lactic acid to accumulate in the body. If possible, the subsequent doses should be based on determination of arterial blood gases and pH. If this is impossible, one-half of the initial dose can be given at ten-minute intervals for as long as the resuscitation effort continues.

(B) Epinephrine is probably the single most important drug for CPR, since it improves myocardial contractility, stimulates spontaneous contractions, elevates perfusion pressure generated during cardiac compression, and, by increasing myocardial tone, helps convert a fine fibrillation to a coarse one that will be more susceptible to defibrillation. The initial dose of 0.5 mg (5 ml of a 1:10,000 solution) should be repeated every five minutes during the resuscitation effort. The action of epinephrine is impaired if the patient is acidotic; hence, the importance of administering sodium bicarbonate at the same time but by a different intravenous route.

(C) Atropine sulfate is a parasympatholytic drug that decreases vagal tone, thereby accelerating the rate of discharge at the S-A node and improving atrioventricular conduction. The acceleration in heart rate, brought on by administration of atropine, increases myocardial oxygen consumption in most instances, an undesirable development in acute myocardial infarction. Thus, atropine is reserved for treating severe sinus bradycardia with hypotension and ventricular ectopic beats, especially following resuscitation. It was not needed in this patient. When it is required, the initial dose is 0.5 mg. The dose can be repeated at five-minute intervals but should not exceed a total of 2.0 mg.

(D) Calcium, usually in the form of calcium chloride, is useful in cardiac arrest due to asystole, but is not usually needed in arrest due to ventricular fibrillation. The dose is 2.5 to 5.0 ml of the 10% solution.

(E) Isoproterenol is a potent inotropic and chronotropic drug, which is used in patients following resuscitation if there is bradycardia with hypotension. Usually atropine is tried first, since isoproterenol is capable of producing myocardial irritability and of increasing the need for oxygen in an area of myocardium that is already ischemic. It is still useful in situations where a cardiac pacemaker is being readied and introduced, as in Adams-Stokes attack with severe bradycardia or asystolic cardiac arrest. The dose for an adult is 1 mg in 500 ml of 5% dextrose in water, producing a concentration of 2 micrograms/ml, titrated at 2 to 20 micrograms/minute for the desired effect.

(F) Propranolol is helpful in preventing recurrent episodes of ventricular tachycardia or recurrent ventricular fibrillation. It should always be tried when lidocaine, in standard amounts, has failed to prevent such recurrences. The dose is 1.0 mg, administered slowly. It may be repeated to a total dose of 3 to 5 mg under careful monitoring.

(G) Dopamine is primarily indicated in cardiogenic shock (see Case 19). The initial rate of infusion should be 2 to 5 micrograms/kg/min; it should be increased gradually, if necessary, to obtain increased blood pressure and urine flow. The 5-ml ampule, containing 200 mg, is added to 250 ml of 5% dextrose or lactate, giving a concentration of 800 micrograms/ml.

(H) Procainamide suppresses ventricular ectopic beats and recurrent ventricular tachycardia, and should be given when lidocaine is ineffective. It is administered in 0.2 to 1.0 gm amounts at a rate not to exceed 25 to 50 mg/min.

(I) Vasoactive drugs, such as levarterenol, are useful in the patient who has been resuscitated but whose blood pressure remains dangerously low. Levarterenol is a potent inotropic agent, but it causes peripheral (including renal and mesenteric) vasoconstriction. For that reason, it is sometimes used successfully in combination with dopamine, which dilates renal and mesenteric vessels. Levarterenol should always be administered through a catheter well advanced into a vein. The drug is titrated as an infusion of 16 micrograms/ml in 5% dextrose in water, or in 5% dextrose in saline solution. This solution is obtained by adding 2 ampules of 4 ml or 8 mg each to 1000 ml of the fluid.

(J) Potent diuretics, namely furosemide and ethacrynic acid, are indicated in the treatment of acute pulmonary edema and may be useful in the treatment of post-resuscitation cerebral edema. Furosemide, 40 mg, is injected slowly over a period of at least one to two minutes. The equivalent dose of ethacrynic acid is 50 mg.

REFERENCES

1. Standards for cardiopulmonary resuscitation (CPR) and emergency cardiac care (ECC). JAMA 227 (Suppl.):833-868, 1974.

2. Manual for Training in Advanced Cardiac Life Support. New York: American Heart Association, 1975.

::

CASE 21: SHORTNESS OF BREATH AND RAPID HEART BEAT WITHOUT EXERTION

HISTORY:

A 67-year-old woman came to the emergency department complaining of shortness of breath and rapid heart beat of 14 hours' duration. A similar episode had occurred two years before and had resolved spontaneously after four hours. She experienced no chest pain with either attack. Radical mastectomies had been done eight years before, and she was receiving chemotherapy, including cyclophosphamide, for widespread bony metastases. No pleuropulmonary metastases had been found on repeated chest roentgenograms, the last having been taken one week before this admission.

Results of the physical examination were negative, except for bilateral radical mastectomy scars and a tachycardia of 160/minute. Blood pressure was 120/80 mm Hg; respirations, 22/minute; temperature, 98.4°F (36.8°C). The rhythm strip (Lead II) is reproduced in Fig. 21.1.

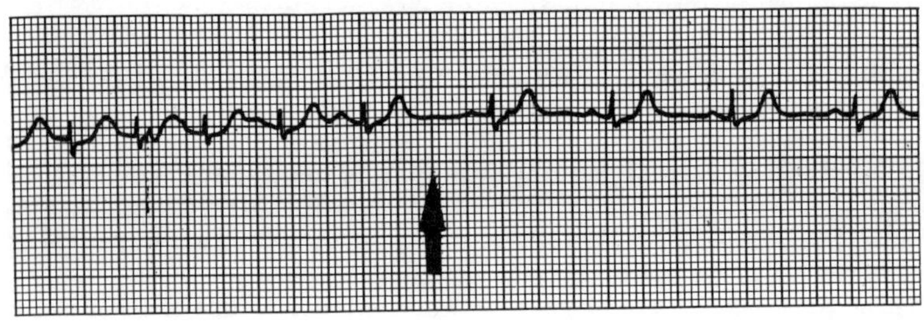

FIG. 21.1: Rhythm strip (Lead II).

QUESTIONS:

1. Analysis of the rhythm strip reveals that it has many of the characteristics of paroxysmal atrial tachycardia (PAT). These include:
   A. Rate of 160 beats/minute
   B. Regular rhythm
   C. Narrow QRS complexes
   D. P waves absent or obscured
   E. Minimal S-T depressions
   F. All of the above

2. Which of the following statements about PAT are true?
   A. It is caused by an accelerated pacemaker mechanism.
   B. It frequently afflicts young patients with normal hearts.
   C. The attacks begin and end abruptly.
   D. The attacks usually last for days, rather than hours.
   E. It can cause severe compromise of the cardiovascular system.
   F. The attack should be terminated quickly if there is underlying heart disease or if cardiac failure, syncope, or anginal pain develop.
   G. It is sometimes difficult to differentiate from ventricular tachycardia.
   H. All of the above

3. Which of the following statements about carotid sinus massage are correct?
   A. It should always be done under electrocardiographic monitoring.
   B. It is useful in differentiating various tachyarrhythmias.
   C. It is useful in terminating atrial or A-V junctional tachycardia.
   D. It may be dangerous in patients with digitalis intoxication.
   E. It should always be tried in patients with sinus tachycardia.
   F. It does not usually cause a change in ventricular tachycardia.
   G. It almost never slows the ventricular rate in patients with atrial fibrillation or flutter.

4. If this patient had not reverted to normal sinus rhythm so readily, what other steps could have been taken?
   A. Other maneuvers that stimulate the vagus nerve
   B. Drug therapy
   C. Cardioversion
   D. Overdrive pacing
   E. All of the above

5. TRUE OR FALSE: A probable cause of the PAT in this patient would have been the Wolff-Parkinson-White (WPW) syndrome.

6. Which of the following are correctly stated regarding the diagnosis of WPW syndrome?
   A. The diagnosis can only be made electrocardiographically.
   B. The P-R interval is short.
   C. The QRS complex is wide, due to the presence of a delta wave.
   D. The delta wave can be clearly seen during episodes of

PAT caused by the WPW syndrome.
E. The typical changes may be absent on a particular ECG.
F. All of the above

ANSWERS AND COMMENTS:

1. (F) All. Paroxysmal atrial tachycardia (PAT) is a run of rapidly repeated premature atrial beats. It is the most common paroxysmal tachycardia; the term paroxysmal refers to its tendency to start and stop suddenly.

(A) The rate usually varies between 160 and 250 beats/minute, but, for any particular patient, it remains the same throughout the attack. (B) The beat is usually regular, although slight irregularity may be present. (C) The QRS complexes are narrow(normal), unless aberrant ventricular conduction or A-V block is also present. If the P-R interval is relatively prolonged, as it often is at rapid rates, the abnormal P wave may merge with the T wave, or may merge with the QRS complex of the preceding beat. In that case, it may be impossible to differentiate between atrial and A-V nodal tachycardia; and the more inclusive term, supraventricular tachycardia, should be used until the differentiation can be made. (E) S-T depression is minimal in this tracing, although it is frequently much greater with PAT. The depression is caused by ischemia, which is caused by decreased coronary blood flow in the presence of increased oxygen demand due to the rapid rate.

2. (B, C, E, F, G) (A) Recent studies have shown that re-entry, rather than accelerated pacemaker, is the mechanism of PAT. This implies a functional longitudinal dissociation between two neighboring areas of myocardial tissue.[1] Re-entry may occur wherever the refractory period of two such areas is significantly different. The attacks, which begin and end abruptly (C), are usually precipitated by a single, appropriately timed, premature atrial beat.

(B) The attacks occur frequently in young persons with normal hearts, and are sometimes, but not always, brought on by emotional or physical stress, or by excessive amounts of caffeine or other stimulants. (D) The attacks usually last for hours, rather than days. The duration of an attack before the patient seeks medical attention depends upon his symptoms and the success he has had in breaking up previous attacks.

(E) Most patients with normal hearts can tolerate a ventricular rate of 160 to 180/minute for up to a few hours, without the development of hypotension or other evidence of cardiovascular collapse. However, if there is underlying cardiovascular disease, this rate would not be tolerated for even one hour. In such patients, the attack must be terminated immediately (F) to prevent the more serious complications of congestive failure, syncope or an anginal attack, with the possibility of more serious dysrhythmias.

(G) It is frequently very hard to differentiate atrial tachycardia with aberrant ventricular conduction from ventricular tachycardia. However, since the mechanism and treatment are different for these two conditions, it is imperative that the distinction be made, if at all possible. Whenever myocardial infarction is suspected or proved, all wide QRS premature beats must be assumed to be ventricular in origin and treated accordingly. Thus, a patient who has runs of 3 or more such beats, which by definition represents ventricular tachycardia, is treated as vigorously as possible with lidocaine and, if necessary, direct current synchronized cardioversion. If the situation seems less urgent, P waves should be searched for; if found, they usually mean a supraventricular origin of the dysrhythmia, regardless of QRS configuration. In the absence of identifiable P waves, the configuration of QRS may help identify the cause, ventricular aberrancy usually being manifested by a right bundle branch block pattern, and an initial QRS vector in the same direction as the normally conducted beats.

COURSE:

This patient was treated first with oxygen, 5 liters per minute, delivered by nasal prongs. When her dyspnea had been so relieved, the carotid sinus was massaged while the heart was monitored electrocardiographically. This massage produced prompt reversion to sinus rhythm at a rate of 110/minute (Fig. 21.2). Her vital signs remained normal throughout. After two

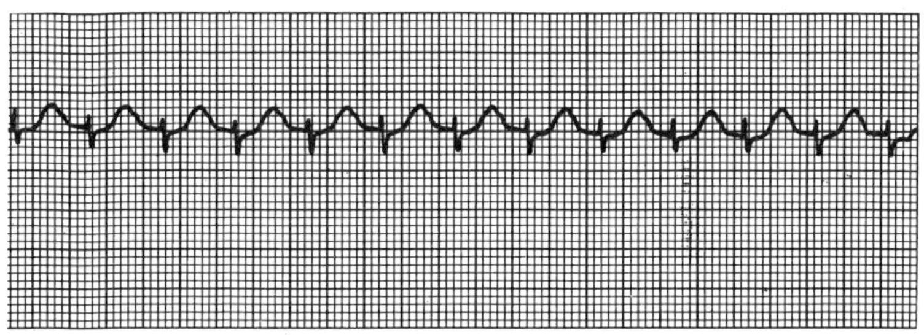

FIG. 21.2: Electrocardiogram showing reversion to normal sinus rhythm, following carotid sinus massage (arrow).

hours of observation, during which time she remained asymptomatic and had no further tachycardia, she was allowed to return home, with instructions to consult her private physician. No underlying cause for the attack was found.

3. (A, B, C, D, F) (A) Carotid sinus massage, or stimulation, is accomplished with the patient semi-erect and under constant electrocardiographic monitoring (or with continuous auscultation of the heart, if the procedure must be done when an electrocardiogram is unavailable). This monitoring will allow immediate discontinuation of the massage on reversion to a normal sinus rhythm. Firm, but gentle, pressure and massage are applied over one carotid sinus for 10 to 20 seconds and then, if necessary, over the other sinus, but never over both at the same time.

(B) Carotid sinus massage is very useful in differentiating the various tachyarrhythmias, especially in patients with regular ectopic tachycardia with wide QRS complexes. In these patients, it is imperative to determine whether ventricular tachycardia accounts for the wide QRS complexes seen on the ECG, or whether aberrant ventricular conduction is present. Any response to carotid sinus massage rules out ventricular tachycardia in most cases, since ventricular tachycardia does not respond to carotid sinus stimulation (F). The treatment for ventricular tachycardia is lidocaine by intravenous bolus, followed by intravenous infusion if the situation is not urgent. Cardioversion by electric shock should be tried if lidocaine fails to work, or if the patient is hypotensive or mentally obtunded.

(C) Carotid sinus stimulation is capable of terminating PAT in about half of the patients. If the patient does respond, he usually does so abruptly, as did this patient (see Fig. 21. 2).

(D) Ventricular fibrillation may result from carotid sinus stimulation if the patient has digitalis intoxication. Digitalis intoxication is the second most common cause of cardiac dysrhythmias, the most common being coronary heart disease. Since nonparoxysmal atrial tachycardia with atrioventricular block is a common manifestation of digitalis toxicity, carotid sinus stimulation should never be used when this condition is present. In the emergency setting, it is seldom possible to differentiate immediately between PAT, which should be treated with carotid sinus stimulation, and nonparoxysmal atrial tachycardia with atrioventricular block. Therefore, it is better not to massage the carotid sinus of any patient who is taking even a small amount of digitalis. Alternate methods of treatment should be sought. Some digitalized patients have died following carotid sinus massage, either from ventricular fibrillation or from ventricular standstill.

(E) Carotid sinus massage should not be used in sinus tachycardia, which may reach 160 beats/minute and should be readily diagnosed by ECG. It may, however, cause transient slowing of this tachyarrhythmia, the cause of which should be treated, such as infection or hyperthyroidism. PAT almost never slows transiently; it will show no response or revert completely. (G) Carotid sinus massage always slows the ventricular rate in atrial fibrillation or flutter, because it increases the atrioventricular block.

4. (E) All. (A) Carotid sinus massage is a vagal maneuver and is usually not the first maneuver tried, even though it was done almost immediately in this patient. Children can be asked to blow up a balloon, which they enjoy doing. This effects a Valsalva's maneuver and frequently terminates PAT. The mechanism is an increase in A-V conduction delay with blockage of the re-entry pattern. Pressure on the eyeballs is effective for the same reason, but is not advisable because of the risk of retinal detachment. Breath holding, coughing, lowering the head between the knees, and gagging with induced vomiting are other mechanical approaches that can be tried and are often successful. Patients who have frequent attacks are able to terminate most of them without direct medical help by learning how to apply one or more of these vagal stimulating maneuvers.

(B) Drug therapy is another means of directly or indirectly stimulating the vagus nerve. Edrophonium (given intravenously at 10 mg in adults) inhibits cholinesterase and prolongs atrioventricular conduction, terminating the dysrhythmia. If it fails to do so, carotid sinus massage is likely to be more effective following its use. The dose in children is 2 mg, or 0.2 ml of the 10 mg/ml solution available at present. A vasoconstrictor drug, such as phenylephrine or metaraminol, can be used to elevate the blood pressure in a normotensive patient and thereby produce a reflex vagal discharge. If the previously mentioned procedures fail, either alone or in various combinations, digoxin or propranolol may be necessary. They should be given with caution, being certain about the diagnosis and paying attention to possible contraindications, especially with the propranolol.

(C) Cardioversion, or (rarely) overdrive pacing (D), may be required to terminate the tachycardia in refractory patients or in those who are tolerating it poorly. Cardioversion should not be attempted in patients taking digitalis, except under the most unusual circumstances. If the dysrhythmia was caused by digitalis, then cardioversion could produce more serious dysrhythmias, such as ventricular tachycardia or fibrillation. At the very least, cardioversion is not likely to be effective in such patients; hence, alternative methods should be tried.

5. (True) PAT is very common in patients with ventricular preexcitation syndrome or the Wolff-Parkinson-White (WPW) syndrome. Also, WPW syndrome is a relatively common cause of the PAT seen and treated in emergency departments, even though the WPW syndrome, itself, is rare, appearing in 0.08% to 0.48% of children and in 0.01% to 0.31% of apparently healthy adults.[2] PAT constitutes 70% to 80% of all dysrhythmias in WPW syndrome. The remaining 20% to 30% are represented by atrial flutter-fibrillation. When the latter is present, the risk to the patient is much greater, in that the ventricular response may be 300 beats per minute, producing syncope or ventricular fibrillation. This is much more likely to occur if the patient has other forms of heart disease, as do 20% to 30% of adults with WPW syndrome.

6. (A, B, C, E) (A) The diagnosis should be suspected in any patient who has a history of palpitation or rapid heart beat or pulse, but the definitive test is the electrocardiogram. There is no characteristic physical finding. Since many previously unsuspected cases of WPW syndrome are detected each year in emergency departments, one should have a high index of suspicion and should order an electrocardiogram for most, or all, high-risk patients, as determined by the history.

(B) With WPW syndrome, the P-R interval is 0.12 seconds or less in adults, 0.10 seconds or less in children, and 0.08 seconds or less in infants. This phenomenon results from a circumvention of the A-V node by the impulse, which passes instead through an accessory pathway called the bundle of Kent. The P-R interval is shortened by the width of a delta wave (see C); the P-S interval remains within the normal range.

(C) The QRS complex is lengthened by the width of the delta wave, which is an initial slurring of the QRS deflection. The delta wave corresponds to the mass of the ventricular myocardium that is depolarized by the impulse which traversed the anomalous bundle. If only a small portion of the ventricular myocardium is activated in this manner, the initial slurring of the QRS complex may be difficult to recognize. Hence, it should always be searched for in all leads whenever a short P-R interval is present, especially in the patient with tachycardia.

(D) The delta wave is usually absent during episodes of PAT, which emphasizes the importance of obtaining a 12-lead ECG after the patient's tachycardia has reverted (or of having access to a previous ECG). On the other hand, the delta wave is visible quite often in patients with WPW syndrome who have atrial flutter-fibrillation, rather than PAT. With atrial flutter-fibrillation, the QRS complexes can easily be mistaken for ventricular tachycardia, and differentiation may depend on the telltale delta wave's being detected.

(E) At times, with WPW syndrome, conduction is only through the A-V node, with no evidence of conduction through the anomalous pathway. At these times, the P-R interval will be in the normal range, and the delta wave will be absent. If the diagnosis is strongly suspected, repeated efforts to find the characteristic changes should be made by repeating the ECG one or more times.

Ambulatory monitoring with the Holter unit is also being used to detect these changes and the supraventricular dysrhythmias, to which patients with WPW syndrome are prone, since many of these dysrhythmias are dangerous, yet asymptomatic.

REFERENCES

1. Tintinalli, J.E. and Fowler, M.: Wolff-Parkinson-White Syndrome. JACEP 6:111-116, 1977.

2. Tonkin, A.M., et al.: Tachyarrhythmias in Wolff-Parkinson-White Syndrome. JAMA 235:947-949, 1976.

::

CASE 22: CHEST PAIN RADIATING TO ARM AND BACK

HISTORY:

A 35-year-old woman reported to the emergency department because of chest pain of 24 hours' duration. The pain radiated into the right arm and down the back. Over the preceding weeks, she had experienced frontal headache and episodes of numbness and tingling of her right upper and lower extremities of several hours' duration. However, there was no weakness of the extremities. She had moderate blurring of her vision and scotomata. She had had nausea but no vomiting.

She had a history of a seizure disorder since age 16 years, hypertension, and repeated urinary tract infections. She had been taking phenytoin and phenobarbital as anticonvulsant therapy, and propranolol (10 mg four times daily) and methyldopa (250 mg four times daily) for treatment of her hypertension. She had taken her last dose of methyldopa six hours before she arrived at the emergency department.

Examination showed that she was alert and oriented, and moderately obese with blood pressure of 208/160 mm Hg. Her optic fundi showed early papilledema and scattered exudates with a few fresh hemorrhages. There was an S-4 cardiac gallop, but no evidence of congestive heart failure. Neurological examination revealed no abnormalities. The results of the remainder of the examination were normal.

LABORATORY DATA:

<u>Electrocardiogram</u>: negative, except for evidence of left ventricular hypertrophy with strain pattern.
<u>Chest roentgenogram</u>: normal, except for evidence of slight to moderate left ventricular enlargement.
<u>Arterial blood</u>:
pH: 7.53
PCO_2: 22 torr
PO_2: 114 torr
bicarbonate: 17.3 mEq/l

The results of her other laboratory tests were not remarkable.

QUESTIONS:

1. The best diagnosis in this patient is:
   A. Myocardial infarction
   B. Hypertensive crisis
   C. Hypertensive encephalopathy
   D. Acute dissecting aneurysm of the aorta
   E. Coarctation of the aorta
   F. Accelerated (malignant) hypertension

2. The proper <u>initial</u> treatment for this patient is which of the following?
   A. Hydralazine intramuscularly
   B. Sodium nitroprusside intravenously
   C. Diazoxide intravenously
   D. Furosemide intravenously
   E. Furosemide orally
   F. Thiazide diuretic orally
   G. Trimethaphan camsylate

ANSWERS AND COMMENTS:

1. (B, F) The first thought of any emergency department physician confronted with an adult patient with radiating chest pain, must be myocardial ischemia, with or without myocardial infarction. If this proves not to be present, he should think next of pulmonary causes and try to rule them in or out. One pulmonary cause that must always be considered is pulmonary embolism, since it signifies future trouble, even a sudden fatality. Chest wall (musculoskeletal) causes of chest pain, although frequent, must usually be diagnosed by exclusion.

Accelerated (malignant) hypertension, which is one form of hypertensive emergency or crisis (B), is the best diagnosis. Malignant hypertension is defined by the presence of marked diastolic hypertension, that is, diastolic pressure above 140 mm Hg.

The early stages of the malignant phase of hypertension may be asymptomatic, although severe headache, acute visual disturbances, as in this patient, and gross hematuria are the usual presenting symptoms. Papilledema, hemorrhage and exudates in the fundi are common and usually precede clinical evidence of renal impairment. Therefore, they should always be searched for, since their detection should lead to the earlier treatment that is essential if the patient is to be prevented from developing rapidly progressive cardiac and renal failure.

Malignant hypertension can complicate any type of hypertension, although it is rare in association with pheochromocytoma and primary hyperaldosteronism. Patients with malignant hypertension develop renal necrotizing arteriolitis and die of uremia within a year or two if they do not receive proper treatment. When malignant hypertension occurs in patients with chronic hypertension, it is usually due to chronic glomerulonephritis, chronic pyelonephritis, collagen vascular disease, or the sudden, rather than tapering, withdrawal of the antihypertensive agent clonidine.

Hypertensive crisis, or emergency, usually refers to a sudden rise in blood pressure to approximately 250/140 mm Hg or higher in a patient with either essential (benign) or accelerated (malignant) hypertension. However, it can occur in patients who were previously normotensive, in which case it suggests acute glomerulonephritis, pheochromocytoma, drug reaction to a monoamine oxidase (MAO) inhibitor, or, where relevant, toxemia of pregnancy.

Hypertensive encephalopathy refers to the acute neurological syndrome of severe headache and mental obtundation, ranging all the way to coma. The syndrome is usually seen in patients with acute glomerulonephritis. The primary underlying pathological condition is cerebral edema, either focal or generalized, as well as multiple small thrombi within the brain. There is usually nausea and vomiting. Seizures may occur and hemiparesis, usually transient, may be present. Rapid reduction of the blood pressure is necessary. In this patient, it is possible that the symptoms in her right extremities, suggestive of hypertensive encephalopathy, were caused by hyperventilation. However, transient cerebral ischemic attacks can cause similar symptoms.

There was no evidence of coarctation of the aorta and no acute dissecting aneurysm of the aorta, although the hypertension and the chest and back pain should certainly cause one to consider the latter possibility in this patient. Her pain was probably caused by myocardial ischemia or relative myocardial oxygen deficiency related to her extreme hypertension.

2. (B or C and D or E) Sodium nitroprusside or diazoxide administered intravenously, usually with furosemide given either orally or intravenously, would be appropriate in this patient. For a patient who has pulmonary edema in association with hypertensive crisis, the furosemide should be given intravenously, rather than orally.

In general, in the treatment of malignant hypertension, a combination of drugs is superior to a single drug of any type, provided the combination is carefully chosen. There is no single drug of choice. The goal is to lower the diastolic pressure to 100 mm Hg within a few minutes to one hour, the interval depending upon the severity of the hypertension, the drug, and the route of administration. Hydralazine intramuscularly (A) accomplishes this goal in many patients with less severe elevation of blood pressure, but it would not be appropriate for this patient.

Sodium nitroprusside was used in this patient, along with furosemide, 40 mg intravenously. The sodium nitroprusside was given by continuous infusion in sterile 5% dextrose in water, at a rate of 1 microgram/kg/min, slowly increased to 5 micrograms/kg/min. Her blood pressure decreased to 184/150 mm Hg in 20 minutes and to 150/110 mm Hg over the next two hours.

The usual starting dose of nitroprusside is 3 micrograms/kg/min, with the dose adjusted to achieve control of blood pressure up to a maximum of 10 micrograms/kg/min. The fine adjustment possible is one distinct advantage of this drug over diazoxide. Careful monitoring of the blood pressure is required during this therapy.

The mechanism of action of nitroprusside is a decrease in peripheral resistance by a direct action on the blood vessels that is independent of anatomical innervation. The action is probably dilatation of the arterioles. Patients who are receiving antihypertensive medications are more sensitive to sodium nitroprusside; these are the ones for whom the lowest dosage is usually satisfactory. If sodium nitroprusside control of hypertension must be maintained for more than a few hours, the level of thiocyanate in the blood should be monitored. The package insert for sodium nitroprusside should be consulted for signs of acute overdosage, the chief manifestation being profound hypotension, as well as for proper treatment of overdosage.

Because of its favorable hemodynamic effect on left ventricular function, sodium nitroprusside is the drug of choice in the patient whose hypertensive crisis is associated with acute left ventricular failure and pulmonary edema.

Diazoxide also decreases peripheral resistance by direct vasodilatation of peripheral arterioles. It is best used by rapid (10-second) intravenous injection of 5 mg/kg up to a maximum dose of 300 mg. The rapid injection is believed necessary, because the drug is quickly bound to albumin. While there have been recent reports of satisfactory reductions in blood pressure with less rapid injection, it would seem better, with our present experience, to continue using the rapid intravenous method.

Side effects of diazoxide therapy are nausea, vomiting and abdominal pain, headache, and palpitation with supraventricular tachycardia. Concomitant diuretic therapy is always indicated, because diazoxide causes sodium retention. In diabetics, supplemental insulin may be required, because diazoxide causes hyperglycemia.

Diazoxide is the drug of choice in hypertensive encephalopathy in association with malignant hypertension. It is also a more convenient drug to use, since close monitoring is less of a problem than with sodium nitroprusside. The hypotensive effect of diazoxide is seen within one to three minutes and lasts from two to twelve hours. Since angina can be precipitated by a rapid drop in blood pressure, diazoxide should be given with caution in a patient with known coronary artery disease. In some instances, an angina-like syndrome has developed with diazoxide therapy in patients with no previous myocardial ischemia.

A thiazide diuretic, given orally, would not be satisfactory treatment for this patient's problem. A more rapidly acting loop diuretic, such as furosemide or ethacrynic acid, is required.

Trimethaphan camsylate has been largely replaced by sodium nitroprusside or diazoxide for the treatment of all hypertensive emergencies, except acute aortic dissection. For the latter, it is preferred over the other two drugs, because its use is associated with decreased cardiac output.

Although parenteral administration of any antihypertensive drug is preferred in the initial treatment of hypertensive emergencies, orally administered antihypertensive drugs should be substituted as soon as possible, beginning, in the case of sodium nitroprusside, before the parenteral drug therapy is stopped, and, in the case of diazoxide, as soon as possible. All patients receiving such drugs should be hospitalized.

COURSE:

This patient was admitted to the hospital after three hours in the emergency department. The same dose of methyldopa was given, but her propranolol dosage was increased to 20 mg four times daily. Her blood pressure was brought under satisfactory control. On the seventh day, she signed out, against medical advice, because of a crisis in her family. Follow-up in the clinic was arranged for one week. Further investigation and treatment of her repeated urinary tract infections were indicated. She was strongly advised to follow a low-salt diet.

::

CASE 23: NEAR-DROWNING

HISTORY:

A 40-year-old man was taken to a hospital after "nearly drowning" in a boating accident on a fresh-water lake. It was not known how the accident occurred or what resuscitative measures were necessary on the scene. The patient was a good swimmer but was known to have been drinking alcoholic beverages before the accident. Just after his arrival at the hospital, he developed ventricular fibrillation and cardiac arrest. He was promptly resuscitated and transferred to our emergency department after vital signs had stabilized. En route, oxygen, 5 liters per minute, was delivered by nasal prongs. There was no history of intrinsic heart disease or diabetes mellitus. He had smoked three packs of cigarettes per day for 15 years and had suffered pneumothorax, due to a ruptured subpleural bleb, two years earlier; the pneumothorax had responded to chest tube drainage.

Examination revealed an alert, asthenic man with the habitus of chronic obstructive pulmonary disease (COPD). He was in mild respiratory distress, using his accessory respiratory musculature, but showed no tracheal tug. Blood pressure was 110/80 mm Hg; respirations, 28 per minute; temperature, 98°F (36.5°C); pulse, 100 per minute and regular. There were a few basal rales, with rhonchi scattered throughout both lung fields. No other abnormalities were noted. There was no evidence, by history or physical examination, of head injury. Electrocardiography revealed no dysrhythmias and no acute changes indicating acute cardiac disease.

LABORATORY DATA:

Urinalysis: within normal limits
Hematocrit: 42.8%
Hemoglobin: 14 gm/dl
White blood cell count: 15,000/mm^3
Serum sodium: 146 mEq/l
Serum chloride: 100 mEq/l
Serum potassium: 4.4 mEq/l
Serum bicarbonate: 29 mEq/l
Blood urea nitrogen (BUN): 13 mg/dl
Blood glucose: 111 mg/dl
Arterial blood:
  pH: 7.42

PO_2: 68 torr
PCO_2: 44 torr

Blood alcohol level: not measured

X-rays: Chest x-rays showed no abnormalities except the changes of COPD, which were also present on x-rays taken previously.

DISPOSITION:

The clinical impressions were (1) near-drowning with subsequent cardiac arrest, post-resuscitation; (2) COPD, emphysematous; and (3) acute alcoholism. He was admitted to a respiratory intensive care unit, where he showed gradual improvement with no dysrhythmias or other complications. He was discharged four days later.

QUESTIONS:

1. TRUE OR FALSE: The term drowning is applied to death from acute asphyxia while submerged in a liquid; near-drowning is used to refer to patients who survive (at least temporarily) asphyxia from submersion.

2. Which of the following factors about this patient are typical of drowning and near-drowning victims in the United States?
   A. Age
   B. Sex
   C. His accident occurred in the summer.
   D. The accident involved a boat on a fresh-water lake.
   E. He had been drinking alcoholic beverages.
   F. Cardiac arrest was due to ventricular fibrillation.
   G. He was a good swimmer.
   H. All of the above

3. TRUE OR FALSE: Hyperventilating before swimming underwater delays the need to come up for air.

4. From the standpoint of pathophysiology, which of the following terms characterize near-drowning?
   A. Asphyxia with hypoxemia
   B. Metabolic and respiratory acidosis
   C. Marked electrolyte abnormalities
   D. Pulmonary edema
   E. Hemolysis
   F. All of the above

5. Unless it is clear that the victim has been submerged for

hours, it is rarely possible to determine at the scene whether his life can be saved. Whenever there is the slightest chance, resuscitation should be attempted. Which of the following should be carried out immediately at the scene of a drowning accident?

A. Remove the victim from the water as soon as possible.
B. Determine if aspiration has occurred.
C. Place victim face down and lift his midsection to remove water from the lungs.
D. Empty the stomach of fluid.
E. Open the airway.
F. Begin mouth-to-mouth ventilation.
G. Check for carotid or femoral pulse.
H. If pulse is absent, start external cardiac compression.
I. All of the above

6. TRUE OR FALSE: After a near-drowning victim is removed from the water and begins breathing again, he may be released to normal activity without further medical observation and treatment.

7. In the emergency facility, which of the following procedures should be carried out immediately and simultaneously in an adult who is receiving only the resuscitative measures outlined in question 5?
   A. Maintain the airway, clearing it further if necessary.
   B. Insert a cuffed endotracheal tube.
   C. Continue ventilation and oxygenation.
   D. Continue cardiac compression if there is no palpable carotid or femoral pulse.
   E. Start intravenous infusions.
   F. Obtain arterial blood for pH and gases.
   G. Administer sodium bicarbonate.
   H. Administer epinephrine.
   I. Connect electrocardiographic electrodes, or use combination electrode-defibrillator paddles, to identify cause of the cardiac arrest and treat accordingly.
   J. All of the above

8. In addition to the initial procedures, which of the following should be done, assuming that the patient has shown no significant improvement?
   A. Insert a central venous pressure line (CVP).
   B. Insert an indwelling urethral catheter.
   C. Insert a nasogastric tube and empty the stomach.
   D. Administer lidocaine.
   E. Obtain a chest x-ray.

F. Obtain other baseline routine admission values, including serum electrolytes, urinalysis and complete blood count.
G. Begin positive end-expiratory pressure ventilation (PEEP).
H. All of the above

ANSWERS AND COMMENTS:

1. (True) The asphyxiation in the early stages is due to reflex laryngospasm, then usually to flooding of the lungs with water; although, in an estimated 10 to 20% of drowning and near-drowning victims, there is no significant or detectable liquid in the lungs. In near-drowning, by definition, the initial resuscitation is successful, but there is no assurance of ultimate survival, since complications, early or delayed, are not uncommon.

2. (B, C, D, E, G) (A) Most drowning or near-drowning victims are younger than this patient. In one series, one out of seven (14%) victims were under five years of age. Overall, in the United States, three-fifths of male, and two-thirds of female, drowning victims are under 20 years of age.[1] In a water-oriented state, such as Florida, 32% of all pediatric (under 13 years of age) accidental deaths in one series were from drowning.[2]

(B) Most victims are male, 85% in some series.

(C) In the United States, well over half of drowning and near-drowning accidents occur in June, July and August.

(D) Most such accidents occur in fresh water, and many of them are associated with recreational boating activities.

(E) Alcohol is a significant factor in 23 to 47% of drowning and near-drowning accidents involving adults. The observation has been made that when a person's blood alcohol concentration is above 0.20%, he is very likely to make no effort to save himself, even if he is a good swimmer. While he may be suicidal under the influence of alcohol, his problem is more apt to be a failure to recognize his danger. The risk of combining alcohol consumption with swimming or boating is compounded when both alcohol and drugs of abuse, in particular hallucinogenic drugs, are consumed or used.

(F) Ventricular fibrillation as the cause of cardiac arrest in near-drowning is unusual. The arrest is usually due to progressive hypoxemia, leading to severe bradycardia and asystole. However, after the patient is removed from the water, cardiac arrest from any cause may occur.

(G) In some series, as many as 35% of victims of drowning or near-drowning were able to swim, and many were considered excellent swimmers.

3. (True) Hyperventilating before swimming underwater, in order to remain under longer, is a very dangerous procedure, but it is still taught by many swimming coaches. It is dangerous because it causes a "wash-out" of carbon dioxide from the lungs, blood and other body stores, thereby delaying the urge to surface and breathe, even though the physical activity of swimming underwater is causing the arterial oxygen tension (PaO_2) to drop rapidly. Unconsciousness occurs with little or no warning and results in reflex breathing, so that the victim aspirates liquid. Even if he is rescued promptly, the low arterial oxygen tension makes resuscitation much more difficult and uncertain, particularly since high concentrations of oxygen are not usually immediately available when the victim is pulled from the water.

4. (A, B, D) (A) The single most important consequence of the asphyxia that characterizes near-drowning is hypoxia, caused by shunting of blood through perfused, but nonventilated, alveoli.[3] The underlying mechanism for this nonventilation after aspiration of fresh water is an alteration of the normal surface tension properties of pulmonary surfactant, with alveolar collapse. The fresh water moves quickly into the blood stream, but the damage is already done by the water. Aspirated sea water remains in the alveoli longer and prevents ventilation. In addition, in both instances, compliance decreases and airway resistance increases, both factors that contribute further to the hypoxia. In the absence of aspiration - and some 10 to 20% of victims are thought not to have aspirated - asphyxiation is possible from reflex laryngospasm or voluntary breath-holding to unconsciousness. (B) Metabolic acidosis is almost invariably present, and respiratory acidosis is usually present, although frequently mild. The metabolic acidosis is caused by an increase in pyruvic and lactic acids, due to anaerobic metabolism. Next to hypoxemia, metabolic acidosis is the most serious aspect of near-drowning and requires rapid and vigorous treatment. (C) Electrolyte abnormalities are <u>not</u> likely to be significant in near-drowning. Their magnitude depends upon the tonicity and the volume of water aspirated.[3] Approximately 85% of drowning and near-drowning victims aspirate less than 22 ml/kg of water, and this quantity of aspirated fluid does not, in itself, produce life-threatening changes in serum

electrolyte concentrations.

(D) If sea water is aspirated during near-drowning, pulmonary edema is the result. The mechanism is the osmotic pressure that draws fluid from the plasma into the alveoli. The extent of this process can cause hypovolemia, so it is very important to differentiate this cause of pulmonary edema from that due to circulatory overload, since the treatment is radically different. This differentiation can usually be made with the help of central venous pressure (CVP) monitoring, although monitoring of pulmonary capillary wedge pressure is also necessary in the more seriously ill patients.

(E) Hemolysis is not a serious problem, unless aspiration of large amounts of fresh water has occurred. Since the hemoglobin concentration determines primarily the oxygen-carrying capacity of the blood, and victims of near-drowning tend to have difficulty with oxygenation, serial hemoglobin and hematocrit determinations are mandatory. If hemoglobin falls significantly, then transfusion of whole blood or packed cells must be considered.

5. (A, E, F, G, H, followed by D) On-the-scene care may determine whether the victim lives or dies. Ideally, the best medical care available anywhere should be administered at the scene. This includes the care, described later, that is available in the best hospital emergency departments and intensive care units, care that is today being taken more and more often to the patient, rather than being provided only after the patient arrives at such a facility. This provision of earlier care will undoubtedly save many more lives in the future than are presently being saved, but will often not be possible. Thus, care rendered by less well-trained persons, under less than ideal circumstances, will remain all too common. For the patient who was submerged only a few minutes, this may be adequate, as he may begin breathing spontaneously as soon as he is removed from the water. However, such a quick recovery cannot be counted upon, and the rescuer(s) should be prepared to follow a protocol for on-the-scene resuscitation and then deliver the patient as soon as possible after stabilization (if stabilization is possible) to the nearest emergency department capable of handling the patient's problem.

(A) It cannot be stressed too strongly that immediate removal from the water is necessary as soon as it is obvious that the victim is unable to surface under his own power. Parts (E, F, G) of the resuscitation effort may be started before the patient is delivered to shore or to a platform or boat, but it is impractical to attempt cardiac compression (H) until the victim is supine and his thorax supported.

There is no dependable way to determine at the scene whether aspiration of fluid into the lungs (B) has occurred, and there is no point in trying to determine it. If it has not occurred, and does not occur during the resuscitation effort, the patient is likely to recover promptly with the care outlined later. Thus, the important point is to prevent any or further aspiration. If fresh water has been aspirated, it will dissipate fairly quickly. If sea water or gastric contents are aspirated, there is no good way to remove them. Lifting the prone victim by the midsection (C), called "breaking" the patient, is usually ineffective and uses up valuable time.

The airway should be opened immediately (E) if the victim is found to be unresponsive when he is placed supine. Even if no debris or other foreign material is present in the hypopharynx, the tongue will obstruct the airway of an unconscious patient in this position. If there is no suspicion of neck injury, as from a diving accident, the head should be hyperextended. Otherwise, the tongue can be brought forward by the modified jaw thrust, that is, by bringing the angles of the mandible forward with both of the rescuer's hands, keeping the neck in the neutral position. If the victim does not begin breathing immediately after this maneuver, mouth-to-mouth ventilation (F) should be started with four quick, full breaths, and be continued with one ventilation every five seconds in an adult and every three seconds in a child. The breaths should be shallower for a child than for an adult. Following the initial four breaths, the carotid pulse should be checked carefully (G); a few seconds may be necessary to be certain whether it is present or absent. If absent, external cardiac compression (H) should be started immediately, with the heel of the hand over the lower third of the sternum. For a single rescuer, the rate should be 80 compressions per minute in an adult, alternated with two quick, full breaths by mouth-to-mouth technique after every 15 compressions. As soon as a second rescuer is available, the cardiac compression rate can be reduced to 60 per minute and a single ventilation interposed after each five compressions, without a break in the rhythm. For a child, the compression should be done high enough on the sterum (middle third) to avoid damage to the liver and spleen, and the rate should be 80 to 100 per minute, with a single breath interposed after every five compressions.

During near-drowning, relatively large quantities of water enter the stomach, and this should be removed (D) as soon as practicable and safe, that is, as soon as the victim's heart is beating and he is breathing spontaneously. Otherwise, this fluid (and other gastric contents, as well) may well up or be vomited into the hypopharynx, enter the lungs of the unconscious victim, and "drown" him a second time, even while he seems to be recovering satisfactorily. It may also complicate cardiopulmonary resuscitation, because ventilation will be difficult. The safest way to remove such fluid is to turn the victim's head to one side and lower the upper part of his body (or raise the lower part of the body) while pressing gently on the epigastrium. If a cuffed endotracheal tube has been inserted (see answer 7), the fluid can be removed even more safely in this manner, since it cannot then enter the trachea. If an esophageal obturator airway has been inserted, the fluid in the stomach can be prevented from coming up and entering the trachea by inflating the esophageal balloon to 30 or 35 ml of air, with the balloon located just below the level of the bifurcation of the trachea.

6. (False) He may not have aspirated any water (although this cannot usually be determined immediately), but he may have severe hypoxemia for a short time. This was undoubtedly the situation with the patient described in this case. It usually doesn't persist for hours or days, but its diagnosis (and that of acidosis) cannot be made on the basis of the patient's appearance or by any on-the-scene clinical examination. Any victim of near-drowning should be kept under close observation and taken immediately to an emergency medical facility for further care. At the very least, he should be given supplemental oxygen by whatever means available, and in the highest concentration possible, until arterial blood gases and pH show that it is no longer needed. In fact, it is accepted practice that all such patients should be admitted to a hospital for at least 24 hours so that such serial studies and continuous monitoring of vital signs can be carried out. One study has shown that 13% of near-drowning victims who were resuscitated and who survived the initial 24 hours died thereafter.

7. (J) All. Resuscitation is a team effort, requiring at least four or five persons right from the beginning. Each must know ahead of time what his or her responsibilities are. (A) The airway may have been only partially cleared at the beginning of cardiopulmonary resuscitation (CPR) at the scene, or it may have become partially obstructed later by mucus secretion or accumulation, or by gastric contents. It should now be cleared with the fingers and with suction, if required.

(B, C) It is absolutely essential to administer high concentrations (100%) if possible) of oxygen without waiting for blood gas reports or any other test results. Even in a near-drowning victim without cardiac arrest, the PaO_2 is likely to be extremely low. Delayed deaths are usually due to this marked hypoxemia. The marked metabolic acidosis that is usually present can largely be alleviated by the better oxygenation, and by the immediate administration of sodium bicarbonate intravenously (see answer G), and the respiratory acidosis alleviated by the improved ventilation. A cuffed endotracheal tube is vital for adequate resuscitation in almost all patients (1) to maintain the airway and (2) to administer oxygen in high concentration by intermittent positive pressure ventilation. The tube must be inserted as expeditiously as possible, since ventilation and cardiac compression should not be discontinued for more than 15 to 20 seconds. A common error is to stop all basic resuscitation procedures as soon as the patient arrives, while someone attempts to insert an endotracheal tube. The procedure done under these circumstances may require 30 to 60 seconds, which is too long, especially if supplemental oxygenation with a bag-valve-mask unit is not carried out first.

(D) In near-drowning with cardiopulmonary arrest, basic CPR is truly only a "holding operation" until advanced life support measures can be applied. In advanced CPR, the cardiac compression is exactly the same as with basic CPR, and it must be done as nearly perfect as possible, and without interruption for more than five seconds for any reason other than insertion of an endotracheal tube. If a central pulse returns, the compressions can be discontinued until the spontaneous heart beat and electrocardiogram can be assessed. However, if the pulse disappears again, the cardiac compressions must be resumed immediately.

(E) The type of intravenous fluid administered is not critical, both Ringer's lactate and 5% dextrose in water being satisfactory. Two separate lines are highly desirable, since one can serve as the CVP monitoring catheter if other veins cannot be cannulated promptly for this purpose.

(F) One of the team members should obtain arterial blood as soon as possible after the patient's arrival, and again as needed, until resuscitation and stabilization are complete. Hospitals that do not yet have the facilities to analyze arterial pH, PCO_2 and PO_2 around the clock are at a serious disadvantage in managing patients with near-drowning.

(G) Sodium bicarbonate, one ampule (44.6 or 50 mEq) given

intravenously immediately, is essential to start correction of the marked metabolic acidosis that is likely to be present. If cardiac arrest has been prolonged, a second ampule given immediately after the first is wise. Thereafter, as a rough guide and as a minimum, one ampule of sodium bicarbonate can be administered for every 5 mEq/l of base deficit present, as indicated by the pH and PCO_2 of arterial blood.

(H) Epinephrine, 5 ml of 1:10, 000 solution intravenously, is vital for the patient with any type of cardiac arrest. If an intravenous route is unavailable, the same dose may be given into a cardiac chamber, or 1 to 2 mg in 10 ml of sterile distilled water may be given directly into the tracheobronchial tree through the endotracheal tube. Epinephrine restores electrical activity in asystole and enhances defibrillation in ventricular fibrillation. It also increases myocardial contractility and may restore myocardial contractility in electromechanical dissociation (the presence of electrocardiographic complexes without effective pulse). The dose must be repeated frequently, even as often as every 5 minutes. Failure to do this is undoubtedly responsible for failure to resuscitate many patients with cardiac arrest from diverse causes.

(I) Many of the newer portable cardiac monitoring units have combination monitor-defibrillator paddles that can be applied to the chest over saline-soaked sponges as soon as the patient arrives. The electrical status of the heart can be read on the oscilloscope immediately, usually minutes before regular electrodes could be applied. If ventricular fibrillation is found, as in this patient, defibrillation can be carried out without a moment's delay. If this initial defibrillation is unsuccessful, one should quickly improve the patient's oxygenation, at least partially correct the metabolic acidosis with sodium bicarbonate, and then repeat the countershock, the power being set at 400 joules (watt-seconds) for an adult.

8. (H) All. (A) As indicated earlier, a series of CVP readings is very valuable in near-drowning from both fresh and sea water for differential diagnosis of pulmonary edema (see answer 4D). The CVP line also serves as a drug access or hyperalimentation route in the event that peripheral veins are not available for cannulation.

(B) Urinary output must be monitored carefully and can be done adequately in a seriously ill patient only by means of an indwelling catheter.

(C) A distended stomach is hazardous even after control of the airway is obtained. It compromises ventilation and circulation, and it may possibly be ruptured by the external cardiac compression. A nasogastric tube should be passed at the earliest opportunity and the stomach emptied. Continuous, low negative pressure should be maintained on the tube thereafter, to keep the stomach empty.

(D) Administering lidocaine by bolus, 1 mg/kg intravenously, followed by 1 to 3 mg per minute intravenously, is excellent practice if defibrillation has been done. Lidocaine depresses myocardial irritability and helps control premature ventricular beats and episodes of ventricular tachycardia, both of which, in this setting, tend to degenerate into ventricular fibrillation.[4]

(E) A chest x-ray, obtained with portable equipment, is needed to ascertain the position of the CVP catheter, as well as to provide a baseline for serial x-rays. There is poor correlation between the degree of hypoxia and the appearance of the initial chest x-ray, in that the x-ray may show no abnormality in the presence of a very low PaO_2. This first x-ray is also useful in ruling out pneumothorax due to fractured ribs sustained at the time of the original injury, or as a complication of cardiac compression.

(F) As indicated earlier, electrolytes are not likely to be abnormal. An exception is serum potassium, which may be elevated due to severe hypoxemia and acidosis, as well as to hemolysis of red blood cells, which occurs after aspiration of a significant amount of fresh water.

(G) PEEP is vital in the nonresponding (or poorly responding) patient, to prevent or reduce pulmonary edema and to relieve intrapulmonary shunting due to atelectasis. The PaO_2 should be kept between 60 and 90 torr if possible. Oxygen toxicity is not a serious risk, unless the inspired oxygen concentration must remain near 100% for 24 hours or longer. A patient who is severely ill following near-drowning cannot be managed adequately without serial measurements of arterial blood gases and pH. If such measurements are not available, the patient should be transferred to a hospital that can provide them.

Even the near-drowning patient who has no cardiac arrest should be admitted to an intensive care unit. Aspiration or "immersion" pneumonitis can best be treated there, if and when it develops. It is one of the life-threatening delayed complications of near-drowning. Bronchoscopy may be indicated in order to remove particles of food from the tracheobronchial tree. Tracheal cultures should be done. A Swan-Ganz catheter should be inserted in the sicker patients for monitoring pulmonary capillary wedge pressure, cardiac output, and function of the right and left sides of the heart.

REFERENCES

1. Statistical Bulletin, Metropolitan Life Insurance Company. Accidental drowning. June, 1972.

2. Rowe, M.I., et al.: Profile of pediatric drowning victims in a water-oriented society. J. Trauma 17:587-591, 1977.

3. Modell, J.H.: The Pathophysiology and Treatment of Drowning and Near-Drowning. Springfield: Charles C Thomas, 1971.

4. Standards for cardiopulmonary resuscitation (CPR) and emergency cardiac care (ECC). JAMA 227 (Suppl.): 833-868, 1974.

::

CASE 24: MULTIPLE TRAUMA

HISTORY:

A 20-year-old man was involved in an automobile accident and transferred by ground ambulance from another hospital 80 miles away.

Before he was transferred, the following procedures were done: oxygen administration established via nasal prongs at six liters per minute; thoracentesis in the left second intercostal space in the midclavicular line, which yielded air and blood; insertion of an intercostal tube, #20 French, at that position connected to underwater seal suction; sand-bag immobilization of the head and neck; continuous intravenous infusion of lactated Ringer's solution; chest wrapping with a six-inch elastic bandage over a gauze roll placed in the left anterolateral position; and intra-urethral insertion of a Foley catheter into the bladder.

EXAMINATION:

The patient was awake and oriented but could not remember details of the accident. His past health had been excellent. He had no known allergies. His blood pressure was 130/90 mm Hg; pulse, 120 beats/minute; respirations, 18/minute. His skin was warm with no cyanosis. There were multiple abrasions over his face, left side of his chest, abdomen and both knees; there were small lacerations of the lower lip and chin and a laceration of the left side of the forehead. Several teeth were broken. The right side of the neck was tender. A flail chest was noted on the left anterolaterally. His abdomen was moderately distended and rigid; bowel sounds were normal. Neurologic examination showed no abnormalities.

LABORATORY DATA:

<u>Hemoglobin:</u> 13.6 gm/dl
<u>Hematocrit:</u> 40.3%
<u>White blood cell count:</u> 37,300 with 55% segmented neutrophils and 28% bands
<u>Urinalysis:</u> 8 to 10 white blood cells and one red blood cell per high-powered field, centrifuged specimen
<u>Serum electrolytes:</u> normal
<u>Blood glucose:</u> normal
<u>Serum lactic dehydrogenase:</u> 900 I.U. (normal range: 60 to

220 I. U.)

Serum glutamic oxaloacetic transaminase: 275 I. U. (normal range: 0 to 40 I. U.)

Serum amylase: 200 Somogyi units (normal range: 50 to 150 Somogyi units)

Arterial blood gas analysis:

pH: 7.31

PO_2: 60 torr

PCO_2: 38 torr

Blood was sent for typing and cross-matching of eight units.

X-rays: An initial cross-table lateral film of the cervical spine, as well as the remainder of the cervical spine series done later, revealed no abnormality. An A-P portable chest film, with the patient semi-erect, showed left hemopneumothorax with multiple rib fractures on the left side. There was no apparent widening of the mediastinum. Abdominal flat films and lateral decubitus films revealed no definite abnormality. No broken or whole teeth were noted in the thorax or abdomen.

Subsequent films of the skull, facial bones, mandible and thoracolumbar spine showed no abnormalities.

OTHER STUDIES: electrocardiogram was normal; abdominal tap yielded gross blood.

QUESTIONS:

1. TRUE OR FALSE: The patient's condition should have been stabilized at the scene of the accident or in the first hospital, no matter how long that required.

2. The first step taken by the emergency department team should be:
   A. Do complete physical examination, with the patient completely disrobed.
   B. Start group O Rh negative whole blood intravenously.
   C. Check the airway to be sure it is open and assist ventilation, if necessary.
   D. Establish a tracheostomy.

TRUE OR FALSE (Questions 3-5):

3. One of the dextran solutions is a good preparation to use in such a patient until blood can be typed and cross-matched.

4. One of the most effective ways of determining adequacy of fluid replacement is to measure the urinary output every 30 to 60 minutes.

5. All needed x-rays could have been taken before definitive therapy for this patient, since his condition was fairly stable.

6. Since partial rupture of the thoracic aorta is such a lethal injury, it must be suspected in all patients with injuries such as this patient had. The following are indications for aortography for definitive diagnosis, <u>except</u>:
   A. Widened superior mediastinum
   B. Fracture of the thoracic spine
   C. Multiple rib fractures with crushed chest
   D. First rib fracture
   E. Posteriorly displaced clavicular fracture
   F. Peripheral pulse deficit
   G. Fractured sternum
   H. Unexplained hypotension

7. Additional important diagnostic or therapeutic maneuvers include the following, <u>except</u>:
   A. Cuffed endotracheal intubation, with assisted ventilation for better oxygenation and for "internal stabilization" of the flail chest
   B. Insertion of a second and larger inter-rib thoracostomy tube and addition of underwater seal suction to both tubes
   C. Insertion of a nasogastric tube
   D. Insertion of a catheter for central venous pressure determination and rapid administration of fluids and blood, if necessary
   E. Tetanus toxoid, 0.5 ml given subcutaneously as a booster
   F. Administration of vasopressors to prevent sudden drop in blood pressure
   G. Elevation of lower extremities 15 degrees, without lowering the head
   H. Electrocardiographic monitoring
   I. Serial arterial blood gas determinations

TRUE OR FALSE (Questions 8 and 9):

8. The small anterior chest tube is adequate to prevent tension pneumothorax, but is not likely to remove air and blood from the left pleural cavity in this trauma victim.

9. Myocardial contusion was no threat to this patient, since he was so young.

10. Flail chest can usually be diagnosed early by all of the following, <u>except</u>:
    A. A high index of suspicion in any victim with chest trauma
    B. History of automobile accident and the presence of multiple injuries
    C. The presence of shock if untreated
    D. Multiple rib fractures, at least some of these in more than one place
    E. The presence of arterial oxygen desaturation
    F. The invariable presence of paradoxical motion on admission to the emergency department

11. TRUE OR FALSE: External stabilization of flail chest (in the form of sandbags or towel clips) has little or no place in present-day treatment, except as a temporary measure.

ANSWERS AND COMMENTS:

1. (False) This case illustrates very well the importance of quickly getting a multiple-injury patient to the nearest medical facility that can provide definitive diagnosis and treatment, including whatever emergency operation may be required. Resuscitation often cannot be accomplished without such an operation. Although intrathoracic, especially pulmonary, hemorrhage can often be controlled without open operation, the reverse is true of intra-abdominal hemorrhage. Undue delay, even for cross-matching in order to administer whole blood, can lead to exsanguination or other fatal complications. For a patient such as this one, the airway and ventilation should be secured; the neck and head should be immobilized; any obvious external bleeding should be controlled (usually by direct pressure); fractures should be splinted; and an intravenous line should be opened and either saline or lactated Ringer's solution started. Then he should be transported to the major care facility by the most expeditious, yet safest, means possible.

2. (C) It is always advisable to check the airway first in a patient with multiple trauma, especially in one having undergone such a long ambulance trip. Mucus secretions, blood and parts of teeth could be lodged in the hypopharynx, producing partial obstruction with the threat of complete obstruction at any time.

A cuffed endotracheal airway and assisted ventilation are advisable in a patient with this degree of chest injury.

Complete examination (A) should be done as soon as possible, but the initial assessment must be brief, with therapeutic procedures being carried out simultaneously, either by the team captain or by other members of the team.

There is seldom justification for starting group O Rh negative blood (B) without typing and cross-matching. The only exception is the patient who has lost a large amount of blood and is already in shock. Even in that situation, the blood should usually be typed (three to five minutes), or an "emergency crossmatch" should be done (30 minutes). As soon as blood can be typed and cross-matched, it should be administered, since shock in a trauma patient is almost always due to blood loss.

Tracheostomy (D) is sometimes required for crushing chest injury, but is used less often now than it was in the past. Initially, the patient can be frequently managed by orotracheal or nasotracheal intubation, but is probably best protected with a cuffed endotracheal tube.

3. (False) With dextran solutions, there is a risk of hypersensitivity reactions and of inducing defects in blood clotting, as well as a risk of interfering with subsequent cross-matching of blood.[4] While blood is being typed and cross-matched, the fluid resuscitation can be increased with lactated Ringer's solution or 0.9% sodium chloride solution ("normal saline"), which may be given rapidly in an amount two to three times as large as the estimated loss.

4. (True) If the hourly amount of urine is 35 to 50 ml, this is a good indication that the kidneys are being perfused well. However, in many seriously injured patients, additional information must be obtained. Steps to be taken include careful checking of the vital signs; repeated examination of the patient as a whole; monitoring of further blood loss, such as from the chest tube; if indicated, repeated peritoneal tap, and lavage if the first one was negative; and exploratory laparotomy, if required. Central venous pressure determination is also a good guide to adequate fluid replacement in most patients with multiple trauma.

5. (False) It is incorrect to send such a patient to the x-ray department and leave him there for several hours to complete

a series of x-rays even with adequate intravenous fluids running. The essential x-rays should be obtained immediately in the emergency department, and the patient taken straight to the operating room if exploratory thoracotomy or celiotomy is necessary. Additional x-rays can be obtained intraoperatively or postoperatively.

It is advisable to immediately obtain a portable cross-table lateral view of the cervical spine, showing all seven vertebrae. Fracture or dislocation of the cervical spine must be detected and treated, or ruled out, before the patient can be moved during subsequent diagnostic, monitoring and therapeutic maneuvers. The other essential x-ray that should be obtained immediately with portable equipment is a chest film, with the patient erect or semi-erect, if possible. This will reveal hemothorax, pneumothorax, or hemopneumothorax and may confirm the presence of multiple rib fractures or draw attention to a flail chest.

Usually, it is advisable to have a flat plate and upright or lateral decubitus film of the abdomen before an abdominal tap is done. In this patient, the tap was done before the abdominal film could be developed, since intra-abdominal bleeding was suspected and immediate confirmation was sought (see Case 25 for definitive management of abdominal trauma).

As can be seen, one of the problems with multiple trauma patients is determining priorities, for both diagnostic studies and therapeutic maneuvers. Davis and associates[1] analyzed a series of 1000 consecutively seen patients with blunt abdominal trauma, many of whom had extra-abdominal injuries as well. They suggested that diagnostic procedures should be limited to those that have proved to be the most productive, and that laparotomy should not be delayed unduly in the patient whose condition is unstable. The abdominal tap may be omitted if the suspicion of intraperitoneal bleeding is high, but, if hematuria is found, an intravenous pyelogram, at the least, should be done before laparotomy.

6. (B) All of the others are relative or absolute indications for aortography.[2] This patient did not have aortography, because of the previously mentioned criteria and because he had only multiple rib fractures and was not in shock. Before exploration of the chest, unless it is necessary on other grounds and is quite urgent, aortography is always wise, since aortic rupture is possible with none of the usual signs. It can even be missed during exploratory thoracotomy for some pulmonary

indication. In the series of 15 patients reported by DeMueles and associates,[2] the overall mortality rate was 73%, largely due to multiple-system injury and missed diagnoses.

7. (F) Vasopressors should not be given to such a patient, except in the most unusual circumstances, because of the following reasons: The patient (especially if a young adult) probably already has maximal vasoconstriction, and these drugs may raise the blood pressure artifically for a short time and give the treatment team a false sense of security; and these drugs are more harmful than beneficial to the patient who needs fluid or blood replacement.

8. (True) A small tube is usually easier to insert; also, it may be the largest size that will go through the trocar and cannula set available where this technique is used; finally, it is quite satisfactory in many instances of spontaneous pneumothorax, where it is almost always air alone that is present in the pleural cavity. However, a small tube is inadequate for the trauma patient who usually has both air and blood in the pleural cavity, as well as a persistent air leak. Usually, for such a patient, two tubes are required, one located anteriorly in the second or third intercostal space, and one located posteriorly in the seventh intercostal space at the mid or posterior axillary line. Both should be large bore, #28 to 36 French, if possible (see Case 11 for technique of insertion of such tubes).

It should be added that the small anterior tube is much better than no tube at all, since tension pneumothorax would otherwise be fatal in some patients en route to the second hospital.

9. (False) Myocardial contusion is a serious possibility in any patient who has contusion of the chest, especially that sustained in an automobile accident in which the steering column may have been involved. Myocardial contusion is a fairly common injury and is often overlooked. The diagnosis is made by daily electrocardiograms and careful electrocardiographic monitoring for the first few days in all such patients. There is no specific treatment available; management is the same as for myocardial infarction.

10. (F) Although this patient had an obvious flail chest, many such patients do not have obvious signs of paradoxical motion when first examined, or even hours or days later, since splinting of the muscles of the chest wall may prevent the false motion considered so characteristic of the flail deformity. This motion is an inward movement of the flail chest wall segment

during inspiration, a normal outward movement of the remainder of the chest wall. There is often a significant degree of contusion of the underlying lung, which adds to the respiratory insufficiency - as lung compliance is decreased, more positive pressure is required to ventilate the lung. It is frequently at this point that the instability of the chest wall first becomes apparent. Needless to say, it is far better to suspect flail chest on the basis of clinical points A through E, and to start treatment, than to wait until the condition becomes apparent.

11. (True) External stabilization of the chest wall probably increased this patient's comfort during his 80-mile trip by ambulance. However, cuffed endotracheal intubation, or cuffed tracheostomy intubation with controlled ventilation, using a volume-cycled respirator, is by far the best method of stabilizing the chest wall.[3] As pointed out previously, treatment should be started as soon as flail chest is suspected.

COURSE:

Abdominal exploration showed rupture of the spleen and transection of the pancreas at the vertebral column. The distal portion of the pancreas and the spleen were removed. The postoperative course was smooth except for persistent air leak in the left lung, which required continuous suctioning for ten days.

REFERENCES

1. Davis, J. J., et al.: Diagnosis and management of blunt abdominal trauma. Ann. Surg. 183:672-678, 1976.

2. DeMueles, J. E., et al.: Rupture of aorta and great vessels due to blunt thoracic trauma. J. Thorac. Cardiovasc. Surg. 61:438-442, 1971.

3. Sankaran, S. and Wilson, R. F.: Factors affecting prognosis in patients with flail chest. J. Thorac. Cardiovasc. Surg. 60:402-410, 1970.

4. Shubin, H. and Weil, M. H.: Bacterial shock. JAMA 235: 421-424, 1976.

::

CASE 25: BLUNT ABDOMINAL INJURY

HISTORY:

An 18-year-old boy was involved in an automobile accident and referred from another hospital fifty miles away.

EXAMINATION:

The patient was alert and oriented. His blood pressure was 110/80 mm Hg; pulse, 120 per minute. There were decreased breath sounds over the left side of the chest but no subcutaneous emphysema. Moderate tenderness was noted over the third and fourth dorsal vertebrae. There was diffuse abdominal tenderness, particularly in the left upper quadrant, with some guarding. No rebound tenderness was noted. Meperidine (Demerol®) had been administered at the referring hospital. Normal bowel sounds were noted. Rectal examination revealed no blood or other abnormalities. There was tenderness over the pubis. Neurologic findings were normal.

LABORATORY DATA:

Hemoglobin: 12.6 gm/dl
Hematocrit: 37.9%
Urinalysis: negative, except for 6 to 8 white blood cells and 6 to 10 red blood cells per high-power field, with several granular casts
Serum electrolytes: within normal limits
Blood glucose: 195 mg/dl, following an intravenous infusion of 5% dextrose in saline.
Arterial blood:
pH: 7.3
PO_2: 75 torr
PCO_2: 39 torr
X-rays: Roentgenograms showed a fracture of the left second and third ribs, with hemopneumothorax on the left, a fracture of the right humerus and of the left clavicle, a compression fracture of the second lumbar vertebra, and an undisplaced fracture of the pubis.

Intravenous pyelography revealed normal bilateral renal function and no extravasation of the dye.

Peritoneal tap with lavage revealed gross blood.

Note: This patient had multiple trauma, as defined and discussed more fully in Case 24. Attention will be directed in this case to the patient's thoracic and abdominal injuries.

In any multiply-injured patient, intra-abdominal injury must be suspected and searched for aggressively.

QUESTIONS:

Regarding blunt abdominal trauma, answer the following three questions true or false:

1. Solid viscera are more frequently injured than hollow viscera.

2. The solid viscus most frequently injured is the kidney.

3. Blood in the peritoneal cavity is usually a sign of significant abdominal injury.

4. The presence of blood in the peritoneal cavity can best be detected by:
   A. Four-quadrant tap
   B. Roentgenographic examination, with the patient in various positions
   C. Serial hematocrit and hemoglobin measurements
   D. Peritoneal tap and lavage
   E. Culdocentesis

TRUE OR FALSE (Questions 5-7):

5. The safest and easiest way to perform peritoneal tap and lavage is to insert a needle through the abdominal wall and inject saline.

6. If the bleeding originates in the retroperitoneal space, a peritoneal tap and lavage will usually be negative.

7. Fractured left ribs indicate possible splenic rupture.

8. The most likely cause of this patient's grossly bloodly abdominal tap is:
   A. Ruptured diaphragm
   B. Ruptured liver
   C. Ruptured spleen

9. TRUE OR FALSE: Insertion of a Foley catheter may be contraindicated in patients with fracture of the pelvis.

10. Other diagnostic and therapeutic procedures in this patient should include which of the following?
    A. Closed left inter-rib tube thoracostomy, with underwater seal suction
    B. Intravenous infusion of balanced salt solution
    C. Cross-matching for immediate whole blood transfusion, if needed
    D. Insertion of a central venous pressure line
    E. Assisted ventilation, with supplemental oxygen as indicated
    F. Nasogastric intubation and continuous suction
    G. Immediate exploratory celiotomy
    H. All of the above

ANSWERS AND COMMENTS:

1. (True) However, the reverse is true in penetrating abdominal injury. In blunt injury, the solid viscera are more likely to be torn by a sharp object, such as the jagged end of a fractured rib, or to be disrupted by a blunt force which impinges the organ against its nearby, relatively unyielding structures, such as the chest wall. The short pedicles that anchor the solid viscera can be torn loose, causing severe bleeding, usually with rapid exsanguination and death.

2. (False) The spleen is the solid abdominal organ most often injured by blunt trauma. Even when normal size, it is vulnerable to any severe blow on the left side of the trunk. When enlarged, as in malaria or lymphoma, the spleen may lie across the entire left side of the body and extend inferiorly as well; it would be difficult for a blow to the left side to fail to damage an organ that large. Finally, whether normal or enlarged, the spleen is pulpy and very vascular, and bleeds quite easily and rapidly.

The liver is the next most frequently damaged solid organ, followed by one or both kidneys.

3. (True) Normally, there should be no free blood in the peritoneal cavity. In fact, blood is irritating to the peritoneum, causing clinical signs of an inflammatory response with an outpouring of leukocytes and the eventual development of adhesions.

4. (D) Peritoneal tap and lavage. As developed by Root and associates,[1] peritoneal tap and lavage is, by far, the most dependable indicator of free blood in the peritoneal cavity. It will reveal even small amounts (50-100 ml) of blood, and any amount

is an indication of injury.

Four-quadrant tap (A) was formerly used almost routinely, but it has certain drawbacks, among them many false-negative results. Roentgenographic examination (B) may suggest the presence of blood within the peritoneal cavity, but the signs, if present, are nonspecific. No such signs were present in this patient. Hematocrit and hemoglobin determinations (C), even when done every hour or so, are not good indicators of active hemorrhage if it is occurring rapidly. Culdocentesis (E) is applicable only in women and is very useful in diagnosing pelvic bleeding, but it is not a substitute for peritoneal lavage for blunt trauma.

5. (False) Following abdominal roentgenographic examination and emptying of the urinary bladder by catheter, the abdomen should be prepared as for any operation. A peritoneal dialysis trocar, with catheter, should then be introduced through a small incision just inferior to the umbilicus. Care is taken not to allow blood to enter the peritoneal cavity through the incision and puncture wound, since such blood would, of course, invalidate the test. Gross blood aspirated through the catheter is an indication for exploratory celiotomy. In the absence of gross blood, the peritoneal cavity is lavaged by introducing 20 ml/kg (up to one liter) of balanced salt solution, after which the patient is turned from side to side. Then the bottle is lowered and the fluid allowed to return by siphonage. If it is impossible to read newsprint through the solution because of the presence of red blood cells, then the test is considered positive for intraperitoneal bleeding. An aliquot of the fluid may be sent to the laboratory for both Gram's stain and Wright's stain to identify bacteria, white blood cells, red blood cells and intestinal contents, the presence of any of which constitutes a positive tap. A blood cell count should also be done. Amylase may also be checked, and, if present, is indicative of pancreatic injury or ruptured stomach or duodenum.

Relative contraindications to peritoneal tap and lavage are (1) a history of previous abdominal operation with possible adhesions; (2) distended loops of intestine, which might be perforated by the catheter; and (3) pregnancy.

Any negative tap and lavage must be disregarded, since the test is meaningful only if it is positive.

6. (True) It will also be negative if splenic or hepatic hemorrhage is confined to the subcapsular space, so-called "delayed" rupture of these organs. However, if a retroperitoneal or subcap-

sular hematoma ruptures into the general peritoneal cavity, obviously the paracentesis and lavage will very likely be positive. The tap and lavage, if negative, may have to be repeated in a few hours, or exploratory celiotomy may be indicated.

Retroperitoneal hemorrhage can be very extensive and dangerous, since it frequently originates from rather large blood vessels. It does not come from rupture of the spleen or liver; but it is frequent, following renal and pancreatic injuries, and in association with pelvic fractures. This patient did have a fracture of the second lumbar vertebra, and retroperitoneal hematoma, usually small, is frequently associated with such fracture. An incidental point is that fracture of a lower thoracic or a lumbar vertebra suggests possible pancreatic or hepatic injury and damage to these organs should be searched for.

7. (True, particularly if the lower ribs are fractured) The usual screening roentgenogram of the chest (usually a single anterior-posterior exposure, using a portable machine) may not show every rib fracture. Even special rib studies may show only a few of the rib fractures present.

Absence of lower rib fractures does not rule out splenic rupture, especially in children in whom the ribs are pliable and don't fracture easily, even from injury severe enough to damage the spleen.

This patient's initial chest roentgenogram showed fractures in only the left second and third ribs. However, subsequent roentgenographic studies showed a fracture in each of the left second through ninth ribs. This emphasizes the importance of having a high index of suspicion of splenic injury in any patient with blunt trauma to the torso.

A good rule to follow is that any patient with evidence of fracture of any of the lower six ribs should be suspected of having an intra-abdominal injury, as well.

8. (C) Ruptured spleen is much more likely than the other answers, although a ruptured diaphragm is a distinct possibility in a patient with injuries such as this patient had. A careful search for diaphragmatic rupture must be made by physical examination and roentgenographic study, as well as at exploratory celiotomy. Complications of unsuspected and unrepaired diaphragmatic rupture are atelectasis and compromised blood supply of the bowel, with possible intestinal infarction and obstruction.

9. (True) Any injury in the area of the pelvis, especially a fracture of the pubis or ischium, may be associated with a torn urethra which does contraindicate insertion of a urethral catheter. Gross blood at the urethral meatus is a frequent sign of such urethral injury which, in the male patient, is usually located in the prostatic or membranous portion of the urethra. Suprapubic bladder drainage would be the preferred approach in such a patient.

10. (H) All. Exploratory celiotomy revealed gross blood in the left upper quadrant and in the pelvis, with laceration of the inferior border of the spleen extending into the hilum. Splenectomy was carried out without difficulty. No other abdominal injury was noted.

COURSE:

The patient's postoperative course was smooth, except for a superficial infection of the abdominal wound, which healed primarily. Open thoracotomy was not required. His fractures were treated successfully by the orthopedic service.

REFERENCE

Root, H.D., et al.: Diagnostic peritoneal lavage. Surgery 57:633-637, 1965.

::

CASE 26: PENETRATING CHEST INJURY

HISTORY:

A 22-year-old woman was stabbed with a steak knife several times over the chest, back, and right buttock. She had no shortness of breath but experienced pain in the right hemithorax on breathing.

Examination revealed a 1-cm-long wound of the right upper, anterior chest, a similar wound of the right infrascapular area, and a 2.5-cm-long wound of the lateral aspect of the right buttock, extending to the ischial tuberosity. Diminished breath sounds were noted over the right upper chest. There was no deviation of the trachea in the neck. The remaining physical findings were normal.

Chest roentgenograms revealed 15% pneumothorax on the right side but no other abnormality.

Arterial blood: PO_2, 73 torr; PCO_2, 35 torr; pH, 7.44; HCO_3^-, 23 mEq/l. The results of all other laboratory tests were normal.

QUESTIONS:

1. Which of the following statements are true of stab wounds of the chest?
   A. All must be assumed to have entered the pleural cavity until proved otherwise.
   B. A nonserious-appearing wound may have produced fatal damage to thoracic organs.
   C. Diaphragmatic and infradiaphragmatic wounds must be considered to be present whenever a stab wound is located below the level of the fourth rib anteriorly.
   D. All of the above

2. TRUE OR FALSE: A general physical examination is not likely to be very helpful in the initial evaluation of the patient with penetrating chest injury.

3. The general principles of initial care of this patient are:
   A. Ensure a patent airway.
   B. Control hemorrhage.

C. Correct the loss of negative intrapleural pressure.
D. Prevent or relieve chest pain by adhesive or elastic strapping.
E. Determine the extent of the injuries.
F. Probe all wounds to see how deep they are.

ANSWERS AND COMMENTS:

1. (D) All. (A, B) Even an ice pick wound through the thoracic wall can be rapidly fatal, the diameter or width of a stab wound bearing no relationship to the degree of injury to vital structures. All wounds of the chest, unless obviously superficial lacerations, must be considered to have entered the pleural cavity until proved otherwise.

The possible internal injuries from the two stab wounds of the chest sustained by this patient are:

a) pneumothorax, with possible tension pneumothorax
b) hemothorax, complicating the pneumothorax
c) laceration of the brachial plexus
d) laceration of the pericardium and myocardium, with hemopericardium
e) laceration of the diaphragm, kidney and liver (C).

Each of these conditions must be ruled out by examination and ancillary studies.

2. (False) All of the factors examined during a routine physical examination are vitally important in the diagnosis and treatment of a stab wound victim. In fact, most of what one needs to know about the patient can be learned during the routine physical examination. Thus, one should never be lax about this phase of the patient's care, although, admittedly, one should not delay the patient's urgent treatment in order to do the most thorough of physical examinations. Any part of the examination that is not done in the first five to ten minutes should be completed as soon as possible, preferably by the first physician to see the patient. The patient should be completely disrobed on arrival, the clothes being cut off if necessary. All parts of the body, the neck and abdomen in particular, since they are contiguous to the chest, must be examined for evidence of injuries. Combined wounds of the chest with either the neck or the abdomen must be looked for.

Very careful inspection is essential to reveal the location and extent of all wounds. This is important in the assessment of the likelihood of internal injuries, by type as well as by organ. For stab wounds and missile wounds, a careful search should also be made for exit wounds.

The degree of expansion of both sides of the chest should be noted and monitored for changes. The point of maximal cardiac impulse (PMI) is often visible, but it should be confirmed by palpation and marked so that any changes in cardiac position can be detected.

Palpation is also useful for determining the position of the trachea at the level of the suprasternal notch, and the presence of subcutaneous emphysema. Fractured ribs may be indicated by point tenderness in a conscious patient, occasionally by crepitation. A flail segment of the chest may be evident at the initial examination, but often may not be apparent until hours or days later, when the splinting chest-wall muscles become fatigued.

Percussion will help determine the presence and level of fluid in the pleural cavity (especially hemothorax), widening of the mediastinum, and the position and size of the heart. The level of both sides of the diaphragm and diaphragmatic motility should be checked if the patient's condition permits, although fluid or blood in the pleural cavity may make this difficult or impossible.

Auscultation should indicate whether the lungs are expanded and are ventilating well, and whether there is partial obstruction of the upper or lower airway. Crepitation in the subcutaneous space, on stethoscopic examination, is often the earliest clue to the presence of subcutaneous emphysema, which indicates damage to the tracheobronchial tree or to the lung parenchyma.

Heart sounds should be checked for loudness, since muffling of these sounds is an early indication of pericardial tamponade. Murmurs, as well as rate and rhythm, should be noted.

3. (A, B, C, E) (A) Whatever is required should be done to ensure a patent airway. Initially, an endotracheal tube is frequently necessary, especially if the patient is obtunded or his respirations are depressed for any reason, such as an overdose of drugs, including alcohol. Aspiration through the tube should be done to remove the excess secretions that are always present in patients with thoracic injuries. At first, positive pressure ventilation should be used cautiously, if at all, since it is apt to cause tension pneumothorax if pneumothorax is present. After tube thoracostomy to relieve pneumothorax, there is less danger from the use of positive pressure ventilation, but excessive force must be avoided.

Even if endotracheal intubation is not needed initially, tracheobronchial suction should be carried out as often as necessary, in order to clear secretions. Otherwise, atelectasis, pneumonitis and other complications are likely to occur. Endoscopic aspiration (laryngoscopic or bronchoscopic) may be necessary if the previously mentioned procedures are not satisfactory.

(B) Hemorrhage should be controlled as rapidly as possible. If the bleeding is into the pleural space, this control can usually be accomplished by closed tube thoracostomy, with a large (#34-38F) tube and underwater seal and suction. If the bleeding is coming from a tear in the lung surface, it will usually stop as the blood is removed and the lung re-expands. However, if the lung is badly damaged or if the bleeding is from a systemic artery where the pressure is higher than in the pulmonary artery system, the bleeding may not stop without open thoracotomy.

(C) The loss of negative intrapleural pressure must be corrected, since even a relatively small degree of pneumothorax is dangerous in the presence of thoracic trauma. Restoration of a negative pressure requires closed tube thoracostomy through the fourth or fifth interspace in the midaxillary line, using a tube large enough to remove blood as well as air, since hemothorax is a fairly common accompaniment of pneumothorax in severe trauma.

Usually, in severe trauma, especially with hemopneumothorax, two large tubes are required, one in the anterior second intercostal interspace in the midclavicular line and the other one in the posterior axillary line in the fifth or sixth intercostal space. Both should be connected to underwater seal suction.

(D) Strapping the chest with adhesive or elastic bandaging is not recommended, because it prevents adequate clearing of secretions by coughing. The exception to this rule is for the patient who has a flail chest in need of stabilization, and for whom the usual treatment of positive pressure ventilation is not yet available, or is not available at all. For relief of pain, intercostal nerve block is far superior to chest strapping and allows the patient to breathe more deeply.

(E) In addition to findings on physical examination, the determination of extent of injuries is based on probabilities, taking into consideration the type, and especially the size, of weapon used, the direction of the blow(s), and the anatomical structures that could have been damaged. Obviously, roentgenograms and other studies are required to rule out injury of both thoracic and cervical structures, as well as abdominal structures.

(F) In general, chest wounds should not be probed if they are more than several millimeters deep, since blind probing within the thorax is potentially extremely dangerous. Wounds other than very shallow ones, especially stab rather than slash wounds, must be assumed to have penetrated the chest wall, and the patient must be managed accordingly.

COURSE:

A closed tube thoracostomy was performed in the emergency department with a #32F silastic tube placed in the right second intercostal space on the midclavicular line. No second tube was necessary. Re-expansion of the right lung was prompt. Her lacerations were sutured and she was admitted to the hospital for observation and further care. No evidence of damage to other structures was found. The thoracostomy tube was removed after 48 hours and her lung remained fully expanded. She was discharged on the third hospital day, with instructions to return to the clinic for suture removal five days later.

::

CASE 27: NECK INJURY FOLLOWING REAR-END VEHICULAR COLLISION

HISTORY:

A 32-year-old woman had stopped her car at an intersection when it was struck from the rear by another car. Her head struck the headrest but not the windshield or the steering wheel. She experienced immediate neck discomfort, which gradually became worse. Four hours later, she reported to the emergency department by car and walked in with her head erect but immobile. There was no history of unconsciousness and no discomfort or weakness in her extremities. Fourteen years earlier, she had had meningitis with no sequelae.

The results of the general and neurological examination were normal except for moderate tenderness of the neck over the spinous processes and lateral muscles, with slight limitation of cervical motion in all directions.

QUESTIONS:

1. The type of injured patient who should be suspected of having an injury of the cervical spine is the patient with:
   A. Head injury
   B. Facial injury
   C. Shoulder injury
   D. Unconsciousness
   E. All of the above

2. TRUE OR FALSE: If a patient with neck injury can walk into the emergency department, as this patient did, he probably does not have a serious neck injury.

3. The most likely diagnosis in this patient is:
   A. Fracture of the spinous processes
   B. Fracture of the odontoid process of C_2
   C. Acceleration or extension-flexion injury of the cervical spine
   D. Mild contusion of the cervical spinal cord
   E. All of the above

4. Management of the conscious patient with history and findings of acceleration or extension-flexion neck injury should consist of which of the following?

A. Routine hospital admission
B. Cervical collar to be worn for three months
C. Analgesics and muscle relaxants
D. Daily physical therapy, including neck traction
E. Careful follow-up
F. All of the above

ANSWERS AND COMMENTS:

1. (E) All. For any patient who is unconscious following a definite or suspected injury (the latter on the basis of sudden syncope or seizure, for example), steps should be taken to rule out an injury of the cervical spine. This can be done by immobilizing the head and neck for the initial resuscitative procedures that are required in every unconscious patient. After the patient's condition is stable, his neck can be examined by roentgenography to rule out bony and, indirectly, ligamentous injuries, including injuries related to intervertebral disc protrusion. Also, any conscious patient who has sustained injuries of the head, face or shoulders, and any patient with obvious neck injury, must be handled as if he had injured his cervical spine and treated accordingly.

It is largely a matter of clinical judgment whether <u>every</u> patient with a history of a seizure or syncope should have roentgenograms made of the cervical spine. A good rule is that if a fall has occurred, an injury must be suspected. Roentgenograms of the spine, especially of the cervical spine, should be made in all patients, including children, who have fallen to a hard surface, as from a height or down steps, and all patients who have been thrown from a vehicle.

2. (False) Many patients with severe neck injury drive themselves to the hospital and walk into the emergency department. This act does not, in itself, rule out a cervical spine injury. Often such a patient will be holding his head tilted to one side or in some other unusual position, and will usually be supporting it with one or both hands. The fact that the patient walks in does not relieve the clinician from his duty to rule out a cervical spine injury. Therefore, the patient should be placed supine, with the neck and head immobilized, until appropriate studies to rule out fracture have been completed.

3. (C) Acceleration or extension-flexion ("whiplash") injury of the cervical spine is the most likely diagnosis. This injury is also called cervical strain or sprain, and is a common problem in most emergency departments. It is also underrated as an

injury by most clinicians. The typical patient has, as did this patient, a history of being in an automobile that is sitting still or moving slowly and is struck from the rear by another vehicle. The head whips backwards, and the patient sustains an injury of the neck, with no blow to the head except against the back of the seat or the headrest.

The mechanism of injury is hyperextension of the neck as the body is thrown forward, followed by hyperflexion of the neck as the body whips back. This produces tears or strains of the ligamentous structures of the neck with, at times, intervertebral disc injury. The extension component of the recoil or oscillating neck motion is the one that causes the injury. Most of these injuries are sprains or strains of the cervical muscular or ligamentous tissues.

The symptoms and findings depend upon the severity of the rear-end collision, as well as the interval following the accident. A properly positioned headrest may give some protection, but one that is too low or too high may do more harm than good. Unfortunately, a snugly fitting lap and shoulder harness gives little, if any, protection from this type of injury, other than preventing the head from striking the steering wheel, windshield, or dashboard.

A detailed general and neurological evaluation should be done routinely in these patients to rule out other injuries and to establish a baseline against which changes can be evaluated.

Cervical roentgenograms of this patient's neck showed no abnormalities except straightening of the normal curvature of the cervical spine.

4. (C, D, E) (A) It is usually not necessary for the patient to be hospitalized, although, in some instances of severe injury, this may be advisable. The patient who cannot be properly treated at home may require hospital care for at least a few days.

(B, C) In any case, bed rest should be prescribed for several days, with analgesics and muscle relaxants as required for comfort and relaxation of muscle spasm. A soft cervical collar gives some neck support, but must not be worn continuously or for more than a few weeks, because psychological dependence develops rapidly in many patients and atrophy of neck muscles can occur.

(D) Physical therapy in the form of heat, usually moist rather than radiant heat, is useful, two to four times daily. Neck traction with halter, rope, pulley and weights is often helpful, especially for patients with more severe injuries. It may be helpful for the patient to go to a physical therapy department for these treatments, although arrangements can usually be made for home care so that the patient does not have to leave his home daily until he is ready to return to work. Such return is usually possible from a few days post-injury up to one to three weeks, depending on the job and the patient. It is advisable for the patient to have a second check-up by his own physician within a few days following his visit to the emergency department, or, in the event that bona fide symptoms persist, to have specialty consultation to determine other causes. These include aggravation of pre-existing cervical spondylosis and a disc injury, either of which may require a longer period away from work and more intensive treatment.

(E) It is vital that all such patients, even if asymptomatic, have specific arrangements made for follow-up care and that these arrangements be documented on the record. Typically, the symptoms, such as pain and stiffness, are milder or absent soon after the accident, but progress or appear for the first time several hours post-injury. For this reason, the patient who is seen within an hour or two after the injury should be treated as if his symptoms will progress.

Other symptoms that may be present, or may appear later, are blurring of vision, vertigo, tinnitus, and aching of the shoulders and upper back, as well as many other vague symptoms that do not seem to fit any traditional pattern. Nystagmus may be present, as may upper-extremity weakness; neither is easy to evaluate. Such symptoms and signs have been attributed to vertebral-basilar arterial spasm, irritation of the cervical sympathetic nerves, or mild brain injury. In the patient who has struck his forehead as well as his occiput, the latter is a distinct possibility. However, regardless of the origin of the real, as well as the nebulous, "hard-to-put-your-finger-on" type symptoms, one should be very cautious about ascribing them to neurosis or other nonorganic mechanisms. Many of these patients consider themselves severely injured and possibly permanently disabled; and reassurance and emotional support, provided from the very beginning of treatment, are necessary if the majority are going to recover.

::

CASE 28: CERVICAL FRACTURE

HISTORY:

A 24-year-old man dove into a river and landed headfirst in shallow water near the water's edge. He was unable to move his lower extremities, but was able to crawl up the bank with his upper extremities. He did not lose consciousness. The paramedic team transported him to the emergency department on a spine board, with his neck immobilized in the neutral position.

Examination on his arrival in the emergency department one hour later revealed poor triceps function and good biceps function bilaterally. There was absence of motor activity below the nipple line and a sensory level anteriorly at C_8-T_1 on the right side and C_7 on the left side.

Roentgenograms of the cervical spine showed a fracture of the superior plate of C_7, with a comminuted fracture located anteriorly, a fracture of the left lateral mass of C_6, and a fracture of the posterior arch of C_7, but no subluxation.

QUESTIONS:

1. Which of the following general statements about diving as a cause of spinal cord injuries are true?
   A. Over three-fourths of all spinal cord lesions from sports are caused by diving.
   B. More than half of the patients with spinal cord injuries from diving are quadriplegic.
   C. Hyperventroflexion is the most frequent mechanism of injury.
   D. Most of the patients do not hit bottom or a submerged object.
   E. There are probably 600 of these serious spinal cord injuries in the United States each year.
   F. All of the above

2. TRUE OR FALSE: In spinal injuries, as in skull injuries, there is an inverse relationship between bony injury and nervous tissue damage.

3. The mechanisms of injury of the cervical spine are which of the following?

A. Flexion with dislocation and fracture
B. Hyperextension
C. Vertical compression
D. Rotation
E. All of the above

4. Although not present in this patient, fracture-dislocation can occur in accidents of this nature. It occurs most commonly at which of the following locations?
   A. C_1 and C_2
   B. C_2 and C_3
   C. C_5 and C_6
   D. C_6 and C_7

5. Proper initial management of a patient such as this one should include which of the following?
   A. Check the airway and maintain ventilation and oxygenation.
   B. Do a careful, but rapid, general and neurological examination.
   C. Check neck flexion and extension.
   D. Obtain roentgenograms of the cervical spine.
   E. Apply skeletal traction (tongs).
   F. Pad all bony prominences.
   G. All of the above

6. The airway and respirations may be compromised in neck injuries. Which of the following are true?
   A. Obstruction of the airway can occur from retropharyngeal hemorrhage with hematoma and swelling.
   B. Respiratory embarrassment or paralysis (apnea) can occur from cord lesions in the midcervical area.
   C. Atlantoaxial dislocation is frequently fatal because of compression of the respiratory center in the medulla oblongata.
   D. The usual causes of airway obstruction also occur in patients with neck injuries.
   E. All of the above.

7. TRUE OR FALSE: If, following spinal injury, a patient has progressive neurological deficit, emergency laminectomy is probably indicated.

ANSWERS AND COMMENTS:

1. (F) All. These grim statistics attest to the seriousness of diving injuries in this country. Diving into rivers, widely practiced in rural areas, is more likely to cause neck injuries than

diving into swimming pools. Obviously, objects such as the river or pool bottom are hit, as in this case, and this does cause injuries. However, it is not infrequent that no object is struck, and the type of wedge fracture produced tends to substantiate the fact that the mechanism is hyperventroflexion as the head strikes the surface of the water. Almost all of the spinal injuries from diving are in the neck, not the thoracolumbar spine.

2. (False) Although it is possible to have extensive damage to the spinal cord without demonstrable bony injury, there is usually a high correlation between vertebral damage and spinal cord injury. One reason is that the vertebrae and their attached soft tissues are usually the agents directly responsible for the spinal cord injury.

3. (E) All. They represent the most common basic mechanisms of injury of the cervical spine. In hyperextension fractures of the cervical spine, the anterior longitudinal ligament may be ruptured, with possible fracture of one or both facets or of the vertebral body. The cord damage frequently results from the sharp edge of the lamina. Spontaneous reduction may occur so that roentgenograms appear normal even though the patient is paraplegic. Any ill-advised hyperextension of the neck, such as in endotracheal intubation, may further damage the cord.

4. (C, D) Fracture-dislocation is the most serious of all vertebral injuries and the one most often associated with spinal cord or root injury. It is more common in the lower cervical region.

The mechanism of dislocation is displacement of one vertebra forward upon another, because of the relatively greater mobility of the upper portion of the spine over that of the lower portion. The displacement is usually accompanied by a fracture, as well as by contusion or persistent compression, of the spinal cord. Spontaneous reduction of the dislocation is common, but the neurological deficit is frequently permanent.

5. (A, B, D, E, F) (A) See question and answer 6.

(B) The rapid, but complete, examination should be done first, with emphasis on the neurological examination. As always, an effort should be made to detect or rule out injuries other than the obvious ones. If hypotension is present, it may be due to spinal cord damage with secondary vasodilation due to sympathetic denervation, or to hypovolemia. If the former, it usually responds to slight elevation of the lower extremities and to intravenous infusion of electrolyte solution. If the latter, the site of the blood loss must be detected, and measures to stop the bleeding and replace the loss must be initiated.

In this patient, head injury occurred but did not seem to be causing any signs or symptoms. No injuries, other than the cervical injuries, were found on subsequent roentgenological study of the head and entire spine, the chest and the abdomen.

Neurological examination, with careful charting of motor and sensory findings, is vital as soon as possible following spinal cord injury. This permits thorough documentation of the progression or regression of any deficit present. Muscle tone and strength, sensory loss, and the presence or absence of both deep and superficial reflexes should be recorded.

(C) Although most of the spinal cord damage occurs at the time of the injury, considerable additional damage to the cord can be done by unwise and careless movement of the patient. This can happen at the scene of the accident, en route to the hospital, or in the emergency department.

At the scene of the accident, fixation of the head and neck should be done immediately, either in the position they were in when the patient was found, or in the neutral position with a head board, spine board, cervical collar or straps, sand bags, or a halter. Such fixation should be maintained until roentgenograms are obtained (D) and skeletal traction with tongs (E) is applied. This means that fixation should be done before the patient is moved at all, if possible, and certainly before he is moved off the spine board. If the patient must be moved from one stretcher to another, he should be moved as a unit, on the spine board, preferably with gentle, continuous cephalad traction being applied on the head by a person who has no other function to perform during the transfer.

It is definitely not safe to remove the immobilization apparatus in order to manipulate the neck to determine if there is limitation of motion or tenderness. <u>Any</u> motion, active or passive, must await at least a lateral roentgenogram of the cervical spine, showing all seven vertebral bodies. If there is any doubt about the interpretation of this film, or if there is any neurological deficit, consultation with both a radiologist and a neurological surgeon should be sought while additional views are being obtained. At least an anterior-posterior and an odontoid view should be interpreted as normal before the neck is manipulated, if the history of injury or the neurological findings are suggestive of damage to the cervical spine or spinal cord. Only after these three views (lateral, anterior-posterior and odontoid) have been declared normal can additional studies, including flexion and extension and oblique views, be made; and those preferably should be made with the consultants in attendance.

(F) Padding, to prevent pressure ischemia, should be placed beneath all bony prominences, especially beneath the thoracic spine, the sacrum, the ischial tuberosities, and the heels.

6. (E) All. (A) One of the indirect points of evidence of an injury of the cervical spine, even with no bony abnormality, is the presence of retropharyngeal swelling. This can become severe enough to interfere with airway patency and require intubation - preferably nasotracheal, but if not possible, then by cricothyreotomy or tracheostomy.

(B) A lesion of the upper half of the cervical cord interferes with, or destroys, the neural control of both the intercostal muscles and the diaphragm, causing apnea. The phrenic nerve is derived from the third, fourth and fifth cervical cord segments; thus injury of the lower cervical spinal cord (below the fifth cervical vertebra, C_5) causes intercostal and abdominal muscle paralysis, but allows diaphragmatic breathing, since the phrenic nerve is intact. However, one should be prepared to assist or control the patient's breathing, since edema, or other changes not well understood, can occasionally ascend to involve some, or all, of the origin of the phrenic nerve. Serial determinations of arterial blood gases and pH are mandatory. Usually, a tracheostomy is indicated, since this form of hypoventilation is likely to persist for days or weeks, even permanently.

(C) Although some patients survive severe dislocation of the atlas on the axis, immediate death is more likely than survival, because both the cardiac center and the respiratory center in the medulla are usually damaged. The mechanism is compression by a part of the first or second vertebra, especially the dens or odontoid process; such compression is possible even when the vertebra is unfractured. In general, the most common cause of early death in cervical spine injury above C_5 is respiratory, rather than cardiac, insufficiency.

(D) All of the usual causes of airway obstruction occur in patients with neck injuries. Even if the patient is conscious, he may be unable to clear his mouth and hypopharynx of accumulated blood, secretions such as saliva, and broken or loose teeth or dentures. Vomiting is likely to lead to aspiration into the tracheobronchial tree because of the patient's inability to turn his head, because of loss of reflexes, or because of the large volume of liquid and solid food particles from the stomach. The usual measures for clearing the airway are required, except that the neck must not be manipulated if it is possible not to do so. During the use of suction for this purpose, not only must the head and neck not be moved by the hospital staff or allowed to move passively, but the patient must be prevented from moving his head or neck, since such movement may produce damage or produce further damage to the spinal cord.

7. (True) This fact reinforces the vital importance of documentation of the results of a thorough neurological evaluation at the scene of the injury and as soon as the patient arrives at the emergency department. Otherwise, slow, progressive deterioration may not be easy to recognize. The urgency lies in the fact that an immediate decompressive operation may prevent further spinal cord damage. A myelogram may be the only study that should be considered preoperatively.

COURSE:

Crutchfield tongs, with traction, were applied in the emergency department. A few hours after admission, a cervical myelogram was done and showed no area of obstruction; however, edema was noted around the spinal cord opposite the lower cervical spine fractures. During the following two weeks in the hospital and the following four months in the rehabilitation center, this patient had repeated urinary-tract infections and repeated episodes of pulmonary embolism. However, at the time he was discharged home, he was progressing well, except for the permanent partial paralysis of his upper extremities and the permanent complete paralysis of his lower extremities.

::

CASE 29: PENETRATING NECK INJURY

HISTORY:

A 53-year-old man was stabbed several times during an altercation in a local bar. A physician arrived with the ambulance, so that an initial diagnosis was made early and treatment was started immediately. A hemopneumothorax on the right side was found; a chest tube with a Heimlich valve was inserted on the right side, and an estimated 1000 ml of blood had been removed from the right pleural space before the patient arrived at the emergency department.

Upon his arrival, the patient's systolic blood pressure was 100 mm Hg by palpation; and his pulse rate was regular at 130/min. There was a 3-cm stab wound in the lower portion of the right side of the neck just superior to the clavicle, a 3-cm stab wound posterior to the middle third of the right sternocleidomastoid muscle, and a 3-cm laceration superior to the right ear. There was a 2-cm laceration on the thenar eminence of the right hand, with loss of function of the flexor pollicis longus muscle, and hypesthesia along the medial aspect of the thumb. The right side of the chest showed no excursion with respiration and was dull to percussion. Breath sounds on the right were absent. The trachea was not deviated. The results of the remainder of the general and neurological examinations were normal.

A roentgenogram of the patient's chest, done at the bedside, revealed a right hemopneumothorax with no shift of the mediastinum.

An additional closed inter-rib tube thoracostomy was done, and suction with underwater seal was applied to both tubes. An estimated 4000 ml of 5% dextrose in Ringer's lactate solution was infused intravenously within the first hour of injury. Over half of this was given at the scene of the injury and en route to the hospital. For this infusion, catheters were placed in both basilic veins and a femoral vein.

QUESTIONS:

1. The initial management of such a patient comprises which of the following?
   A. Probe the wounds to determine their depth and direction.
   B. Open and secure the airway.

C. Do a brief examination to rule out other injuries.
D. Control bleeding by gentle pressure, if possible.
E. Rapidly administer electrolyte fluid or blood intravenously.
F. Prepare the patient for immediate operation under general anesthesia.

2. The structures that can be damaged by a penetrating wound of the neck are which of the following?
   A. The spine and spinal cord
   B. Blood vessels
   C. Lungs
   D. Larynx and trachea
   E. Esophagus
   F. Neurogenic tissue
   G. Thoracic duct or right lymphatic duct
   H. Thyroid or parathyroid glands
   I. Muscles
   J. Intracranial contents
   K. Maxillofacial tissues
   L. All of the above

3. In addition to airway obstruction and hemorrhage, other immediate or delayed complications of penetrating neck injuries are:
   A. Cerebrovascular accident due to vessel damage
   B. Air embolism
   C. Massive aspiration of blood
   D. Infection with abscess formation
   E. Esophageal fistula
   F. All of the above

4. TRUE OR FALSE: As opposed to penetrating injuries, blunt injuries of the neck are not likely to produce severe injury or to be followed by complications.

ANSWERS AND COMMENTS:

1. (B, C, D, E, F) (A) The general rule is that any wound that penetrates the platysma muscle must be explored in the operating room, with the patient under general endotracheal anesthesia, <u>not</u> in the emergency department by anyone, for any reason, with the finger or with any instrument. To do otherwise is to run the risk of producing uncontrollable hemorrhaging from a large vessel that had stopped bleeding, obstructing an airway that was previously open, and damaging other structures not damaged by the original injury.

Instead, the patient should be prepared for operative exploration under general anesthesia (F) at the earliest possible time. Almost without exception, anterior and lateral neck wounds require such exploration, so there is no excuse for wasting time with special procedures or studies of any type. One exception to this rule is the case of a patient who is bleeding so rapidly that immediate control in the emergency department is required. Another exception is the patient whose airway is so seriously compromised that endotracheal intubation, cricothyreotomy or tracheostomy is essential before the patient can be moved. Obviously, if the emergency department is equipped with major surgical facilities, equipment and personnel, the patient does not need to be moved to another operating area at all, or at least, does not need to be moved initially.

(B) The opening and securing of the airway is the first and most important single step, since the airway may already be obstructed, or may suddenly become blocked by swelling of the surrounding tissues (as by hematoma), or by mucus, blood or other foreign material in the trachea. Assisted ventilation should be provided and oxygen should be administered if there is any clinical evidence that hypoxemia or hypercarbia is present, or is likely to develop. Later, the oxygen flow and ventilation should be adjusted on the basis of serial arterial blood gas and pH determinations.

(C) The brief initial physical examination allows the physician to determine the extent of the wounds and their location. Also important is the detection of any evidence of injury to the spinal cord, brachial plexus, or cranial nerves. This baseline examination is important, and the findings should be documented so that changes can be detected.

Also, other injuries must be ruled out or found and treated, since they may be more serious than the neck injury. An example is massive hemopneumothorax, as in this patient, especially if tension pneumothorax is also present.

(D, E) Not all patients with penetrating neck injuries will be bleeding actively when they arrive at the emergency department. However, it is not unusual for a patient to exsanguinate from a relatively small wound of the neck at about the time he arrives in the emergency department. Light pressure can be used to control the bleeding, at least temporarily. It is sometimes difficult to estimate the amount of blood lost before the patient's arrival. The safest rule is to suspect blood loss of moderate to severe degree, such as this patient had, and to administer fluid of the electrolyte type, blood substitutes, or whole blood as rapidly as possible, at first. This should be done through at least two intravenous lines, plus a central venous line.

If the injury is near or at the root of the neck, the central venous line should be inserted through a femoral vein, as in this patient, in order to avoid leakage of the fluid at the point of disruption of tributaries to the superior vena cava.

2. (L) All. The listing of these tissues found in or near the neck was done to remind you that they are crowded into a very small space where damage to any of them may be life-threatening. This patient is a good example of this problem, in that the wound at the base of his neck proved to have lacerated the internal jugular and subclavian veins and the apex of the lung, as well as the clavicular head of the sternocleidomastoid muscle. All other vessels and the nerves were intact. Following repair of the vessels, a careful search was made for damage to the subclavian artery and the brachial plexus, but these structures were intact.

This patient also illustrated the fact that patients do not always fit the neat categories we try to assign them to, such as "pure" head injury, neck injury, chest injury and abdominal injury. Penetrating injuries are particularly difficult to categorize, since they may traverse any tissues in the immediate or surrounding area, including the least expected ones. This is particularly true of gunshot wounds, the missile of which may penetrate, or be deflected by, bony structures. Adjacent tissues, especially of the cervical spinal cord, not traversed by the missile may be damaged by a shock wave phenomenon, and this damage may be delayed for hours or days. This fact becomes important in assessing the patient's prognosis, at best, a somewhat difficult exercise in the emergency department setting.

3. (F) All. Although these do not represent all of the complications, they account for most of the deaths from penetrating neck injuries. The overall mortality for patients with penetrating neck injuries in civilian life is 5 to 10%. In some series where all such wounds are explored immediately, the figure is as low as 2%.

4. (False) If small wounds can be deceptive as to the extent of damage, blunt injuries are frequently even more treacherous. Almost all of the structures in, and adjacent to, the neck can be damaged by an injury that produces little or no external sign of trauma. A high index of suspicion must be maintained, based

on the history of the injury and a careful examination, as well as a period of observation, the latter preferably in the hospital. Special procedures are usually required to rule out damage to the larynx, trachea, carotid arteries, spine, and spinal cord, which are the structures most often injured by blunt neck trauma.

COURSE:

This patient developed recurrent right pneumothorax following removal of both chest tubes on the fifth hospital day. This was corrected by insertion of another tube for two more days, after which his recovery was complete.

::

CASE 30: CLOSED HEAD INJURY

HISTORY:

A five-year-old girl fell backward off of her bicycle, hitting the back of her head against the ground. She was immediately drowsy and slightly confused. She did not vomit and was not unconscious.

Examination one hour later revealed a drowsy child with no amnesia and no disorientation. There was slight tenderness over the right occipital area but no laceration. There was no hemotympanum, no ecchymosis of the eyelids, no tenderness, no bogginess or discoloration of the mastoid area on either side, no nuchal rigidity, and no tenderness over the neck.

QUESTIONS:

TRUE OR FALSE (Questions 1 and 2):

1. A patient such as this does not need skull roentgenograms, since a fracture is most unlikely.

2. All patients with skull fractures must be treated.

3. In a patient with blunt head injury, cervical spine roentgenograms should be obtained under which of the following circumstances?
   A. In any unconscious patient
   B. In a patient with multiple injuries sustained in a vehicular accident, especially maxillofacial injuries
   C. In extension-flexion neck injuries
   D. When the head injury was due to a fall on the head
   E. When there is pain or tenderness of the neck in a conscious patient
   F. When there is evidence of cervical cord or nerve root damage
   G. All of the above

4. Basal skull fracture is characterized by which of the following?
   A. It can be easily demonstrated roentgenographically.
   B. Bleeding or leakage of cerebrospinal fluid from the ear is an indication of fracture of the petrous portion of the temporal bone.
   C. Bleeding or leakage of cerebrospinal fluid from the nose

is often indicative of basal skull fracture.

D. Ecchymosis of the upper eyelid or mastoid region is suggestive of such a fracture.

E. Basal skull fracture may be suggested by signs of cranial nerve damage.

F. Pneumocephalus is one of the roentgenological signs.

ANSWERS AND COMMENTS:

1. (False) A patient with a significant head injury does, in every instance, require diagnostic roentgenograms of the skull. The matter hinges on the meaning of the word significant. A patient with a minor blow to the head, confirmed by a reliable history and followed by no loss of consciousness and no neurological signs or symptoms, does not necessarily need skull roentgenograms, especially if he is a child. In this patient, the slight drowsiness and earlier confusion constituted neurological signs, albeit very minor ones. Before the physician decides not to obtain skull roentgenograms, he should consider the medicolegal side of the question. He should discuss the matter with the patient or the responsible party so that the decision to omit the roentgenological studies will be a mutual one. In the emergency department setting, if the patient or the family insists that roentgenological studies be done, it is almost always better to do them.

One criterion for this decision is whether the presence of a fracture would change the treatment.

This patient illustrates the problem well, in that skull roentgenograms showed that she had a basal skull fracture of the middle fossa which did not communicate with the sinuses or the ear. There was not much likelihood of a cerebrospinal fluid fistula developing, but it was important to know that the fracture was present, for both medical and medicolegal reasons. The patient's condition did require that she be hospitalized for observation.

A contrecoup injury is one remote from the point of impact of the head and is usually due to sudden deceleration of the moving head. Contrecoup injury is caused by the brain striking against the skull and edges of the dura, especially at the sphenoid ridge or against the free edge of the tentorium cerebelli. Such brain damage can occur whether the patient has a skull fracture or not.

2. (False) Skull fractures, unless compound or depressed, rarely, in themselves, require treatment. Compound fractures of the

cranial vault require operating room care with thorough cleansing, debridement and closure of the wound; most depressed skull fractures, as discussed in Case 31, should be elevated.

3. (G) All. In most instances, the cervical spine should be checked by at least a horizontal beam exposure (called cross-table lateral view) before the patient is moved from the stretcher or spine board on which he arrived. Until all seven cervical vertebrae are "cleared" by the radiologist or the attending physician, the head should be kept immobilized by straps or sandbags or both. Five to ten per cent of unconscious trauma patients will have a neck injury.

This patient's cervical spine roentgenograms, which included a view of the odontoid process, revealed no abnormalities. From the type of head injury she had sustained, there was a good possibility that she could have fractured one of the upper cervical vertebrae, especially the odontoid process. However, this and other bones of the upper cervical spine seem somewhat "protected," particularly in a child, although a fracture or other injury must be ruled out even in the presence of negative findings on physical examination.

4. (B, C, D, E, F) (A) It is usually <u>not</u> possible to see a basal skull fracture on a roentgenogram. Therefore, the possibility that such a fracture may be present in any patient with blunt head injury must be kept in mind during the diagnostic period. On the other hand, the presence of air in the cranial vault (pneumocephalus), on the roentgenogram (F), is diagnostic of basal skull fracture communicating with one of the paranasal sinuses or the ear.

(B) In view of the difficulty in detecting basal skull fracture by roentgenography, a careful search for physical evidence of such a fracture must be made. Blood behind the tympanic membrane (hemotympanum) must be checked for, the cerumen being removed from the external auditory canal, if necessary, for good visualization. Blood or cerebrospinal fluid coming from the external auditory canal must be interpreted as representing a basal skull fracture through the petrous portion of the temporal bone; the tympanic membrane, in this instance, is usually ruptured. Obviously, bleeding from the external ear, including the canal, must be differentiated from bleeding from within the skull. If it appears that the blood or cerebrospinal fluid is coming from the middle or inner ear, there should be no probing or irrigating of the external auditory canal, for the obvious reason that infection could thus be introduced into the cranial cavity.

(C) Bleeding or leakage of cerebrospinal fluid from the nose has the same significance; that is, a basal fracture is present, in this instance, a fracture of the anterior fossa communicating with one or more of the paranasal sinuses.

Nasal bleeding alone, without cerebrospinal fluid, is usually caused by a direct blow on the nose, usually with a fracture of the nasal bone compounded to the inside of the nose instead of the outside, although it may be compounded in both directions. If cerebrospinal fluid in the nasal or aural drainage is suspected, it can usually be detected by the ring test. A drop of the bloody fluid is placed on a piece of filter paper and allowed to spread. The spinal fluid makes a larger ring than the blood, since it penetrates the paper faster and farther from the center of the original drop. The fluid should also be tested with Dextrostix®, because glucose in the nasal secretion is diagnostic of cerebrospinal fluid rhinorrhea.

(D) When present, ecchymosis of the eyelids is a helpful sign. Usually the upper lid on one side shows this change, but sometimes both upper and lower lids do so bilaterally. Ecchymosis of the eyelids may indicate a basal skull fracture in the anterior or middle fossa, even if no cerebrospinal fluid fistula is present. In a patient with multiple injuries, the possibility must not be overlooked that a direct blow to, or contusion of, the eyelids may have caused the ecchymosis.

Another useful physical sign is bogginess or bluish discoloration of the mastoid area on one side, called Battle's sign. It is usually an indication of a basal fracture in the middle or posterior fossa.

(E) At times, the only evidence of a basal fracture is cranial nerve damage. This fact highlights the importance of a carefully performed neurological examination. The patient may have lost his sense of smell, a disorder often overlooked in the "routine" neurological examination. An impaired sense of taste at the tip of the tongue, damage to the fifth cranial nerve at its emergence from the skull and peripheral facial nerve paralysis are examples of the nerve deficits that may point to a basal skull fracture not otherwise demonstrable.

Fortunately, most patients with head injury seen in the emergency department have sustained relatively mild trauma and do not require extensive studies or hospitalization for observation or treatment. They do, however, require a very careful work-up including, usually, roentgenograms of the skull, as well as a period of observation in the emergency department. Before they are sent home, they require detailed verbal and written instructions on the circumstances under which they should return to the emergency department for re-examination. A "head sheet" listing these criteria should be a standard item in every emergency department.

::

CASE 31: DEPRESSED SKULL FRACTURE AND EPIDURAL HEMATOMA

HISTORY:

A 19-year-old man was in an automobile accident, sustaining a scalp laceration over the vertex. This was sutured in a community hospital, where skull roentgenograms were made, and showed a 3-cm wide depressed fracture of the left frontal bone. He was transferred to this hospital for evaluation of the fracure. It was uncertain whether he had been unconscious.

His level of consciousness was depressed, but he was able to give his name on being aroused. Otherwise, the results of the general and neurological examination were normal.

COURSE:

He was operated upon shortly after arrival, and the bone fragment (depressed one centimeter) was elevated. A moderately large epidural hematoma in the left frontal region was evacuated. His postoperative course was uncomplicated.

QUESTIONS:

TRUE OR FALSE:

1. Scalp lacerations should never be closed before the full series of skull roentgenograms are completed and interpreted.

2. The best way to record the level of consciousness is to use the terms <u>stupor,</u> <u>semicoma</u> or <u>coma.</u>

3. Which of the following are true about depressed skull fractures?
   A. They can be present either with or without scalp laceration.
   B. They are always associated with neurological symptoms and findings.
   C. Palpation of the scalp is always diagnostic.
   D. All require elevation of the depressed fragment.
   E. They are often followed by post-traumatic seizure disorders.

4. Epidural hematoma has which of the following characteristics?
   A. It is always due to arterial bleeding.

B. It is usually associated with fracture of the temporal bone.
C. There is 25% to 50% mortality.
D. The lucid interval is pathognomonic.
E. All of the above

ANSWERS AND COMMENTS:

1. (False) In general, scalp lacerations should be repaired promptly to stop bleeding, which may be profuse, and to convert a contaminated open wound into a clean closed wound. There is no objection of obtaining skull roentgenograms before the wound is closed, provided a light pressure dressing can be applied, to prevent both further bleeding and further contamination. If the patient has multiple injuries, investigation of these may have to take precedence over repair of scalp wounds, since closure of the scalp wound may require an hour or more. Until cervical spine roentgenograms are completed (or at least a satisfactory lateral view is obtained), one should be wary of manipulating the neck, even to apply a circumferential pressure dressing. In such a case, the wound may have to be left open and covered loosely while such studies are being completed.

2. (False) Responsiveness to the spoken voice is the preferred way to record and follow the level of consciousness of a head-injured patient. It is far superior to use of the ill-defined terms <u>stupor</u>, <u>semicoma</u>, and <u>coma</u>. If there is no response to the spoken voice, then one should try painful stimuli, such as pressing over the supraorbital nerve, pressing over the sterum, or pinching, the latter especially useful for testing for facial grimacing and active motion of the extremities.

3. (A, E) (A) Depressed fracture of the skull can occur in the absence of a scalp laceration or other visible defect in the scalp. Examples are when a patient strikes his head against a small blunt object, such as the corner of a table or when his head is struck with a hammer or pipe. Depressed fractures are usually caused by high velocity injuries, whereas linear fractures tend to be produced by low-velocity injuries. Usually, considerable force is required to depress the skull, and any patient with a history of a firm blow to the head should be suspected of having a depressed fracture, whether signs of scalp damage are visible or not.

If both a laceration and a depressed fracture are present in the same area of the scalp, one must assume that a compound depressed fracture has occurred with all of the risks of infection, not only of the wound, but also of the meninges and underlying brain.

(B) Fractures of the skull, including depressed fractures, are often not associated with neurological symptoms or signs. It is paradoxical that a patient with a depressed skull fracture may have few, if any, symptoms, whereas a patient with no skull fracture at all may be profoundly unconscious. This emphasizes the importance of treating the patient and not the fracture. This rule is especially important in the case of head-injured patients.

(C) Although the history may be helpful in determining the type of fracture likely to be present, the diagnosis must still be made by roentgenological studies. Physical examination, especially digital palpation, may also be misleading. All emergency department physicians have been misled at least once by the fact that a subgaleal hematoma can give the impression of a depressed fracture when it has a soft center and a firm rim. Therefore, one should exercise restraint when telling the patient or family about an "obvious" fracture before a definitive roentgenological examination has been completed.

(D) Whether a depressed skull fracture requires elevation is a matter of judgment on the part of the neurosurgical consultant. In children, depressed fractures almost always require operation for repair of the torn dura and elevation of the fracture. This is because focal epilepsy usually follows untreated depressed fractures, especially in children (E).

In adults, the decision about operative elevation is based on the size of the depressed segment, the depth to which it is depressed and the area of the skull in which the depressed fracture occurs. A small fragment is more likely than a large one to require elevation if it appears to be sharp, since it is likely to tear the dura and damage the brain. A depressed fragment of any size that lies over the motor strip, and one that is depressed more than a centimeter, should be elevated. All compound depressed fractures, such as this patient had, must be operated upon in order to clean up the superficial wound and the damage to, and contamination of, the dura and underlying brain.

4. (B, C) (A) Epidural bleeding is either venous or arterial, but most commonly venous. However, the most dangerous epidural hematomas are produced by bleeding from a major artery, usually the middle meningeal artery.

Except in conjunction with a depressed skull fracture, venous epidural hematomas are small and limited to the area of the fracture. This is because the dura mater in adults adheres firmly to the inner surface of the skull. Children are more likely than adults to develop epidural bleeding from diploic veins or dural sinuses.

(B) Epidural hemorrhage is usually associated with a fracture of the skull, usually a fracture of the squamous portion of the temporal bone where the groove for the middle meningeal artery is located. Any fracture that crosses this groove should lead one to suspect an epidural hematoma. Roentgenographic or echoencephalographic evidence of a shift of the midline toward the contralateral side confirms this suspicion. On this basis, along with historical and neurological evidence of a rapidly expanding intracranial mass lesion, the patient should be taken immediately to the operating room for craniectomy and control of the bleeding. Delay will almost inevitably lead to early death, due to compression of the midbrain and then the brainstem, with respiratory arrest.

However, in some adults and up to 25% of children, there is no demonstrable skull fracture, the shearing force between the skull and the dura mater accounting for the vascular tear. Two reasons for the larger percentage in children with epidural bleeding in the absence of skull fracture seem to be (1) that, in the child, the dura mater adheres more loosely to the skull and (2) that the skull in children is more elastic. Therefore, one should not fail to consider the diagnosis of epidural hematoma in the absence of a skull fracture, especially if other findings are suggestive of this condition.

(C) At least 25 to 50% of these patients die; almost 100% die without treatment.

(D) The so-called lucid interval of a few minutes to a few hours refers to the period following initial unconsciousness, during which the patient seems fairly alert, complaining only of headache. It is <u>not</u> pathognomonic of epidural hemorrhage, since it is also seen at times in patients with subdural or intracerebral hemorrhage. The danger of this interval is that bystanders, and even emergency department personnel, will misinterpret it as a sign of improvement and not take proper steps to obtain urgent treatment. Once progressive loss of consciousness, pupillary dilatation with fixation to light (usually on the side of the hematoma), and hemiparesis or decerebrate rigidity occur, the time until death is short; and life-saving surgery, comprising at least burr holes and evacuation of the hematoma, must be performed immediately.

In that connection, it should be pointed out that the pupils should not be dilated pharmacologically in the emergency department setting, since such dilation will make subsequent evaluation difficult. The progressive or sudden dilation and unresponsiveness of previously normal pupils is a strong indication of continued intracranial bleeding, and is, therefore, too important a sign to be masked pharmacologically. Dilation of the pupils of a head-trauma patient, in order to look for papilledema, is almost never justified, since (1) this sign is seldom present in the emergency department; (2) it would probably not effect a change in treatment if it were present; and (3) a second physician, seeing a patient with dilated pupils and head trauma, may do unnecessary burr holes because he does not know that the pupils had been dilated intentionally.

::

CASE 32: PENETRATING HEAD INJURY

HISTORY:

A 23-year-old man was shot in the left side of the head with a .22-caliber hand gun. He was unconscious, but breathing, when found a few minutes later. He was taken to the emergency department, where he responded to painful stimuli with decerebrate rigidity. His respirations were regular at 16/min; blood pressure, 130/82 mm Hg; pulse, 56/min and regular. There was a 1.5-cm wound of entrance over the parietal bone, 6 cm superior to the orifice of the external auditory canal. No exit wound was found. His right pupil was widely dilated and did not react to light. The results of the remainder of the examination were normal.

Skull roentgenograms showed a defect in the left parietal bone and the bullet lodged in the midportion of the right cerebral hemisphere.

QUESTIONS:

1. The following are true about penetrating wounds of the head, except:
   A. Eighty percent of patients with through-and-through head injuries die at once or within a few minutes.
   B. Loss of consciousness always occurs.
   C. Focal or focal and generalized seizures occur in the early phase of the injury in 15 to 20% of cases.
   D. The prognosis for productive life is poor in most survivors.
   E. Cerebral edema is likely to be a serious problem in the early post-injury or postoperative period.

2. Although this patient's prognosis seems hopeless, he does illustrate many of the principles involved in the management of patients with penetrating head injury. What initial steps should be taken in the diagnosis and treatment of this patient's problem?
   A. Open and maintain the airway.
   B. Assure adequate respiratory exchange and oxygenation.
   C. Call for a neurosurgical consultation.
   D. Determine the anatomical extent of the injury.
   E. All of the above

TRUE OR FALSE (Questions 3-6):

3. A lumbar puncture should usually be done on a patient with penetrating head injury for diagnosis and to relieve the increased intracerebral pressure.

4. In penetrating head injuries where the object is still protruding, immediate removal by the emergency physician is advisable.

5. A small object, such as an ice pick, is not likely to cause extensive cerebral damage.

6. In a patient who arrives conscious, following penetrating head injury, monitoring the level of consciousness is the single best way to follow his progress.

ANSWERS AND COMMENTS:

1. (B, D) (B) In penetrating head injury, the skull and brain may be only minimally displaced if the injury is due to a small, low-velocity missile, or other object, that punctures the skull. The patient may remain conscious, or he may fall down due to momentary unconsciousness. The degree of anatomical injury is what determines whether he becomes unconscious and, if so, whether he regains consciousness. Because of the extent of his injury, this patient became unconscious immediately and remained so.

(D) Many patients who have sustained a penetrating head injury recover and live useful and productive lives. Most require anticonvulsant therapy for one to two years, although some require anticonvulsant therapy for the rest of their lives.

2. (E) All. (A, B) The most common cause of death in head-injury patients is hypoxia. This means that the primary emergency department effort should be aimed at opening and maintaining the patient's airway and assisting his ventilation, if necessary. Oxygen should be added initially, but whether it is continued depends upon blood gas and pH determinations, tests that should always be done in a comatose patient with head injury. Almost invariably, the patient who is unconscious from a head injury should have endotracheal intubation with a cuffed tube. This prevents aspiration of gastric contents, such aspiration being a common cause of airway obstruction and pneumonitis. It also allows suctioning through the tube for removal of the excess tracheobronchial secretions that are usually present.

(C) There is not likely to be any initial response to the previously mentioned resuscitative procedures in a patient such as this one. However, the decision on what type of treatment, operative or expectant, to be started is a decision to be made by a neurosurgical consultant, not by the emergency department physician alone.

(D) The anatomical extent of the injury often determines whether operative treatment should be carried out. If surgical exploration is to be done, it should be started as soon as possible. This patient's decerebrate rigidity was an indication of extensive midbrain and brainstem damage; further damage would have been produced by surgical debridement of the missile tract, whether the bullet was removed or not. Also, extensive cerebral edema was sure to develop, whether the operation was carried out or not. This edema would almost certainly cause progressive neurological damage, due to herniation of the brainstem through the foramen magnum, this mechanism leading rapidly to respiratory arrest and death.

Admission to the intensive care unit for expectant care was all that was recommended by the neurosurgical consultant. The family was approached about organ donation. This is a step that should always be considered, since most transplant organs, especially the kidneys, are currently being obtained from patients with this degree of craniocerebral damage.

If a patient with a penetrating head injury of this severity is not breathing when he arrives in the emergency department, it is difficult to decide whether or not to start resuscitative measures. In the pre-hospital phase, there is no question about what to do; all patients should be given the benefit of the doubt and resuscitative efforts begun. However, when the patient arrives in the emergency department, it is more difficult for the physician to decide within the first few seconds just how vigorously he should act in getting the patient to breathe spontaneously, and how long he should persist in the artificial ventilation, including whether he should place the patient on a respirator. The possibility of organ donation may influence this decision.

3. (False) Lumbar puncture is almost never needed for diagnosis in the emergency department for any type of head injury. In a patient such as this one, lumbar puncture is absolutely contraindicated because of the likelihood of temporal lobe herniation through the tentorial incisura, or herniation of the cerebellar peduncles or brainstem into the foramen magnum. The former was probably already present in this patient.

4. (False) The emergency department is not the place for removal of a protruding object that has penetrated the skull. Bleeding can be profuse and uncontrollable if the object has punctured an artery or a dural venous sinus. This problem is best taken care of in the operating room by the neurosurgeon. However, the emergency department physician should immobilize the foreign object so that it cannot be accidentally dislodged or pushed farther into the skull or brain.

5. (False) Extensive damage may be caused immediately, depending upon the depth and direction of the object, as well as the possibility that it may have been moved in an arc or circle beyond the point of entry. Also, the injury may be overlooked completely; or, for example, if the object has punctured the eyelid, it may be believed to have only produced a puncture wound or laceration, when, in actual fact, it has penetrated the brain through the roof of the orbit. Meningitis is a common sequel, the organism depending upon the degree of contamination of the penetrating object. Such a small penetration of the bony orbit may not be visible on initial roentgenograms, if indeed, such a study is requested at all. Special views, including tomographic views, would be required to demonstrate the bony injury in most instances. Also, computerized axial tomography may be needed to demonstrate the brain damage. A high index of suspicion is needed for any type of puncture wound about the face or head so that appropriate studies will be obtained.

6. (True) It is advisable to start a neurological examination check sheet with the baseline observations, and repeat them every 10 to 30 minutes, while the patient remains in the emergency department. The response to spoken voice or to painful stimuli represents the best estimate of the level of consciousness, which, in turn, is the best single method of detecting deterioration in the patient's condition. Determination of vital signs and the other elements of the full neurological examination is also important, and the findings should be recorded serially.

COURSE:

This patient was admitted to the intensive care unit for expectant treatment and died a few hours later. No organ donation was permitted.

::

CASE 33: FACIAL FRACTURES

HISTORY:

A 20-year-old man was a passenger in the back seat of an automobile which struck a telephone pole at high speed. He was not wearing a seat belt and was thrown forward, striking his face against the back of the front seat. He may have been unconscious for a short time, since he stated that he "woke up" in the ambulance. His general health was good, and he had no history of any serious illness or injuries.

The results of the examination were negative except for the following: small pieces of broken glass in his hair and on his face; a 2-cm laceration of the right upper eyelid; multiple superficial lacerations of the forehead and face with several puncture wounds, and some avulsion-type lacerations with skin loss; tenderness and moderate swelling of the left eyelid, contusions of the left cheek with moderate swelling, but no bony deformity; and contusions of both knees. The eyes and eye movements appeared normal.

Roentgenograms of the skull, facial bones, mandible, cervical spine, chest and knees showed no abnormalities other than a "tripod" (trimalar) fracture of the left maxilla and zygomatic bone, with opacification of the left maxillary sinus (antrum).

QUESTIONS:

1. Initial treatment encompasses all of the following, <u>except</u>:
   A. Special attention to the upper airway
   B. Pharyngeal suctioning
   C. Narcotics and sedatives for pain and restlessness
   D. Immediate tracheostomy
   E. Clamping of all bleeding points
   F. Immediate repair of all lacerations

2. Which of these general statements about fractures of the facial bones are true?
   A. All fractures of the facial bones, regardless of location and degree, require reduction and fixation.
   B. The fractures are always obvious on preliminary clinical and roentgenological examination.
   C. A Water's projection is a vital part of the roentgenological examination.

D. Fractures involving the orbital-maxillary complex are usually indicated by blood in the maxillary sinus.
E. All of the above

TRUE OR FALSE (Questions 3 and 4):

3. For both cosmetic and functional reasons, maxillofacial injuries have first priority in the care of multiply-injured patients.

4. The most commonly fractured facial bone is the nasal bone.

5. Which of these statements are true regarding mandibular fractures?
   A. The most frequent fracture site is the midbody at the mental foramen.
   B. Most mandibular fractures are bilateral.
   C. Mandibular fractures are usually indicated clinically by malocclusion of the teeth.
   D. Hypesthesia or anesthesia in the distribution of the mental nerve is an indication of fracture of the condyle.
   E. Mandibular fractures are frequently difficult to diagnose on initial roentgenograms.
   F. The chief goal of treatment of mandibular fractures is restoration of normal dental occlusion.

6. Which of these statements are true regarding maxillary fractures?
   A. Malocclusion of the teeth is a useful clinical sign for diagnosis.
   B. Hypermobility can be demonstrated by grasping the anterior maxilla with the thumb and index finger, and attempting to move it in or out.
   C. Le Fort I, II, and III represent a convenient classification of maxillary fractures.
   D. All maxillary fractures must be definitively treated immediately.
   E. The coexistence of mandibular and maxillary fractures, due to blunt trauma, usually contraindicates open reduction.
   F. All of the above

7. Which one of the following statements is true regarding zygomatic fractures?
   A. Checking for loss of sensation of the face is of no help in clinical evaluation of zygomatic fracture.
   B. The "tripod" or trimalar fracture is fracture of the

zygomatic-frontal suture, the zygomatic-maxillary suture, and the zygomatic arch.

C. An isolated depressed fracture of the zygomatic arch almost never occurs.
D. Reduction of a displaced fracture of the body of the zygomatic bone can usually be done under local anesthesia and should be done immediately.
E. All of the above

8. Which of the following statements are true about an isolated fracture of the orbital floor?
   A. Such a fracture is popularly called a "blowout" fracture.
   B. The globe may be injured as well.
   C. Unfortunately, there are no clinical symptoms and signs of a blowout fracture.
   D. The roentgenological signs of a blowout fracture are usually obscure.
   E. All blowout fractures require surgical correction.

9. TRUE OR FALSE: Diplopia is a common symptom in facial fractures.

ANSWERS AND COMMENTS:

1. (C, D, E, F) (A, B, D) Special attention should be given to the airway in all such patients; this is the first priority. Foreign bodies, clotted blood, loose teeth, or broken pieces of teeth or dentures, or simply accumulation of saliva or mucus, can cause either partial or complete airway obstruction at the scene, en route to the hospital, or at any time thereafter.

An oropharyngeal or nasopharyngeal airway is a help in patients, such as this one, who do not require endotracheal intubation. If only an oropharyngeal or nasopharyngeal airway is used, careful continuous attention should be directed to the patient's airway, since obstruction below the artificial airway, such as from edema or hemorrhage, can occur after the airway has been inserted.

However, the most common cause of obstruction of the airway in obtunded patients is the tongue, which falls back against the pharyngeal wall. These obtunded patients are the ones who have the most trouble handling secretions. Either an orotracheal or nasotracheal tube should be inserted in all such patients, along with suctioning used as needed.

With extensive mandibular fractures, the tongue tends to obstruct the pharynx, even in a fully conscious patient whose jaw has been brought forward to prevent this. The reason seems to be that unstable fracture fragments prevent the tongue from following the mandible forward, as it usually does. In that event, a towel clip, suture, or even a safety pin may be placed through the tongue near its tip. It should be placed in the midline in order to reduce the tendency to bleed. Traction on the tongue then usually keeps the airway open. If these maneuvers, plus an oropharyngeal or nasopharyngeal airway, fail to obtain or maintain an open airway, other causes of obstruction in the hypopharyngeal and glottic areas should be sought.

Tracheostomy (D) is no longer indicated immediately in patients with facial fractures and contusions such as this patient had, but is still indicated in the patient with severe crushing injuries of the mid-face that will severely compromise the airway and require prolonged care, including multiple operations. If the upper airway is seriously compromised and endotracheal intubation is not technically feasible, emergency cricothyreotomy may be necessary. In that case, tracheostomy should be performed within the next few hours.

(C) Narcotics and sedatives are contraindicated, since, by depressing respirations, they may cause hypoxia. Also, many patients who are anxious, agitated, and asking for pain medication are already hypoxic, and they become much calmer when ventilation and oxygenation are improved. Vomiting and aspiration are constant threats in these patients; narcotics increase the likelihood of both. It should be remembered that pain from facial injuries is usually relatively mild, and most patients do not require narcotics for this type of facial pain.

Narcotics and sedatives are also contraindicated because they interfere with continuous monitoring of the central nervous system (by repeated neurological examination) and of the abdomen (by repeated examination for tenderness).

(E) Control of bleeding has high priority, but clamping or ligating bleeding points in lacerations of the face is unwise, because it may damage branches of the facial nerve or other nerves, or salivary gland ducts. The use of gentle pressure to control bleeding is much safer and is usually successful. One can then proceed with the necessary work-up, including roentgenograms, before taking the patient to the operating room for repair of all lacerations. A compromise may be required, of course, in the patient whose bleeding cannot be controlled by pressure, whose condition is unstable, or who has other injuries. However, relatively blind clamping or ligating of bleeding points in the emergency department, especially in a struggling patient, is to be condemned.

(F) Although repair of lacerations of the face may be safely deferred for up to 24 hours, the lacerations within the mouth may require immediate attention because of brisk or persistent bleeding. Usually, the need for immediate care can be determined at the time the airway is cleared, and a few mucosal sutures can be applied if bleeding persists and does not stop with pressure or packing, as around an airway or endotracheal tube. At times, the lacerations are deep and direct visualization of these wounds or through-and-through wounds is required, preferably in the operating room with the patient under general endotracheal anesthesia. For less extensive lacerations, local anesthesia is preferred and can be used in most patients, including children.

The reason repair of lacerations of the face, scalp and neck can be safely deferred longer than most lacerations in other parts of the body is the better blood supply to the head and neck. It allows satisfactory primary healing and decreases the tendency toward infection. It is axiomatic that patients whose wounds are repaired late, and with primary closure, require prophylactic antibiotic therapy (see Case 36 for more information about repairing facial lacerations).

2. (C, D) Any patient with a blow to the face must be considered to have a fracture until this possibility is ruled out.

Displacement of most fractures of limbs and torso is caused by the pull of the attached muscles. However, in facial fractures, except those of the mandible, the displacement is produced by the trauma itself.

(A) Not all fractures of the face require manipulation. If there is no displacement or only minimal displacement, and if the fracture is stable, it can usually be left alone.

The extensive, comminuted fractures of gunshot wounds are frequently best managed by packing, with secondary reduction and fixation to be considered later, after all infection has subsided, if this proves to be necessary. Too early attempts at reduction and fixation, especially with metal or with bone grafting, will lead to osteomyelitis or necrosis of the bone.

(B, C) Fractures of the facial bones are not always obvious on preliminary clinical and roentgenological examination. The emergency department physician must know the involved pitfalls, as well as the clues, that require further special study and consultation. Some of these are listed in the discussions that follow.

Although, in any patient who has severe facial injury, a fracture of the skull and cervical spine must be ruled out by appropriate roentgenograms, the emergency department physician must not be so concerned about possible craniocerebral injury and neck injury that he overlooks facial bone fractures. Even if he suspects such fractures, he will miss them if he fails to request, or the consulting radiologist fails to take, the necessary roentgenograms, or if those taken are of poor technical quality, due, for example, to the patient's failing to cooperate and hold still.

The single most important view for any patient who has a probable facial injury is the Water's projection. This, along with the usual lateral projections, will show most fractures of the face. Then tomograms can be used to outline the exact location and extent of the fractures. If tomography is not available, stero Water's views may be used routinely for the same purpose, although they are not always as definitive as tomograms. Special views are required for special bones, such as the nasal bone, the zygomatic arch, the mandible, or the alveolar ridge, but for screening, the Water's view cannot be surpassed and must always be done (see answer 5E for discussion about panoramic views for mandibular fractures).

(D) The maxillary sinus usually shows clouding when there is a fracture of the maxilla or floor of the orbit. This usually indicates hemorrhage into the maxillary sinus, provided acute and chronic sinusitis and mucocele can be ruled out by history and physical examination, and provided the clouding is not due to overlying soft tissue swelling. One of the clues to the need for further investigation is this clouding of the antrum - it always requires careful study of the floor of the orbit, usually by tomography, as well as careful clinical examination of the eye, including the extraocular movements. At least one lateral roentgenological projection should be with the brow up, in an effort to demonstrate an air fluid level in the antrum or the other sinuses.

3. (False) The only exception is that adequate attention be paid to the upper airway. Otherwise, craniocerebral injuries, neck injuries, and chest and abdominal injuries take precedence over maxillofacial injuries. However, care should be taken to control bleeding, due to the maxillofacial injury, by packing, if

possible, or by clamping or ligating vessels if unavoidable. Further contamination of the wounds must be prevented. Blood replacement should be arranged as needed, since it is not unusual for a patient with only facial and scalp lacerations to arrive at the emergency department with a hematocrit of less than 20%.

4. (True) The nasal bone is subject to fracture any time a person falls forward or whenever he is struck in the face by a hard object. Next in frequency of facial bone fracture are the mandible, the zygomatic-malar bones, and the maxilla. It is not unusual to see patients with at least one fracture of every major bone of the face, especially patients having been involved in high-speed automobile accidents.

For injuries of the nose, diagnostic roentgenograms should include lateral views with soft tissue technique and a superior-inferior projection.

The timing of treatment of nasal fractures depends somewhat upon the amount of edema present. If the patient is seen immediately, reduction and external splinting (the latter largely for protection from refracture) can be done at that time. However, if marked edema is already present, making accurate alignment of fragments difficult or impossible, it is best to wait a few days until the edema has subsided. Compound nasal fractures should be treated promptly by wound repair, with immediate or delayed reduction of the fracture.

Whether compound or closed, nasal fractures in children require careful reduction and protective dressing at the time of injury. This is to prevent abnormalities of growth with subsequent deformity.

5. (B, C, F) (A) As to frequency, fractures of the mandible are divided roughly into equal thirds, as follows: (1) fractures of the condylar neck; (2) fractures of the coronoid process, angle and ramus; and (3) fractures of the body of the mandible, including the alveolar ridge, plus the anterior portion of the mandible.

(B) Most mandibular fractures are bilateral, a frequent combination being a fracture at the mental region of the mandibular body on one side, with a fracture of the condyle on the opposite side. This is an important point for the physician to remember, and the less easily detected condylar fracture must be looked for. Special views and techniques may be required.

(C) Malocclusion is a helpful sign pointing to fracture of the mandible. The patient may say that his teeth don't fit together as they did before, or it may be easy to demonstrate separation of the teeth in full-bite attempt. Malocclusion is one of the most important signs to look for in clinical diagnosis of facial fractures (see answer F).

Clinical examination of the mandible for fracture involves putting the index finger in the mouth, and the thumb outside the mouth over the mandible, and checking for false motion, for palpable fractures, and for tenderness. If both sides are to be examined at the same time, the thumbs can be placed inside the mouth, with one or more of the other digits placed on either side around the mandible outside the mouth.

(D) Hypesthesia or anesthesia in the distribution of the mental nerve (sensation of the lower lip and chin) is indicative of a fracture of the body of the mandible, where the nerve (a branch of the inferior alveolar nerve) emerges at the mental foramen. It is not indicative of a fracture of the condyle.

(E) Fractures of the body of the mandible are almost always easily seen on initial films of the usual type (posteroanterior, both obliques, and an anteroposterior Towne's projection). However, fracture of the condyle or of the coronoid process may be impossible to demonstrate without special views. The emergency department physician must have a high index of suspicion for fractures in this portion of the mandible if he is to arrange for tomographic and other special studies. Even better than the previously mentioned routine, where available, is the panoramic view, which shows all parts of the mandible quite well.

(F) Restoration of normal dental occlusion is the goal of management of mandibular fractures. These fractures should usually be handled by a specialist, since in-hospital care and careful follow-up care are required. This is true of most fractures of the bones of the face, since both function and appearance are strong considerations in the management of these patients.

6. (A, B, C) (A) Malocclusion is a helpful sign in maxillary fractures, as it is in mandibular fractures. In the case of maxillary fracture, there is an open anterior bite. This should always be sought, since the initial roentgenological studies may be equivocal. In that case, the open anterior bite can be a guide to what additional special views or studies are needed. Even a minimal bite discrepancy, not present before the trauma, is highly suggestive of a displaced fracture of either the maxilla or

the mandible or both. Although malocclusion is by far the most important indication of a displaced fracture of the jaws, it may well be missed in the emergency department in the rush to get the patient to the x-ray department.

(B) Hypermobility of the maxilla can easily be demonstrated by grasping the anterior segment with the thumb and index finger. Any motion when this part of the face is pushed or pulled on is indicative of a maxillary fracture.

(C) The Le Fort classification indicates the height of the maxillary fractures. Most Le Fort fractures are bilateral, and all are associated with excessive mobility of the maxilla at the nasal bridge and zygomatic bones. Le Fort I is a fracture at the level of the floor of the antrum, with separation of the alveolar process from its attachment to the facial bony structure. Le Fort II is at the level of the orbit; only the medial section of each infraorbital rim moves with the anterior segment of the maxilla when it is pushed or pulled. Le Fort III is through the orbital area; the hypermobile segment includes the whole of each infraorbital rim.

The Le Fort system does not include vertical fractures, pure alveolar fractures, or displaced zygomatic fractures. Combinations are possible, such as a Le Fort II fracture on one side and a Le Fort III fracture on the other side.

(D) Fractures of the maxilla are not usually first priority when multiple injuries are present. Treatment may be delayed for one to two weeks, if necessary, depending upon the extent of the deformity. However, the patient should be under the care of an appropriate specialist, preferably in the hospital, at least for the first few days. Delay of repairs beyond seven to ten days may allow early fibrous union of the fracture, especially of the fine bones of the orbital floor, making reduction difficult.

The displaced fracture is reduced through re-establishment of dental occlusion, and the reduction is maintained until healing takes place. The methods used for such maintenance of reduction are beyond the scope of this discussion.

(E) Coexisting maxillary and mandibular fractures due to blunt trauma usually require, rather than contraindicate, open reduction and fixation. This emphasizes the importance of full diagnosis of the location and extent of all facial fractures when the patient is first seen.

7. (B) The zygomatic bone makes up the prominence of the cheek, which is the malar eminence. The lateral wall and floor of the orbit are extensions of the zygomatic bone, as is the anterior portion of the zygomatic arch. Damage to any part of the zygomatic bone may leave an unacceptable cosmetic deformity, which may at first be obscured by soft tissue swelling. Roentgenological studies required for proper management include a submental vertex projection.

(A) Loss of sensation of the dental alveoli of the maxilla and of the upper lip is characteristic of injury of the ipsilateral infraorbital nerve, due to fracture of the body of the zygomatic bone. Other signs of fracture are flattening of the cheek (although this may be obscured by soft tissue swelling), subconjunctival hemorrhage, and disturbance of extraocular muscle function, especially with diplopia.

(B) The "tripod" or trimalar fracture is of the zygomaticofrontal suture, the zygomatico maxillary suture, and the zygomatic arch. The body of the zygoma is frequently displaced posteriorly.

(C) An isolated depressed fracture of the zygomatic arch is common, usually being caused by a direct blow. This possibility must be considered in any facial or head injury, and appropriate clinical and roentgenological studies must be carried out. Soft tissue swelling may so obscure the usually obvious deformity that neither inspection nor palpation will reveal it. If the depression is severe, having the patient attempt to open his mouth reveals a mechanical block in front of the coronoid process of the mandible. Even less depressed fractures usually produce unacceptable deformities after the swelling subsides. It is important to obtain a submental vertex roentgenological projection when such a fracture is suspected, since elevation of the fracture should be accomplished within a few days or as soon as the patient's general condition permits.

(D) Reduction of displaced zygomatic bone fractures, except of the arch, requires general anesthesia. Various methods are available for maintenance of the fracture. Reduction can be deferred until the patient's condition stabilizes, during which time careful observation should be maintained.

8. (A, B, D, E) (A) A blow that is evenly distributed to the orbit causes the thinnest part of the orbit, the floor, to give way. This isolated fracture of the floor of the orbit is called a blowout fracture. It cannot be detected by palpation; frequently,

there are no positive physical findings. Blowout fractures not infrequently occur in the presence of other maxillofacial fractures.

A fracture of the floor of the orbit that also involves the infraorbital rim is, strictly speaking, not a blowout fracture. Differential diagnosis involves a careful and gentle check for physical signs, such as "stepping" or notching, or other irregularity, as well as for tenderness.

The floor of the orbit is also the roof of the maxillary sinus (antrum). This means that any clouding of the antrum that is thought to be related to acute trauma may represent an orbital injury.

(B) As important as it is to rule out an injury of the globe, this is often not handled well in busy emergency departments. The examination steps available in the emergency department may be limited to testing visual acuity, ophthalmoscopic examination, and the usual tests of extraocular motion and pupillary reaction. Although this may be sufficient in many patients, immediate or early follow-up examination by an ophthalmologist should be arranged if there is any suspicion, by history or examination, that the globe has been injured (see Case 35). In the meantime, the roentgenological studies to detect fracture should be completed. This patient had no evidence of injury of the globe and no evidence of entrapment of extraocular muscles.

(C) In many patients, there are clinical clues to the presence of such a fracture. Pain is likely to be present, but tenderness along the orbital rim is not always present. The two most important clinical indications of a blowout fracture are the presence of diplopia (which can occur in certain other facial fractures as well; see answer 9) and lack of mobility of the eye. If the diplopia becomes manifest when the patient looks up, this is an excellent indication of a blowout fracture. Nausea may be present constantly, or only when the patient experiences double vision.

Limitation of motion of the eyeball, if present, is caused by incarceration of the inferior rectus muscle or the inferior oblique muscle or, rarely, both muscles in the fracture. If such limitation is suspected, this can be tested by the ophthalmologist using the forced duction test, which is attempting to move the globe into the extremes of its range of motion. This finding may not appear for several days, so it must be actively pursued by the clinician on follow-up visits.

Enophthalmos is another helpful sign but it is seldom present in the acute phase because of swelling and hemorrhage. Enophthalmos is backward displacement of the eyeball and is caused by prolapse of the orbital fat into the antrum, along with the fracture fragments. Unfortunately, it usually appears after several days or weeks when the orbital reaction clears, and may be missed by all concerned unless a careful search for it is made. Also, it may be missed when the eye is more prominent than normal (proptosis), due to the presence of severe swelling and hemorrhage.

Finally, hypesthesia or anesthesia in the distribution of the infraorbital nerve (the dental alveoli and the upper lip) may indicate injury to that nerve in the floor of the orbit. However, a fracture of the zygomatic bone must be ruled out as the cause before one assumes that a blowout fracture is present from this sign alone.

(D) Some of the patients who have blowout fractures present with none of the previously mentioned signs and symptoms. In such patients, the history, a high index of suspicion, and the obtaining of special roentgenological studies (including tomograms) represent the best hope of correct diagnosis.

The roentgenological signs of a blowout fracture are often absent on conventional films. In other instances, a soft tissue mass may be seen extending into the maxillary sinus from the floor of the orbit. Tomograms usually reveal the soft tissue mass more clearly, and one or more spicules of bone may be seen, which represent the thin orbital floor projecting into the antrum.

(E) Many blowout fractures that are not apparent clinically require no operative correction. If operation is required, it can be delayed for seven to ten days with no ill effect.

One approach to repair is the one illustrated in this patient (see Course). Many specialists prefer a transcutaneous approach through the lower eyelid, with care being taken not to damage the optic nerve by dissecting too far posteriorly, or by placing an orbital floor support too far back if one is required.

In summary, the reason blowout fractures are so important is that they are fairly common and they can be missed so easily, even with excellent roentgenograms of the orbital area.

9. (True) Diplopia, or double vision, is a symptom about which

the patient should be asked in a careful, non-leading manner. However, diplopia can be tested for, and, if found, quantitated. It may be present in trimalar, blowout, and Le Fort III fractures. Interpretation should be done carefully, along with complete neurological examination, since the diplopia may be due to cranial nerve injury, rather than to extraocular muscle damage, entrapment or displacement of the eyeball. In other words, it may not be a symptom of the fracture itself, or it may be present in the absence of facial fracture.

COURSE:

This patient had repair of all his facial lacerations in the emergency department, following the principles outlined in Case 34. The eyelid laceration did not extend through the tarsus or through the edge of the eyelid. Healing was prompt and the cosmetic result excellent. No foreign body was found in any of the facial wounds.

On the second hospital day, left antrotomy, via the Caldwell-Luc approach, was carried out. Multiple fractures of the anterior wall of the antrum were noted. The comminuted fragments of the floor of the orbit were elevated and the antrum was packed. Healing was complete and there was no evidence of infection. Subsequent roentgenograms showed normal position of the orbital floor, and there was no displacement of the eyeball or extraocular muscle imbalance postoperatively. He was able to return to work in four weeks.

::

CASE 34: FACIAL LACERATIONS

HISTORY:

A 17-year-old boy was thrown over the handlebars of his bicycle when it ran into a car. He had been drinking alcoholic beverages. He had a 3-cm, full-thickness laceration of his tongue near the tip on the right side, a 2-cm laceration of the mucosal surface of the lower lip, and a 2-cm, irregular, superficial laceration of the chin; the right lateral incisor and left central incisor were chipped and the right central incisor was loose.

The chin laceration was closed with 6-0 nylon in one layer; the mucosal laceration of the lip was closed with 4-0 chromic catgut, and the tongue laceration was closed with 3-0 chromic catgut, placed as horizontal mattress sutures in the deeper layers and interrupted, inverted sutures of both the superior and inferior surfaces.

He refused any treatment for his dental injuries and was advised to see his own dentist at the earliest opportunity.

Penicillin V potassium, 500 mg, was prescribed for eight days, and he was to be seen in the plastic surgery clinic in four days for follow-up care, including removal of the sutures in the wound of the chin.

This patient and the patient presented in Case 33 illustrate the problems of laceration repair in an emergency department.

QUESTIONS:

1. TRUE OR FALSE: In the emergency department, the important thing is to get the laceration closed, with revision of the scar later, if necessary.

2. Which of these general statements about soft tissue injuries of the face are correct?
   A. Debridement should be conservative, and all possible viable tissue should be saved.
   B. Most extensive lacerations or those involving special structures should be repaired in the operating room.
   C. A special effort should be made to find and remove any foreign bodies.

D. Lacerations may be suitable for open reduction of underlying fractures.
E. All of the above

3. Repair of wounds of the face should follow which of the following principles?
   A. Eliminate dead space by careful anatomical approximation of divided muscle and subcutaneous tissues.
   B. Use subdermal absorbable sutures, and fine nylon or silk sutures, to approximate the skin.
   C. Undermine normal skin if needed to prevent wound tension.
   D. Warn the patient or family that later revision of the scar may be necessary.
   E. Apply pressure dressings to prevent hematoma formation and decrease edema formation.
   F. All of the above

TRUE OR FALSE:

4. Repair of simple lacerations usually should not have priority over the other more life-threatening injuries.

5. All traumatic lacerations are contaminated.

6. All sutures in most wounds can be removed in one week.

7. For the best cosmetic effects, wound repair should be started in the center and the gaps at each end then filled in.

8. All hair near a wound should be shaved before a wound is repaired.

9. Clear paper tape, such as Steri-Strips(TM), is useful in closing some wounds.

ANSWERS AND COMMENTS:

1. **(False)** Although the possibility of revision of scars by plastic surgeons and other specialists does exist, it is no excuse for slipshod primary repairs in the emergency department. It is important for the primary physician to differentiate those lacerations that he can repair as well as anyone else from those that should be referred immediately to a specialist. This case will outline some of the principles of plastic repair, but the technique, itself, can only be learned by <u>supervised</u> practice and by experience. Repair of facial lacerations should never be delegated to the least experienced staff member just because

such repair is so time-consuming, or in order to provide that person with experience, especially if this experience is unsupervised.

It is far better that the initial closure be done correctly than that it be done immediately. This is particularly true in the case of the more extensive wounds, especially those on the face. A few hours delay is not harmful, and this should be explained to the patient.

As in the matter of who should repair the laceration, the decision about whether the patient should be taken to the operating room is an important one. It requires mature judgment on the part of the emergency department physician and the consultant. Local conditions often dictate taking almost all patients with major lacerations to the operating room. These include hospital rules about the use of various types of anesthesia in the emergency setting, the availability of good lighting, and the possibility of obtaining and maintaining a clean atmosphere in the emergency department. The principles that have to do with the repair itself, and the location of the wound, will be touched upon in the following discussions. Most of these apply to wound repair in other parts of the body, as well.

2. (E) All. (A) Although all devitalized tissue must be removed to prevent infection, it is important to debride as conservatively as possible in order to save all viable tissue.

(B) For both cosmesis and function, it is important that extensive lacerations of the face be repaired in the operating room by a trained surgical team. This applies to lacerations of the edge of the eyelids, the nasolacrimal apparatus, the parotid gland or duct, any laceration in the area of the facial nerve, and wherever there is significant tissue loss. Repair of lacerations near joints requires special attention, since simple closure of a wound that has actually entered the joint may cause septic arthritis later.

(C) The most frequent foreign material in facial lacerations from automobile accidents is glass. Since glass may not show up on conventional roentgenograms, special soft tissue techniques, or the use of xerography, should be ordered where available. However, the most important steps are to look and feel carefully for such foreign material and to irrigate the laceration well at the time of repair. This should be done under optimal conditions, e.g., good lighting, adequate assistance, and an unhurried atmosphere, with the patient calm and quiet. These are difficult to achieve in most busy emergency departments.

(D) Before lacerations of the face are repaired, the bony injury should be known, since reduction of the underlying fracture may need to be accomplished through the laceration. This may prevent having to make a separate wound for open reduction if later attempts at closed reduction fail. The trend is toward immediate definitive care of all facial fractures, especially compound fractures, except those comminuted fractures of shotgun injury (see Case 33).

3. (F) All. (A) The three levels of a deep wound that will hold sutures are the fat-fascial junction, the fat-dermal junction, and the dermis just below the dermal-epithelial junction. Failing to approximate these separate layers, and leaving dead space in the depth of the wound invites disaster. It will allow blood (hematoma) or serum (seroma) to collect and will most likely lead to infection.

(B) The edges of the wound should be brought close together first with fine absorbable sutures in the subdermal layer, to help reduce the tendency of the scar to spread as it heals. The skin should be sutured with fine (6-0 or smaller) monofilament material, such as nylon, and the sutures should be placed close together with the skin edges accurately approximated. The sutures should be separated by no more than one-eighth to one-sixteenth of an inch, and should be one-eighth to one-sixteenth of an inch from the wound margin. Care should be taken not to tie the sutures too tightly. Usually, vertical mattress sutures are not required, but one should not hesitate to use at least a few of them if the skin edges tend to invert or markedly evert. Slight eversion of wound edges is necessary, so that the final scar will not be depressed below the skin level. Both wound edges should be at exactly the same height. Under no circumstances should one of the wound edges be allowed to roll under the other edge. Such a wound will not heal primarily, is more subject to hematoma and infection, and, because of the unevenness of the edges, will produce an unacceptable scar.

The knot should be buried if the last row of deep sutures is close to the skin surface, that is, if the dermal-epidermal layer is quite thin. This is to decrease the foreign body reaction from the knot, thereby reducing the risk of infection. The technique is to move the needle from deep to superficial on the first side, and then from superficial to deep on the other side, making sure that the two bites are symmetrical, that is, that they are in the same layer of tissue and at the same depth and width from the wound edge. When the suture is tied, the knot flips over to the deeper side, making it farther away from the skin surface.

The skin sutures should be placed so that the depth is greater than the width, in order to produce the slight eversion that is needed. To reverse this relationship is to encourage or actually cause the wound edges to invert, which will produce a more noticeable scar after final scar tissue contracture has taken place.

The needle should emerge from one wound edge equidistant from where it was inserted in the other side of the wound. Also, the depth of the bite must be the same on both sides. In other words, the suture placement must be as nearly symmetrical as possible.

The first loop of the suture should be pulled to whichever side of the wound tends to be more depressed, and it should be locked before the final knots are placed. This tends to elevate the low side to the level of the other side. It is not necessary to lock all of the sutures on the same side of the wound just in order to make the wound look nice. As many as four to six knots may be required to prevent subsequent loosening and possible untying; the latter is particularly a hazard with nylon sutures.

By all means possible, stitch marks, stitch holes and cut-over marks must be avoided. Not only are they unsightly, but they are difficult to remove by revision of the scar. Closing wounds under tension, using suture material too large, taking needle bites too far back from the wound edge, and leaving the sutures in too long all contribute to this gross deficiency in wound care.

(C) If there is any tension on the wound, it must be relieved by careful subcutaneous undermining of the edges of the wound. Wounds closed under tension tend, at worst, to disrupt, and, at best, produce unsightly scars. Another way to relieve tension is to close the deeper layers separately with absorbable suture material. If tension on the skin edges is still present, the sutures should be placed closer together and closer to the wound edge, not the reverse, as is sometimes taught and practiced.

(D) There is no argument about whether the patient or his family should be warned about the possible need for revision of the scar in 12 to 15 months, or at some later time. Generally, as has been mentioned, consultation with a plastic surgeon or other appropriate surgical specialist is advisable before repair of extensive wounds in special locations (such as the lips, the eyelids, or the area around the medial canthus) is undertaken. Split-thickness skin grafting will be required if skin loss is extensive, and some wounds require complete excision with closure in a straight line. The general rule should be to seek consultation or assistance, or to refer the patient if the repair is beyond the emergency physician's skill, or if it requires more time than he is able to devote to it and still be available to care for other emergency patients. In certain patients, or for certain types and locations of wounds, even the most expert primary repair will be followed by excessive hypertrophy of the scar, even keloid formation.

(E) If possible, pressure dressings should be applied, but early (one to three days) change of the dressings should be arranged in most instances.

4. (True) Although it should be self-evident that potentially life-threatening conditions take precedence over soft tissue wound repair, this principle is often violated in emergency departments. An example is taking time to repair a laceration of the face or ear in a patient who has thoracic and abdominal injuries with internal bleeding. At the very least, the major injuries should be diagnosed and, if possible, corrected or controlled <u>before</u> the soft-tissue wounds are sutured.

5. (True) All traumatic lacerations are contaminated by skin bacteria and bacteria on the instrument or weapon of injury. Further contamination occurs after injury if the wound has been exposed or has been touched or dressed with an unclean object. Gross contamination occurs at times when well-meaning patients or friends apply liquid, ointment or other material, even soot, to the wound.

If there is crushed tissue present, it must be identified and debrided. However, there are locations where debridement causes more problems than it alleviates, locations such as the lip, the free edges of the nares and of the eyelids, and certain other parts of the face.

In some instances, the entire crushed or dirty wound should be excised with primary closure of the resulting clean wound. There are special techniques for this, and one should generally defer to the consultant for such a repair. The same can be said about special techniques of plastic closure, such as the dog-ear maneuver, W-plasty, S-plasty, and Z-plasty.

6. (False) It is a sure indication of an inexperienced emergency

department physician if he advises all patients to have their sutures removed in a week. In some wounds, as of the face, this is much too long. In some, as of the leg or foot, this is much too short. Besides the location of the wound, the type of suture material used affects this matter. However, it has less to do with the depth and length of the wound than most people think, provided multilayer closure is used when indicated. Often, sutures should be removed in stages, with an early return visit scheduled for inspection and removal of sutures that are too tight, and for removal of a drain if one is left in. The remaining sutures may be removed at one or more subsequent visits.

7. (False) If key points are present, such as the vermilion-cutaneous border of the lip or a sharp angle, the first sutures should be placed at these points in order to align the wound edges. In a straight, elliptical wound, as on the abdomen or thigh, the skin repair should be started at the ends, working toward the center. The sutures used to approximate the deeper layers must be approached in the same manner, with care being taken not to get the skin layer out of alignment.

8. (False) Shaving hair from around the wound is helpful in most instances; it facilitates the cleansing of both the wound and the surrounding skin. However, this shaving should be done conservatively in some parts of the body, including the scalp. Eyebrows and eyelashes should be shaved or clipped only if there is no way to avoid it: eyebrows may not regrow properly, if at all, and leaving them in place may help to align the wound edges.

9. (True) The use of clear or paper tape strips is becoming more and more popular, either as a substitute for sutures in superficial wounds or as a supplement to the suture closure of a wound. These strips can also be used to hold the skin edges in exact approximation and avoid inadvertent wound disruption, as in children, following early removal of skin sutures. For the patient who refuses suture repair - not an uncommon experience in an emergency department - such material can serve as a reasonably satisfactory substitute, provided the wound is not too deep.

COURSE:

The final result is not known on this patient, but at his initial return visit, he was doing quite well, with all wounds healing satisfactorily.

::

CASE 35: INJURY TO THE EYE

HISTORY:

A 15-year-old boy was playing football when he was struck in the right eye by another player's finger. He experienced immediate pain in the eye and blurring of his vision. He was not rendered unconscious.

The findings on general and ophthalmological examination were negative, except for swelling and bluish discoloration of the lower eyelid, and blood layered in the inferior portion of the anterior chamber of the right eye. Pupils, extraocular movements, and fundi showed no abnormality. Uncorrected visual acuity in the right eye was 20/40 and in the left eye 20/20 (Rosenbaum near-vision card): his uncorrected vision by history had been 20/20 bilaterally.

QUESTIONS:

1. TRUE OR FALSE: A small amount of blood in the anterior chamber is not serious and the patient can usually be treated on an ambulatory basis.

2. Which of the following general statements concerning eye injuries are true?
   A. The most common cause of eye injuries in childhood is a thrown object.
   B. If the eyelids or the globe are lacerated, an intraocular foreign body must be ruled out.
   C. The two true ocular emergencies are chemical burns of the eyeball and central retinal artery occlusion.
   D. Most patients with laceration or penetration of the globe should be given antimicrobial medication parenterally, as soon as possible.
   E. All of the above

3. TRUE OR FALSE: A black eye (periorbital ecchymosis) often masks serious damage.

4. Which of the following general statements about evaluating eye injuries in the emergency department are true?
   A. It can usually be left for an ophthalmologist to do later.
   B. Special equipment not available in most emergency departments is required.

C. Determination of visual acuity must be done first.
D. The history is not likely to be helpful in diagnosis.
E. Improper handling of the eye during examination can make an injury worse.
F. It is not advisable to dilate the pupil routinely in the emergency department in order to make the examination easier and more complete.

5. Which of the following statements about ocular foreignbodies are true?
   A. They represent the most frequent cause of eye injury.
   B. Their most common site is on the tarsal plate beneath the upper lid.
   C. They should not be removed until after visual acuity is checked and recorded.
   D. Fluorescein staining is of little value in their diagnosis.
   E. Irrigation should be the first means tried to remove them from either the cornea or the conjunctiva.
   F. They can usually be removed from the cornea without sterile topical anesthetic being applied.
   G. They are best removed with a sterile, moistened, cotton-tipped applicator stick.
   H. The rust ring, associated with certain metallic foreign bodies, will gradually fade and may safely be left alone

6. TRUE OR FALSE: Chemical injuries or "burns" of the eye, like third-degree cutaneous burns, are usually painless.

ANSWERS AND COMMENTS:

1. (False) The patient must be hospitalized and kept at bed rest for several days, preferably under the care of an ophthalmologist. Blood in the anterior chamber of the eye (hyphema) is usually due to blunt trauma to the globe, which causes cleavage of the ciliary body. Hyphema must be suspected and searched for in every patient who has a history suggesting contusion of the orbit or the globe.

Diagnosis can usually be made by inspection of the eye, using a penlight with a focused beam. The blood is either bright red or dark red. It canbe missed if it ispresent in the anterior chamber in small amounts, the examination is performed cursorily, or the physician does not recognize it as blood or understand the significance of its presence.

Occasionally, swelling of the eyelids will prevent an adequate initial examination of the eye, even by an ophthalmologist. However, the consequences of missing the diagnosis of hyphema, for whatever reason, are serious. Secondary hemorrhage is a threat in all patients, regardless of the size of the hyphema. Other serious complications are profound staining of the cornea with blood pigment, which can permanently impair vision, and secondary glaucoma. For these reasons, all patients with hyphema, regardless of its size, must be treated in the hospital by an ophthalmologist. In addition to being placed on absolute bed rest with his head elevated at about 60°, the patient should have patches on both eyes, be sedated, and be given an antiemetic to prevent vomiting, since vomiting may precipitate secondary hemorrhage. Other treatment that may be required is use of a miotic to increase the outflow of blood as it increases the outflow of aqueous fluid in glaucoma, and the use of an osmotic diuretic, usually glycerol or mannitol. If these measures fail to control the increased intraocular pressure, paracentesis is required. Irrigation of the anterior chamber with instillation of fibrinolysin may be helpful if elevated intraocular pressure persists.

If a hyphema is suspected but cannot be verified, the patient should be checked again by the primary physician or seen in consultation by an ophthalmologist in one to three days. During this interim, he should be confined to bed and wear bilateral eye patches. If this approach is not feasible, or if he cannot be depended upon to follow it, his admission to the hospital for observation, including daily examination, is probably indicated.

2. (E) All. (A) Children are usually unaware that direct trauma to the eye can cause serious damage, and thus often fail to try to avoid such trauma. The most common injuries in this age group are from thrown objects, such as a ball or a rock, followed in frequency by mechanically projected objects, such as an air rifle pellet, an arrow, or a stone from a slingshot.

(B) Intraocular foreign bodies may be overlooked unless there is a clue to their presence from the history or the examination. Their presence must be included whenever the eye appears to have a lacerating or penetrating injury, however small.

The cornea, if penetrated, simulates foreign body sensation when the eyelid moves over the site of injury. Any hemorrhagic area in the bulbar conjunctiva should be suspected as the point of entrance of a foreign body, even in the absence of a history of an injury, since some penetrating eye injuries are almost painless when they first occur.

(C) There are many urgent eye injuries and diseases, but none quite so demanding of immediate treatment as these two. However, all patients with eye injuries should be given high priority in an emergency department. See answer 6 for a discussion of chemical injuries of the eyes and Case 36 for a discussion of central retinal artery occlusion.

(D) For all lacerations or penetrations of the globe, the patient should be given antimicrobial medication parenterally, as soon as possible. No one has an eye to spare, and the loss of vision due to a preventable infection is particularly tragic. Often forgotten, but extremely important, is the advisability of administering tetanus prophylaxis in such patients.

3. (True) Although swelling of the lids following trauma can make evaluation of the globe difficult, it is always necessary to rule out occult injuries, such as rupture of the lens capsule, dislocation of the lens, tearing of the choroid with choroidal hemorrhage, and retinal detachment. Complications such as traumatic iridocyclitis, must be detected or ruled out. Since some of these require careful determination of visual acuity and ophthalmoscopic examination for diagnosis, they should be looked for, when possible, before the eyelid swelling becomes severe. The eyelid swelling may also mask orbital injury, as mentioned in Case 33. One sign of a blowout fracture (fracture of the floor of the orbit) is enophthalmos, which may not be detected if severe eyelid swelling is already present. On the other hand, the only clinical sign of a blowout fracture may be the swelling and discoloration of the lids. Therefore, whether or not the globe can be examined satisfactorily on the initial visit, an orbital fracture must be ruled out by appropriate roentgenological studies, and arrangements must be made for consultation and follow-up examination. In addition, a fracture of the base of the skull may be manifested only by ecchymosis of the eyelids. Thus, in a patient with a black eye induced by trauma, roentgenograms of the skull, as well as of the face, are usually indicated. Since basilar skull fracture is often undetectable on routine roentgenological studies, special studies may be required.

4. (C, E, F) Much of the following applies to examination for any eye problem, but it is specifically directed toward the examination in the presence of eye injuries.

(A) The examination must be done as soon as possible by either the emergency department physician or the ophthalmologist, preferably both. Patients with eye injuries should be given high priority and checked, at least briefly, as soon as they arrive. This should assure adequate screening and prompt diagnosis and management for those patients whose eye injuries are unexpectedly severe. It also prevents a false complaint of deterioration of visual acuity while the patient waits for a definitive examination.

(B) The equipment and supplies needed for proper diagnosis and management of the vast majority of eye injuries and diseases in the emergency department are relatively simple. At a minimum, there should be: an eyechart for determining visual acuity; a penlight; an ophthalmoscope; applicator sticks for everting the upper lid; a topical anesthetic; sterile fluorescein strips; a hypodermic needle (#27) on a 5-ml syringe for removal of foreign bodies from the corneal surface; sterile irrigating solution; a magnification loupe; and eye patches and metal shields. A blue light is useful for looking for injury of the conjunctiva and cornea following fluorescein staining, but is not essential. The emergency department physician should develop expertise in using this equipment and in evaluating what he finds. In many places, a slit lamp is available in the emergency department or in a nearby clinic. A Schiotz or other tonometer, if available, should be used for determining intraocular pressure.

(C) The ideal time to check visual acuity is as soon as the patient arrives. Visual acuity should be checked in the best way possible, as in an ophthalmologist's office, using a well-lighted chart or projected letters or symbols appropriate to the patient's age and intelligence, preferably the usual 20-foot distance away. However, modification must be made according to the circumstances and the equipment available. A nonambulatory patient with possible multiple injuries may have to be tested with a near-chart only, such as the Rosenbaum Pocket Vision Screener held 14 inches from the eye, as was used in this patient. For patients unable to see the largest character on the chart used, visual acuity may have to be estimated by determining ability at finger counting (F.C.), hand movement detection (H.M.), or light perception (L.P.), in decreasing order of acuity. If the patient is unable to see at all, the term "no light perception" is preferable to "blind," which is confusing, since "blind" is used clinically for various stages of loss of sight.

Visual acuity should be determined for each eye separately, with and without correction, if this is feasible. If glasses are worn but are unavailable, a card with a pin hole, held in front of the eye being tested, is a fair substitute for the correction of glasses. The best corrected vision for each eye is the most important item to record.

This testing has considerable medicolegal significance and should never be omitted in the emergency department, unless the patient will be seen immediately by the ophthalmologist, and possibly not even then.

(D) The history is likely to be the most important part of the etiological diagnosis, and it can be definitive for the anatomical diagnosis, since the circumstances of the accident usually suggest the nature of the injury.

(E) Improper handling of the patient, especially the eye itself, can convert a trivial injury into one that is serious enough to eventuate in blindness.

At no time should the globe be pressed directly, including when the upper lid is everted. Even the pressure of severe blepharospasm must be avoided in a patient suspected of having a penetrating ocular injury. To examine the eye, the upper lid can be elevated by pushing up on the brow against the superior orbital rim, and the lower lid can be retracted by gently pressing against the inferior orbital rim and pulling the eyelid down. Instillation of a drop or two of sterile topical anesthetic solution in the eye will relieve most of the pain and blepharospasm, allowing adequate examination in most instances.

In areas where an ophthalmologist is not readily available, it is often better to do nothing for a patient with a severe eye injury than to do a wrong thing that would jeopardize his sight. The specialist should be contacted by telephone or radio for advice and assistance, even when consultation will be delayed for hours. This failure to treat his injury, and the reason for the delay, must be explained to the patient and family.

There is no easy way to examine the uncooperative patient, whether a child or an adult. If justified by the suspected seriousness of the eye injury, sedation (even general anesthesia) should be used.

(F) Although circumstances vary widely in emergency departments, routine dilatation of the pupil is unwise. There are risks involved, and the additional information gained does not justify those risks. This maneuver may precipitate an attack of glaucoma or cause an acute glaucoma attack to become worse, unless one has ruled out this possibility by measuring intraocular pressure. (Digital pressure may be useful for screening but is not sufficiently accurate for this purpose.) As mentioned in Case 31, in the patient who has sustained head injury as well, dilatation of the pupils may mask neurological changes or make them impossible to evaluate.

5. (A, B, C, E) (A) Foreign bodies lodged on the globe or the eyelids represent the most common cause of eye injury. The vast majority of these can be removed in the emergency department, with the patient referred to an ophthalmologist for a follow-up visit within one to three days.

(B) The most common site of a foreign body is on the medial portion of the tarsal plate of the upper lid.

(C) As discussed in answer 4C, visual acuity should always be checked before any manipulation or treatment of the eye is done, with the exception noted in answer 6.

(D) Fluorescein staining shows up corneal irregularities, including abrasions, lacerations and foreign bodies. This examination is enhanced by the use of magnification, such as one gets from a loupe or an ophthalmoscope. Fluorescein strips are much preferred to the solution (except in individual vials), since solution used over and over often harbors pseudomonas organisms, which can destroy a cornea within hours. Putting a drop of sterile saline or water on the tip of the strip is better than touching the dry strip to the sclera and waiting for tears to wet it.

The use of a blue light is optional for finding foreign bodies in the eye, as well as abrasions of the cornea. However, since such lighting highlights a fluorescein-stained area of the eye by making it bright yellow, it is well worth having a pocket flashlight with blue light or a Wood's light in the emergency department. A piece of blue cellophane over the end of a penlight is frequently a satisfactory substitute.

(E) Following the recording of visual acuity, the single most important step in examining the patient for foreign body is eversion of the upper and lower lids. This is done for the upper lid by asking the patient to look down, grasping the eyelashes with the fingers of one hand, and laying a cotton-tipped applicator along the outside of the lid without pressing on the globe. The upper lid can be turned upward over the applicator, which can then be removed, leaving the lid everted at the level of the superior border of the tarsal plate. The undersurface of the lid can then be inspected carefully for debris or a discrete foreign body, and it and the cul de sac can be inspected and irrigated well. Rarely, a foreign body can lodge in the upper cul de sac and be difficult to remove by irrigation or by forceps. For this location, double eversion of the upper eyelid may be required.

Normally, there is immediate relief after removal of the foreign body, but discomfort may persist if the cornea has been scratched. In any case, antibiotic drops or ointment should be prescribed, and the patient should be warned that at least a few hours of persistent pain should be expected.

(F) Sterile topical anesthetic is almost always required for removal of ocular foreign bodies, except possibly those that wash out easily. It may be required in a patient who has severe blepharospasm due to pain, nervous tension, or fright, or may be required even before an eyelid can be everted. In any case, the cornea is too sensitive in most patients to allow removal of a foreign body without one or more drops of an anesthetic. To a lesser degree, the same can be said about a conjunctival foreign body.

Any sterile ophthalmic anesthetic is satisfactory, but usually one of the following is used: tetracaine hydrochloride 0.5%; proparacaine hydrochloride 0.5%; or benoxinate hydrochloride 0.4% to 1%. A second dose may be required after a few minutes in some patients, especially for removal of foreign bodies from the cornea. In children, premedication may also be required.

(G) Oblique, focal illumination with a penlight can be used to cast the shadow of a corneal foreign body onto the iris. Once a corneal foreign body has been detected, a cotton-tipped applicator stick should not be used to remove it, since this method damages or removes too much corneal epithelium. Rather, irrigation should be tried first, since it can be done in some patients without topical anesthesia and since there is always some additional trauma during mechanical removal of a foreign body imbedded in the cornea. Unfortunately, few imbedded objects will yield to irrigation alone. If irrigation fails to dislodge an object, a small (#27) hypodermic needle (on a small syringe) or a special spud may be used under magnification, with minimal damage to the epithelium. It must be remembered that while the cornea is tough, it is also very thin (1 mm). A loupe frequently provides sufficient magnification, although a slit lamp may be necessary for removal of deeply imbedded objects. Use of the latter allows better control and removal of less epithelium, and helps prevent perforation into the anterior chamber, which must be avoided at all costs.

Careful, even daily, follow-up should be arranged as long as there is a possibility of infection with scarring. Even a small corneal scar in the pupillary area can distort vision (see answer H).

Local antibiotics, such as chloramphenicol ophthalmic drops 0.5 to 1.0%, should be instilled hourly for several hours, then every 4 hours for several days. The reasons are that every foreign body leaves a corneal wound that is subject to infection, and the foreign body itself may have carried virulent organisms.

A short-acting cycloplegic may be indicated to reduce the effects of secondary iritis. The same is true for corneal abrasion without foreign body. Usually, tropicamide 0.5 to 1%, or cyclopentolate 0.5% drops, is used for several days, although a single initial dose is all that is used by many clinicians.

An eye patch is seldom required following removal of a foreign body. It may encourage infection, and the use of the medications just mentioned is far more important than having the eye covered.

Regardless of the means used to remove the foreign body, the examiner must be sure that every foreign body has been removed. If left in the eyeball, even a small foreign body may cause permanent loss of vision or loss of the eyeball, as well, from hemorrhage, infection or detached retina. Ocular foreign bodies are frequently multiple, and if one is removed from the conjunctiva or the cornea, the examiner should not immediately conclude that that takes care of the matter. If a foreign body is found on the cornea, it is still necessary to evert the upper lid and look for additional foreign bodies. If a topical anesthetic has been used, the patient will no longer feel any discomfort on blinking, and a retained, undetected foreign body may damage his cornea or lid before the anesthetic wears off. Also, it is inconvenient to all concerned when a patient has to return to the emergency department to have additional foreign bodies removed.

(H) A rust ring is a halo of corneal staining that surrounds certain metallic foreign bodies, chiefly iron. If possible, the ring must be removed at the same time the metallic foreign body is removed. An unremoved rust ring continues to irritate the eye and can cause corneal scarring. However, the emergency physician should not damage the cornea unnecessarily in order to remove the rust ring, since it can be removed safely 24 to 48 hours later by an ophthalmologist using special equipment, such as a dental burr under slit lamp magnification.

6. (False) The patient usually has severe pain and requires a narcotic, as well as a topical anesthetic, for relief and to allow him to cooperate during examination and treatment.

Any ocular chemical burn is serious, in that it can result in permanent corneal scarring and visual loss. Thus, a chemical burn of the eye is a true emergency. No preliminaries, such as obtaining a detailed history or doing a full examination, should be allowed to delay treatment, which is immediate, prolonged, and copious irrigation. This is one of the instances when visual acuity should not be tested before any ocular manipulation is carried out. A lid speculum is very useful for irrigating the eye.

Acids precipitate tissue protein, and this tends to localize the damage to the area of contact. A pH of less than 2.5 (as contrasted with a pH of 7.0 for tears) is likely to seriously damage ocular tissue, although buffering by the surrounding tissue proteins helps to counteract that damage. Examination shows redness and edema of the conjunctiva, with an opaque corneal epithelium. However, as this superficial layer sloughs, the underlying corneal stroma is usually clear. In other words, further penetration is not the rule, unless the acid is very strong and present in large amounts.

Initially, an alkali burn appears innocuous, but alkali continues to penetrate and the release of hydroxyl ions causes the injury to progress. The true extent of an alkali burn is not apparent for three or more days. The higher the pH (especially a pH of 11.0 to 12.0), the worse the damage. Scarring of the cornea is due to combination of the chemical with the lipids of the cellular membranes of the cornea; this softens the tissues, allowing more rapid penetration into the deep corneal layers and even the anterior chamber. Ammonium hydroxide is especially damaging to the cornea.

Calcium oxide, in the form of lime or plaster, is a common cause of damage, since undissolved lime adheres to the cornea and bulbar conjunctiva and dissolves slowly, thereby causing prolonged damage even after seemingly minor burns.

Therapy for all types of chemical burns (acid, alkali and unknown) is copious irrigation of the eye with any type of nontoxic liquid available, preferably water (as in the home or on the job) or physiological saline (as in the emergency department). The irrigation should be continued for at least 30 minutes, using at least 2 liters, or until the pH of the conjunctival fornices (as tested by nitrazine paper) has returned to 7.0. Any particles of the chemical must be removed mechanically if they cannot be washed out.

Local and systemic antibiotics are also indicated to decrease infection, which is always present. For this reason, corticosteroids are of questionable value, although they may make the patient more comfortable.

In addition, a cycloplegic should be instilled as soon as the initial irrigation is completed. Recently cysteine and other collagenase inhibitors have been found to be of value in preventing one of the most dreaded complications, perforation into the globe.

COURSE:

This patient was admitted to the hospital and progressed satisfactorily with no complications. The hyphema was gradually resorbed. A long-term follow-up note was not available.

::

CASE 36: ITCHING, BURNING, AND SWELLING OF LEFT EYE IN A 3-YEAR-OLD GIRL

HISTORY:

A 3-year-old girl was brought to the emergency department with a three-day history of itching, burning and swelling of the left eye. There was no definite history of trauma, but there was a questionable history of a bee sting of the upper lid. Because of itching and burning, she had rubbed her eye a great deal. She had no known allergy to medications and had no other allergic history.

Examination was not remarkable except for periorbital erythema and swelling, with mucopurulent discharge coming from the palpebral fissure of the left eye. The conjunctiva was diffusely hyperemic.

Gram's stain and culture of the exudate showed, respectively, gram-positive cocci in short chains and beta-hemolytic streptococcus. The diagnosis was bacterial conjunctivitis and periorbital cellulitis.

The patient was seen by an ophthalmologist, who started treatment with neomycin-hydrocortisone-polymyxin B, two drops four times daily in each eye, and nafcillin, 125 mg orally every six hours. When she was rechecked in the eye clinic two days later, she was much improved, but her mother was advised to continue the medications for a total of 10 days and to bring the child back for another checkup.

The emphasis of the following questions and answers will be on some of the eye diseases that require urgent diagnosis and treatment.

QUESTIONS:

1. Which of the following are true about conjunctivitis?
   A. It is very common and it may be acute or chronic.
   B. It is caused primarily by bacteria.
   C. It always affects both the bulbar and palpebral conjunctivae
   D. It is always bilateral.
   E. It is extremely painful.
   F. It almost always impairs vision.
   G. It is seen at all ages.

2. Treatment of bacterial conjunctivitis comprises the routine use of which two of the following?
   A. Topical antibiotic solution or ointment
   B. Systemic antibiotics
   C. Warm compresses
   D. Topical corticosteroid treatment
   E. Eye patch

TRUE OR FALSE (Questions 3 and 4):

3. Conjunctivitis is not likely to be confused with more serious eye disease.

4. Even in the absence of a history of trauma, a subconjunctival hemorrhage is usually a sign of serious eye disease.

5. Which of the following are true about dacryocystitis?
   A. It is found only in the acute form.
   B. It is always bilateral.
   C. It is almost always associated with obstruction of the nasolacrimal duct.
   D. It occurs only in adults.
   E. It is usually caused by Staphylococcus pyogenes, Diplococcus pneumoniae or Hemophilus influenzae.
   F. Its cause can usually be determined by stained smear and culture of the purulent discharge.
   G. Topical antibiotics are sufficient for treatment.

TRUE OR FALSE:

6. Central retinal artery occlusion presents as a unilateral, painless loss of vision and occurs in elderly persons.

7. Detachment of the retina is frequently characterized ophthalmoscopically by a translucent fold that bulges inward.

8. Temporal arteritis is not a primary disease of the eyes but can seriously threaten sight.

9. Orbital cellulitis requires immediate diagnosis and treatment to prevent complicating cerebral abscess.

10. The most common and the most important systemic disease leading to visual impairment, even blindness, is diabetes mellitus.

ANSWERS AND COMMENTS:

1. (A, B, C, G) (A) Conjunctivitis is the most common eye disease in the western world. It varies in severity from mild hyperemia to membranous changes indicating severe necrosis. Acute conjunctivitis is the type we are most concerned with in this case study and discussion, although patients with subacute or chronic conjunctivitis are occasionally seen in emergency departments in this country.

(B) There are many causes of acute conjunctivitis, including irritants, such as smoke or smog, as well as allergic (atopic) causes. These must be considered in the differential diagnosis, but the most important causes are microorganisms. These include various bacteria, such as beta-hemolytic streptococcus (especially in children, as in this patient), gonococcus, staphylococcus, pneumococcus, and meningococcus. Viral causes are herpes simplex types 1 and 2, adenovirus types 3 and 7 (pharyngoconjunctival fever), as well as adenovirus types 8 and 19 (epidemic keratoconjunctivitis). Chlamydial causes are trachoma (rare in the United States), inclusion conjunctivitis, and lymphogranuloma venereum.

The lay term "pink eye" usually refers to an epidemic form of acute conjunctivitis, caused by pneumococcus in temperate climates and Hemophilus aegyptius in hot climates.

Bacterial acute conjunctivitis is the most common and the most treatable form in the western world. The most dangerous of the bacterial conjunctivitises is that caused by Neisseria gonorrhoeae, since it may lead to corneal ulceration, even perforation.

Clinical differentiation of the different types of conjunctivitis is limited, but the following points may be helpful: (1) The purulent discharge is likely to be profuse with bacterial conjunctivitis. Tearing is increased considerably in viral conjunctivitis. The presence of preauricular adenopathy points more toward a viral cause, since that sign is unusual in bacterial conjunctivitis. Itching is a prominent feature in atropic or allergic conjunctivitis. The injection or hyperemia of the conjunctiva is similar in type and degree in all of the acute conjunctivitises. (2) Viral conjunctivitis is suggested if the stained smear (Gram's or Giemsa stain) shows predominantly monocytes. Whereas bacterial conjunctivitis is characterized by bacteria and polymorphonuclear cells, a fungal conjunctivitis is characterized by hyphae on a potassium hydroxide (KOH)-stained preparation. In allergic conjunctivitis, eosinophils are likely to predominate.

(C) Both bulbar (globe) and palpebral (eyelid) involvement are almost always present, although one or the other may predominate.

(D) Although acute bacterial conjunctivitis is often bilateral, it usually begins in one eye. It spreads to the other eye in the absence of treatment and in the presence of poor hygiene. Allergic conjunctivitis is usually bilateral at all stages.

(E) Acute conjunctivitis causes almost no actual pain, although itching, even stinging, and heaviness of the eyes are frequent.

(F) Vision is usually not impaired, an important differential point among eye diseases. Careful checking of the best corrected visual acuity must be emphasized at this point. Visual acuity should be checked in some manner the first time the patient is seen and each time thereafter. If no chart is available, the ability to read newsprint indicates at least 20/40 or 20/50 vision. If the patient normally wears glasses and they are available, the eyes should be checked with and without them. The use of a card with a pinhole, to substitute for glasses, helps rule out visual loss due to lack of glasses or to improper glasses. If the patient's vision improves on looking through a pinhole, a refractive error is present. If not, disease or injury of the eye as a cause of the decreased vision must be looked for.

(G) Acute conjunctivitis occurs at all ages and is especially serious in the newborn, being capable of causing blindness within 24 hours. This applies mainly to the gonococcal type, but the staphylococcal and chlamydial (inclusion blennorrhea) types are also serious. Gonococcal ophthalmia neonatorum is rare where silver nitrate prophylaxis is practiced.

2. (A, C) (A) An antibiotic solution or ointment should be used routinely, but systemic antibiotics (B) are not usually required. This child's disease was an exception, because it was feared that her eyelid cellulitis had caused orbital cellulitis, although the usual mechanism of this condition is spread from an infected paranasal sinus (see question and answer 9).

Another exception is inclusion blennorrhea, which should be treated with systemic tetracycline or sulfonamide, or both, in children and adults (eyedrops of tetracycline or sulfonamide in newborns).

One very important exception is gonococcal conjunctivitis, in which topical therapy alone is <u>not</u> recommended. If it is in a neonate, gonococcal conjunctivitis requires penicillin G crystalline (not aqueous procaine), 50, 000 units/kg/day intravenously or intramuscularly in two to three doses for seven days. The infant should be in the hospital. Even larger doses are required if complications, such as meningitis or septicemia, have developed. Saline irrigations of the eyes and penicillin, tetracycline, or chloramphenicol eyedrops should be used.

For childhood gonococcal ophthalmia, hospitalization is also required and treatment should include crystalline penicillin G, 75, 000 to 1, 000, 000 units/kg/day in four doses for seven days, saline irrigations and instillation of penicillin, tetracycline or chloramphenicol eyedrops. For older children, aqueous procaine penicillin G can be used, given intramuscularly 75, 000 to 100, 000 units/kg/day in two doses for seven days. If the child is allergic to penicillin, erythromycin may be substituted in the dose of 40 mg/kg/day in four oral doses for at least seven days.

For adults with gonococcal conjunctivitis, the treatment is topical penicillin G ointment, plus probenecid, 1 gm orally; the probenecid is to be followed in 30 minutes by 4. 8 million units of aqueous procaine penicillin G. Follow-up doses of ampicillin, 500 mg orally or intramuscularly, are also indicated, preferably given in the hospital, where constant observation for allergic reaction is feasible and where one is sure of compliance with this regimen. For adults who are sensitive to penicillin, oral and topical tetracycline should be used in the same treatment schedule as for genitourinary gonorrhea, plus topical or systemic therapy with erythromycin, 0. 5% ointment or liquid.

When topical antibiotics alone are used, the choice between drops and ointment is partly a matter of personal preference, partly a matter of convenience. Ointment is easier to manage in small children; drops are preferred by most adults. Drops are prescribed as two drops every one to two hours at first, then every four to six hours; ointment may be substituted at bedtime. Ointment tends to last longer, but the medication may not be released as well as from solution.

Penicillin used topically may produce penicillin sensitization, so should be avoided when possible. Sulfacetamide, 10 to 30% ophthalmic solution, is the preferred treatment for conjunctivitis due to Hemophilus influenzae or Hemophilus aegyptius, and is reasonably safe and effective for most other bacterial causes of conjunctivitis. Since it is only used topically, it is preferred over sulfonamides that are used systemically (1) to avoid sensitization of the patient and (2) to avoid development of organisms resistant to other sulfonamides.

Erythromycin 0.5% is the drug of choice in conjunctivitis due to pneumococcus, streptococcus, sensitive staphylococcus, and Moraxella lacunata. Neomycin is a common ingredient in many ophthalmic mixtures. It is commonly used in combination with polymyxin B and hydrocortisone, as in this patient, in order to widen its spectrum of activity. However, it readily causes sensitization and may cross-react in the future with other aminoglycoside antibiotics used systemically.

To repeat, a definitive diagnosis must be made before treatment with an antibiotic is started. Otherwise, the wrong medication may be used, or urgent, specific treatment for acute glaucoma or other noninfectious conditions may be delayed. An exception is infection with Pseudomonas aeruginosa, which is capable of causing corneal ulceration within a few hours. When Pseudomonas aeruginosa is the suspected cause of conjunctivitis, topical gentamicin (also useful against other gram-negative organisms) should be started immediately, combined with parenteral gentamicin in most instances.

(C) In the presence of mucopurulent ophthalmic discharge, warm compresses are helpful in soaking up the debris and in relieving excessive tearing and itching. They should be used for 15 minutes, four times a day.

(D) Corticosteroids should not be used routinely in a patient with acute bacterial conjunctivitis; in fact, they would seldom be indicated. However, a combined corticosteroid-antibiotic solution was used in this patient with satisfactory results. The steroid, if safe for the condition, helps relieve the itching and pain that cause the patient to scratch and rub the eyes, possibly producing further injury. A general rule is that an inflammation of the eye serious enough to require steroids is serious enough to be referred to an ophthalmologist. The risk of misdiagnosis of inflammatory eye disease is too great to make the use of steroids safe under the circumstances of emergency department treatment. However, for allergic conjunctivitis, steroids are very useful for both symptomatic and definitive management. Any patient who is receiving topical ophthalmic steroids in any form must be followed up carefully, since the treatment is not entirely free of complications.

(E) An infected eye, whether having conjunctivitis or otherwise, should not be patched, with the possible exception of one infected with herpes simplex keratitis. The reasons are that a patch promotes, rather than controls, infection, and makes topical antibiotic medication very difficult or impossible.

3. (False) Other causes of a red eye are often difficult to differentiate from conjunctivitis. These must be ruled out by appropriate examination before therapy is instituted, since the consequences of using too little therapy or the wrong therapy can be serious. In short, acute conjunctivitis must not be confused with iritis (anterior uveitis), acute glaucoma, or corneal ulceration, since the treatment of each of these is different and is also different from that of conjunctivitis. They are far more serious than most cases of conjunctivitis, although some inflammations, such as keratoconjunctivitis, involve both tissues.

If the clinician is not sure that a patient's red eye is due to conjunctivitis, he should seek immediate or early consultation with an ophthalmologist. Even if the differential diagnosis can be made in the emergency room with a slit lamp (required in confirmation of acute iritis) and other aids, the patient still must be treated, as well as followed closely, by an ophthalmologist. In addition, keratitis (inflammation of the cornea, with or without ulceration) constitutes a threat to vision, and patients with this condition require specialty care from the earliest time the diagnosis is suspected.

Another example is acute glaucoma, which is usually of the angle-closure type or is secondary to some other eye disease or injury. In acute glaucoma with extremely high intraocular pressure, optic nerve damage can occur within 24 to 48 hours and may be permanent. For this reason, the patient with symptoms and signs indicative of or suggesting acute glaucoma must be referred immediately to an ophthalmologist.

Acute glaucoma is extremely painful, a helpful point in differentiating it from conjunctivitis. The discomfort is in the globe and surrounding area. Some patients complain only of headache, nausea, and vomiting, causing the clinican to think of systemic viral infection or other cause, and not of the severe eye disease that acute glaucoma represents. Treatment consists of pilocarpine 4%, two drops in each eye every 15 minutes for several hours, as well as an osmotic agent, oral glycerol. If the patient fails to respond to this treatment, surgical intervention is imperative.

4. (False) As mentioned in Case 35, when a subconjunctival hemorrhage is present, an intraocular foreign body must be ruled out. However, most such red eyes are due to spontaneous

hemorrhage and do not require any special treatment since they usually clear spontaneously over two to three weeks. Cold compresses (which should be changed to warm compresses after 24 hours) may hasten resolution of the hematoma.

5. (C, E, F) (A) Dacryocystitis is inflammation of the lacrimal sac located near the medial canthus. Both acute and chronic dacryocystitis occur. The latter is usually caused by Candida albicans; and, while its treatment is not urgent, it should be treated, since it is capable of causing acute recurrent episodes, presumably due to superimposed bacterial infection.

(B) Acute dacryocystitis is usually unilateral but may be bilateral. (C) Obstruction of the nasolacrimal duct is almost always present and presumably causative. Relief of the obstruction is necessary in order to obtain clearing of the infection.

(D) The disease occurs mainly in adults over 40 years of age, but may occur both acutely and chronically in infants whose nasolacrimal ducts fail to canalize.

(E) The acute process is almost always due to one of the bacteria listed, and they can usually be suspected from the Gram's stain of the discharge and confirmed by culture (F).

(G) Systemic antibiotics are necessary for treatment, the oral route being satisfactory in most instances. Penicillin, 500 mg (800, 000 units) every six hours, or ampicillin, 500 mg every six hours, can be used, either one to be continued for at least seven days. For patients allergic to penicillin (except children under eight years of age and pregnant patients), tetracycline, 250 mg every six hours, is a satisfactory substitute. If all three drugs are contraindicated and if the organism is sensitive to it, erythromycin, 250 mg every six hours, may be used.

A topical antibiotic ointment is optional, although chronicity can be masked by its use. It should never be used alone. It is frequently used to decrease the chance of secondary conjunctivitis and keratitis. These two conditions are rare as complications of dacryocystitis; however, if a corneal ulcer occurs, as it does occasionally in the presence of pneumococcal dacryocystitis, both systemic and topical treatment must be vigorous, and removal of the ductal obstruction is urgent. Warm compresses should be applied for 15 minutes, four times a day. Opening (by probing) and dilatation or re-routing (dacryocystorhinostomy) of the nasolacrimal duct is indicated, since recurrence is common.

A related condition, dacryoadenitis, is inflammation of the lacrimal gland located near the lateral canthus. It is either viral or bacterial in origin. In addition to being caused by the bacteria listed under E mentioned previously, it may be a complication of gonococcal conjunctivitis, requiring culture for identification and specific therapy. Warm compresses are indicated for relief of pain and promotion of drainage. Incision may be required.

6. (True) Occlusion of the central retinal artery is a true emergency, since permanent damage to the retina can occur within 30 to 60 minutes. This condition must be suspected in any patient with a history of sudden, complete, painless loss of vision in one eye. The patient is usually elderly. The characteristic ophthalmoscopic findings are bloodless arterioles, pallor of the optic disc, edema of the macula with the appearance of a "cherry-red spot," and "boxcar" segmentation of the blood in the retinal veins.

Treatment is not satisfactory in most instances, but it should be undertaken immediately. Minutes after onset, suddenly decreasing the intraocular pressure by incising the limbus at the edge of the cornea may restore blood flow in the central retinal artery. Unfortunately, such rapid diagnosis and treatment are not usually possible. Anticoagulants may also be tried, and some clinicans have found vasodilators to be helpful. Massaging the globe for several seconds through the closed eyelids and then suddenly releasing the pressure may help, if done within the first one to two hours of onset.

Thrombosis of the central retinal vein is another cause of unilateral, slow, painless loss of vision. Diabetic retinopathy and hypertensive retinopathy can be differentiated, as they are always bilateral. Fibrinolytic agents should be tried, but anticoagulant therapy is of no proven value.

7. (True) Retinal detachment is characterized by sudden loss of vision and a shower of floaters or "lightning flashes" or "a curtain coming up (or down) in front of my eye." It constitutes a true ocular emergency. The most common location of a retinal tear is the superior nasal quadrant. Usually, the detached translucent fold gives the appearance of a billowing cloud, which ripples when the patient moves his head. Often a retinal hole may be seen. The detachment may progress rapidly or slowly, and it frequently involves the macula. Treatment is surgical, and the patient must immediately be referred to an ophthalmologist when the condition is suspected.

8. (True) Temporal or cranial arteritis, also called giant cell arteritis, is a rare disease. It usually occurs in patients over 60 years of age and is manifested by blurring of vision, scotomata, or pain over the temples. It specifically affects the medium-size arteries of the external carotid system, but it is usually more widespread. The intimal layer, particularly, is infiltrated by giant cells with obstruction of the vessels; such infiltration is accompanied by severe pain over the temporal arteries. Ischemic optic neuropathy leads to severe visual impairment, possibly permanent total blindess, if early treatment is not instituted.

The diagnosis is made on the basis of an erythrocyte sedimentation rate of 60 to 100 mm in one hour, although, in the early stages of the disease, the rate may not be elevated much, if at all. Arterial biopsy confirms the diagnosis.

Steroids should be given in large doses and maintained in smaller doses for many months or years. Even with adequate and prolonged treatment, blindness in one or both eyes may occur.

9. (True) Orbital cellulitis is inflammation of the orbital tissue surrounding the globe and is usually secondary to acute purulent sinusitis, caused by pneumococcus, streptococcus or staphylococcus.

Some eye diseases are misjudged by the emergency department physician as being more serious than they really are. This is one disease that is liable to be misjudged in the opposite direction, and with disastrous results. One reason is that the sinusitis may have been relatively asymptomatic or associated with only a dull headache. The spread is by direct extension, and the orbital cellulitis may seem to be of sudden onset.

Treatment is immediate hospitalization and intravenous administration of large doses of antibiotics. Incision and drainage through the upper eyelid may become necessary for complete resolution. Complications are meningitis, cavernous sinus thrombosis, osteomyelitis, and cerebral abscess.

10. (True) The ocular complication of diabetes mellitus, diabetic retinopathy, is a change in the retinal blood vessels. It occurs in both juvenile- and maturity-onset diabetes and is a leading cause of blindness in the western world. The incidence and severity of this complication of diabetes increases with the duration of the disease; it is invariably present in patients with juvenile-onset diabetes by the third or fourth decade

of life. Poor control of the diabetes seems to hasten development of the retinopathy, although good control may not stop its progression.

Such patients are frequently seen in emergency departments when they have an acute exacerbation of their basic disease or of the ocular complications. Often, noncompliance with treatment protocols is responsible for the acute deterioration. Management should be handled jointly by the primary physician and the ophthalmologist.

::

CASE 37: TWISTED ANKLE IN A 13-YEAR-OLD GIRL

HISTORY:

A 13-year-old girl turned her left ankle while playing basketball. When she reported to the emergency department one and one-half hours later, she had a painful swelling over the lateral aspect of the ankle, but walked into the emergency department with only a moderate limp.

EXAMINATION:

There was marked swelling and tenderness over the lateral malleolus and moderate swelling over the medial aspect of the ankle. All ligaments were grossly intact. There was no other evidence of injury.

QUESTIONS:

TRUE OR FALSE (Questions 1 and 2):

1. From a carefully performed physical examination, it is usually possible to determine the presence or absence of a fractured ankle in a child.

2. If the patient walked into the emergency department, she should be allowed to walk to the x-ray department to have her films made.

3. Which of the following is the least important anatomical structure regarding ankle sprains and fractures?
   A. The tibia
   B. The fibula
   C. The talus
   D. The cuboid
   E. The lateral collateral ligament
   F. The medial collateral ligament

TRUE OR FALSE (Questions 4-6):

4. Since roentgenographic examination is to be done, it is not necessary to do a careful physical examination of the injured ankle.

5. Stress films are useful only if a fracture is found on routine roentgenological studies.

6. The differential diagnosis in this patient is epiphyseal injury (ankle fracture) and ligamentous injury (ankle sprain).

ANSWERS AND COMMENTS:

1. (False) Even with the most complete history and physical examination, it is almost impossible to rule out a small fracture or an epiphyseal fracture without roentgenological examination. Therefore, every patient with an ankle injury should have roentgenological studies done after the physical examination is complete. Conversely, even with easy access to roentgenological examination in most emergency departments, it is still very important to do a careful physical examination, because routine roentgenograms will not yield direct evidence of ligamentous injury. Such injury may be just as serious as bony injury (see question and answer 6).

Ligamentous injury of the ankle varies in severity and in the number of ligaments involved. It is never sufficient to diagnose ankle sprain alone, if it is possible to specify the particular ligament involved and the severity of the injury.

2. (False) Although she may be able to walk to the x-ray department, she should never be allowed to do so. For instance, she may fall and hurt her ankle further, with no record having been made of the original type and extent of injury.

A patient with a sprained ankle should be met at the car or ambulance, or at least at the registration desk, and be brought into the examination area in a wheel chair or on a stretcher. That is for humanitarian, as well as for medicolegal, reasons. Other immediate first-aid procedures for patients with possible sprains, fractures or dislocations of the ankle are application of ice packs, elevation of the injured part, administration of an analgesic or narcotic if indicated, and application of a splint, such as an air splint, if appropriate. The reason for those measures is the unavoidable delays in obtaining roentgenological studies and orthopedic consultation in some busy emergency departments. The pulses distal to the injury should be monitored carefully.

3. (D) The cuboid (D) is a lateral bone in the tarsus and is not directly involved in ankle injuries. The tibia (A) contributes the medial malleolus to the ankle mortise, and the fibula (B) contributes the lateral malleolus. That mortise is the most important mechanical feature of the ankle, but it is the talus (C) that is the key to understanding, as well as to managing, ankle

fractures. Being convex from back to front and concave from side to side, with rounded edges, the talus allows rotary rocking and tilting motions. The concave surface of the talus fits into the convexity of the weight-bearing surface of the tibia. Although the talus, itself, is seldom fractured, it may be subject to excessive rotary motion that tends to fracture or dislocate the tibia and the fibula. On the other hand, because of its stability, the talus is used as a mold for reshaping a fracture of the ankle joint.

(E) The lateral collateral ligament of the ankle is far more frequently injured than the medial collateral ligament. The lateral collateral ligament consists of the calcaneofibular ligament, and the anterior and posterior talofibular ligaments. The anterior talofibular ligament is the most important of the lateral ligaments. It is that ligament that is injured in the majority of ankle sprains, largely because it is tensed in plantar flexion, and most sprains occur in that position.

The calcaneofibular ligament is the next most injured ligament, and it is injured as the foot is forced into slight dorsiflexion. The posterior talofibular ligament is only rarely involved in ankle injury.

(F) The medial collateral ligament comprises the four parts of the deltoid ligament: the anterior tibiotalar, the tibionavicular, the tibiocalcaneal, and the posterior tibiotalar ligaments, in that order from front to back. The medial collateral ligament lies on the medial side of the ankle and is much less often involved in ankle sprain than the lateral group.

The remaining ligaments of the ankle are those that attach the tibia to the fibula at their distal ends: the anterior tibiofibular ligament, the posterior tibiofibular ligament, and the interosseous membrane (tibiofibular syndesmosis). They become very important when the foot is in dorsiflexion, since the talus widens within the mortise in that position, tending to separate the distal tibia and fibula. Those ligaments are ruptured only in the presence of a severe ankle injury, when the talus is rotated externally and the tibia is rotated internally, forcing the malleoli apart.

4. (False) The physical examination is at least as important as the roentgenographic examination. From his first contact with the patient, the clinician should be thinking about what he will do for the patient if the roentgenographic studies are negative. The answer to that question depends almost entirely upon a carefully performed physical examination.

The setting for the examination is important. When all beds and stretchers are occupied in the emergency department, the patient is frequently seated in a chair in the hall with his feet on the floor. That is an awkward position for the examiner, to say nothing about the patient, who should have had his injured extremity elevated, packed in ice, and splinted, if that is indicated. Optimally, the patient should be on a stretcher or examining table, as for other types of injuries, so that a more adequate examination can be done.

The examination should start with a search for other injuries, which are not infrequently present with the more severe ankle sprains. Examples of areas of associated injuries are the upper extremity on the same side, the lower spine, the pelvis, and the hip and knee on the same side.

Examination of the ankle should follow a general outline:

a) Inspection should reveal any obvious deformities, such as swelling or displacement.

b) Palpation should reveal specific areas of tenderness, provided the examiner begins the palpation away from the area of maximal swelling. That part of the examination should include checking the Achilles tendon, the posterior tibial pulse, the dorsalis pedis pulse, and the foot, especially the head of the fifth metatarsal. Proximal compression of the tibia and fibula is an excellent method of testing the integrity of the interosseous membrane.

c) Palpation of the ankle, itself, should include feeling for the anterior capsule and joint line, the distal anterior tibiofibular ligament, the posterior talofibular ligament, the calcaneofibular ligament, and the anterior talofibular ligament, the one that is most commonly injured. That examination should reveal the area of maximum tenderness, which, in turn, should help identify the specific ligament(s) injured.

d) Stress testing of the ankle (testing for instability) comes last. It is an excellent means of indicating possible disruption of ligaments, but it may not indicate which ligaments are involved if only partial tearing or stretching has occurred.

   Stress testing begins with determining the degree of excursion of the talus in the ankle mortise (the anterior drawer sign). The tibia is fixed with one hand and the foot is displaced forward while slight plantar flexion is maintained. If that passive motion is possible, a marked degree of ankle instability is present, indicating rupture of the anterior talofibular ligament and the calcaneofibular ligament.

The talar-tilt sign is also useful for detecting tears of those two ligaments. It is done by rotating the foot into a varus position, with the leg firmly fixed with the other hand. If excessive mobility is possible, one or both of those ligaments are probably disrupted. Conversely, talar tilt is impossible when an isolated tear of the anterior talofibular ligament is present, because such a tilt is prevented by the central fibers of the calcaneofibular ligament.

5. (False) Usually, stress films are not necessary if a fracture is obvious. However, they are very helpful in diagnosing an epiphyseal fracture, which does not show up well or at all on conventional x-rays. They are also useful in detecting the location and extent of ligamentous injury in a patient whose films are negative but who has evidence of significant joint damage. They are required to indicate instability of the talus within the ankle mortise.

To do stress films usually requires anesthesia, either local or general; although, in the first hour or two postinjury, some patients will permit adequate manipulation of the joint so that satisfactory studies can be done. Such was the case with this patient.

Stress films are often necessary for both right and left ankle joints and in exactly the same projections. That is true even for adults, since the comparison views may be required to establish a particular patient's normal anatomy and function. One set of bilateral stress films should be lateral views made in the position of testing for the anterior drawer sign. The other set should be anterior-posterior views, with each foot rotated into a varus position, as in the talar-tilt position described previously. If injury of the medial collateral ligament is suspected, stress films, with the foot rotated into valgus, may be indicated.

It is not just an academic exercise to determine which ligaments are involved. Rather, that information dictates the proper form of treatment. For example, it is possible to make a patient's injury worse by applying an elastic bandage and fitting the patient with crutches when a short-leg cast or even open repair of disrupted important ligaments is indicated.

6. (True) In a child in early adolescence, such as this patient,

an epiphyseal injury would seem more likely than a ligamentous injury, since sprains are relatively uncommon in children. One reason for this is that the ligaments are relatively stronger than the epiphyseal plates to which they attach. For example, a force which, in adults, results in a sprain of the lateral collateral ligaments, usually produces a Type I epiphyseal injury (see below) of the fibula in children. It was that fracture that was suspected in this patient. However, routine roentgenological views revealed no fracture, and stress films with comparison views showed no epiphyseal fracture and no disruption of the ankle ligaments.

Epiphyseal injuries are categorized by the Salter-Harris classification I-V, the numbers having reference to the extent and direction of the epiphyseal damage.

Type I is a slip fracture at the most vulnerable area of growing long bones, the epiphyseal plate. By definition, there is no tear of the periosteum in this injury.

Type II is a fracture in which a fragment of the metaphysis breaks off and slips over with the epiphysis. There is an associated periosteal tear. A Type II fracture is the most common type of childhood fracture involving the epiphyses. It is caused by bending forces of just the type that cause most ankle injuries.

Type III is a vertical break that splits off a fragment of the epiphysis at the epiphyseal plate. If closed reduction fails to produce anatomical alignment, open reduction is always indicated.

Type IV is a vertical fracture through the epiphyseal plate, involving both the epiphysis and the adjacent metaphysis. An operation is usually indicated for a Type IV fracture.

Type V is a compression injury that causes direct damage to the cartilaginous cells of the epiphyseal plate. The cellular injury may be temporary, allowing growth to continue. If it is permanent, it almost always leads to severe disturbances in growth of the bone.

It is clear that all patients with epiphyseal injuries should be under the care of an orthopedist for both immediate and long-term care.

COURSE:

This patient was seen by an orthopedic consultant who treated her injury with padded elastic bandaging, elevation, ice packs, and non-weight-bearing ambulation with crutches. She was to be checked again in 24 hours.

::

CASE 38: HAND INJURY

HISTORY:

A 23-year-old woman amputated the distal end of her right index finger in an electric fan. She had received her last tetanus toxoid booster at least ten years before.

EXAMINATION:

Examination showed a clean laceration through the tip of the finger at the level of the distal fourth of the nail. The tip of the phalanx was exposed and protruded slightly. The volar flap was slightly longer than the dorsal level of amputation. No roentgenological examination was done.

TREATMENT:

She was given a tetanus booster injection. After the finger was anesthetized with a 1% lidocaine digital nerve block, the tip of the phalanx was ronguered away and smoothed. The volar flap was defatted, and brought up to the end of the nail, and sutured in place with 5-0 monofilament nylon.

Penicillin was prescribed for six days, and the wound healed satisfactorily.

QUESTIONS:

TRUE OR FALSE (Questions 1-5):

1. This patient should have had a free full-thickness skin graft applied instead of the shortening procedure that was done.
2. The hand is the most commonly injured part of the body.
3. In repairing lacerations of the hand, epinephrine should be added to the anesthetic solution if bleeding is likely to be a problem.
4. A roentgenological examination is not required if all of the damage to the hand appears to be to the soft tissues.
5. Crushing injury of the fingertip usually does not require treatment.

6. Which of the following are true regarding minor injuries to the hand?
   A. An adequate sensory examination should be accomplished before any regional anesthesia is used.
   B. The goal is obtaining a closed wound at the earliest possible time.
   C. Probing of all deep wounds of the hand should be carried out as a supplement to functional testing.
   D. All of the above

7. TRUE OR FALSE: Almost all hand injuries can be handled in a well-equipped emergency department.

8. Examination of the more seriously injured hand should be based on which of the following basic principles?
   A. It should be complete.
   B. It should be done and recorded by the first physician who sees the patient.
   C. It should be done before any anesthesia is used.
   D. A rubber band tourniquet should be applied to each finger that is bleeding so that blood will not interfere with proper examination.
   E. Spurting vessels in the palm should be clamped in order to allow a more adequate examination.
   F. All of the above

9. TRUE OR FALSE: Maintenance of the position of function of the hand is important only following major fractures of the hand.

10. Which of the following apply to replantation of severed fingers?
    A. Almost 75% of the replanted digits can be expected to survive.
    B. The most difficult technical problem is venous reconstruction.
    C. Incomplete amputations are more satisfactory to correct because of the intact veins in the remaining skin bridge.
    D. If the patient is a candidate for replantation, the amputated part should be placed immediately in saline solution.
    E. All of the above

ANSWERS AND COMMENTS:

1. (False) This type of repair is called revision of amputation of

the tip of the finger. If the amputation is fairly clean, that is, with little or no crushing element to the injury, as in this patient, the repair can almost always be done in the emergency department. The rationale for this form of treatment is that the protruding bone has to be removed anyway, which will cause a shortening of the finger. Fortunately, in this patient, the volar flap was longer than the dorsal portion; after the fat was removed down to the undersurface of the dermis, it served as an attached full-thickness skin graft to cover the tip of the finger.

2. (True) The hand is the most commonly injured part of the body, and the crushed or amputated fingertip is the most common of hand injuries. Approximately one out of every ten patients treated in an emergency department has a complaint referable to the hand. Thus, from 10 to 15 patients with hand complaints may be seen in an emergency department during a 24-hour shift. That is reason enough for emergency department physicians to become familiar with the proper management of hand injuries and diseases.

Injuries to the soft tissue of the hand include contusions and abrasions, lacerations, penetrating injuries, and perforating injuries.

Blunt trauma is suggested by the finding of a contusion or abrasion. Just how severe the blunt force was is more likely to come out in the history than on the basis of the physical findings. In any case, one should always look for injury to deep tissues with that type of injury, since the damage often is not apparent on initial examination.

Abrasions, in particular, are frequently very dirty wounds, and failure to remove all of the debris can lead to unsightly tattooing. Such cleansing requires regional or general anesthesia in most patients.

Lacerations are usually straightforward, both in their diagnosis and treatment. The important thing is not to overlook injury to deep structures. One should not hesitate to extend the wound, in order to get a better look at underlying structures which may have been only partially severed.

Penetrating injuries are those that extend only partly through the hand, whereas perforating injuries pass all the way through. Examples of the latter are impaling injuries caused by a metal rod or sliver of wood, as well as gunshot wounds. An unusual, but serious, hand injury is an accidental high-powered injection of a foreign material, such as grease or paint. That leads to compartmental pressure that is higher than arterial blood pressure, and the result is ischemia. Also, the foreign body reaction is immediate and severe. Unless the compartment involved (for example, the digit, palm or wrist), is decompressed with fasciotomies, necrosis requiring amputation usually occurs. The importance of this injury to emergency physicians is that its serious nature is not usually apparent, and the patient could be sent home without benefit of surgical consultation and definitive in-patient care.

3. (False) Epinephrine should never be used in finger or toe injuries, because of the risk of ischemic nerve damage and necrosis of the involved digit(s).

4. (False) In most instances of hand injury, a roentgenological study should be done to rule out an unsuspected fracture, as well as to search for a foreign body. Roentgenograms are particularly important for crushing injuries of the fingertips, where the extent of injury is almost always impossible to determine from external examination. Also, for infections that may have been present for days or weeks, a roentgenological study is essential as a baseline study for future comparison, as well as to rule out any bony changes such as early osteomyelitis.

5. (False) Appropriate treatment is always indicated for a crushing injury of the fingertips. Treatment consists of removing the nail if it is almost totally avulsed, evacuating a subungual hematoma if present and the nail is to be preserved, splinting of any fracture of the distal phalanx, and antibiotic therapy, if a compound fracture is present.

Because of the extreme pain of a subungual hematoma, care should be taken in evacuating the blood. That evacuation can be done in most patients with a red-hot paper clip, best held in a hemostat, with only about one-eighth of an inch of the clip extending beyond the jaws of the instrument. That arrangement prevents the end of the clip from going too far inward after it penetrates the nail. Equally satisfactory is the use of a sharp-pointed scalpel blade, which makes a hole in the nail without discomfort, provided it is rotated back and forth carefully with minimal pressure.

6. (A, B) (A) If an adequate sensory and motor examination is not done before regional anesthesia is carried out, it is possible that a nerve laceration, especially of a sensory nerve, will be overlooked.

(B) The goal should always be to get the wound closed as soon as possible, as a protection against secondary infection and disability. Large skin defects should be covered, at least temporarily, by an appropriate graft, probably a partial-thickness graft. Of course the grafting is delayed until all damaged underlying structures have been repaired, unless some of them require delayed repair.

(C) Functional testing is usually adequate for assessing the damage; and probing deep wounds of the hand is contraindicated, because it may cause further damage and may introduce organisms that can cause secondary infection.

7. (False) Certain hand injuries or diseases should not be treated definitively in the emergency department; rather, they must be treated in the operating room. Those include most severe injuries, especially in children, such as transection of tendons, and puncture wounds that may have damaged nerves or other tissues. Most minor hand injuries can be treated in any well-equipped, well-staffed emergency department.

8. (A, B, C) (A, B) The examination should be complete, and both a gross description and functional evaluation must be recorded before any treatment is carried out. One reason for the complete examination is that the surgeon can go directly to the area of the injury and avoid unnecessary exploration which, in itself, takes time and can cause additional injury.

(C) It is almost never advisable to inject a local anesthetic in order to assess the function of the hand or the extent of injury present. Even in children, the tendon function can be assessed without anesthesia, although diagnosis of partial severance of a tendon may not be possible until the wound is explored in the operating room. All of the major nerves must be tested for both sensory and motor function before any anesthetic is used. Otherwise, it will be impossible to diagnose the injury properly.

One exception to that rule is when stress roentgenological films are required. In that case, the functional, as well as the roentgenological, appearance should be described, both before and after the anesthetic is used.

(D) Under no circumstances should a rubber band tourniquet be applied during the examination phase, since it may damage nerves that were not damaged by the original injury. For the same reason, it is not even advisable to use that type of tourniquet during the definitive repair. One further reason that militates against the tourniquet is that it may be overlooked when a bulky dressing is applied, either while the patient waits for the consultant or after definitive care has been rendered, and such retention of the tourniquet might cause loss of the finger. A small penrose drain is better than a rubber band; and, in itself, is less likely to cause damage and is less likely to be overlooked. The ideal solution to excessive bleeding is the placement of a pneumatic tourniquet on the arm to occlude the brachial artery. Under no circumstances should any tourniquet be left on longer than absolutely necessary, the maximum, even in the operating room, being an hour.

(E) Spurting blood can almost always be stopped by direct pressure, thereby avoiding the use of a tourniquet and avoiding probing the wound and clamping blindly. The last two procedures are dangerous and cannot be condoned.

9. (False) The position of function of the hand must be maintained after every procedure in which the hand is splinted. That includes almost all surgical procedures, since even the application of a bulky dressing (almost always indicated for other than minor wounds) constitutes a form of splinting. The position of function is extension of the wrist 30 degrees, flexion of the metacarpophalangeal and interphalangeal joints 10 to 15 degrees, and abduction of the thumb slightly away from the palm. In addition, the forearm should be neutral between pronation and supination, and the elbow should be flexed to approximately 90 degrees.

One reason that it is so important to maintain the position of function is that most patients with hand injury maintain the position of injury or the position of rest. The latter is the opposite of the position of function, and involves flexion of the wrist, extension of the digits, pronation of the forearm, and extension of the elbow. Function will be severely compromised if the extremity is left in that position for very long, especially if it is splinted, thus making exercise difficult or impossible.

It is always the mark of an amateur in hand care when the patient leaves the emergency department with the treated hand in the position of rest, rather than in the position of function.

After treatment, the injured hand should be elevated to prevent swelling and to decrease pain. That means, for example, when the patient is sitting, that the elbow should be higher than the shoulder and the hand should be higher than the elbow.

10. (E) All. Replantation is an exciting new field in surgery, and emergency department physicians play a vital role in that field.

::

CASE 39: PAINFUL INFECTION OF THUMB

HISTORY:

A 52-year-old man reported to the emergency department when the pain from a three-day-old infection of his left thumb had become unbearable. He knew of no injury to the thumb, and there was no personal or family history of diabetes. He was allergic to penicillin.

There was a small abscess at the base of the left thumb nail along the radial aspect, with moderate redness and swelling along the entire base of the nail. The base of the nail was elevated from its bed. There was no epitrochlear or axillary lymphadenopathy, and no red streaking of the hand or forearm to suggest lymphangitis.

A digital nerve block was done with lidocaine 1%, and the abscess was opened. Because pus was found beneath the base of the nail, it was necessary to remove four millimeters of the proximal part of the nail across its entire width.

QUESTIONS:

1. Which of the following statements about paronychia are true?
   A. Trauma is usually the cause.
   B. Simple incision and drainage is never adequate treatment.
   C. Roentgenological examination of the finger is always indicated.
   D. A Gram's stain and culture should be done in every instance.
   E. Antibiotic therapy is required in all cases.
   F. The abscess may involve the nail matrix, the nail bed and the phalanx.
   G. All of the above

2. Another type of fingertip infection is a felon. Which of the following are true about this condition?
   A. It is an abscess of the closed space of the fingertip.
   B. The causative organism is usually staphylococcus.
   C. The most common complication is flexor tenosynovitis.
   D. Treatment is early incision and drainage.
   E. Antibiotics are not usually necessary.
   F. All of the above

ANSWERS AND COMMENTS:

1. (A, F) (A) Although minor trauma is usually the precipitating cause of paronychia, most patients do not recall a specific injury. Children who bite their fingernails, especially a hangnail, are prone to develop one or more paronychias, often with mixed organisms.

(B) Simple incision and drainage is sufficient for the well-localized abscess with no extension beneath the base of the nail. This may even be possible without anesthesia by separating the eponychium from the base of the nail. In this patient, the abscess extended beneath the proximal end of the nail, so a portion of the nail was removed for adequate drainage. In making the longitudinal incision along one or both sides of the base of the nail, care should be taken not to extend the incision as far proximal as the extensor tendon insertion, since that might allow spread of the infection in the form of pyogenic tenosynovitis or arthritis.

(C) Roentgenological examination of the finger is not usually necessary, unless there is a history of trauma with possible fracture of the phalanx or an imbedded foreign body. However, if the infection has been present for several weeks, a roentgenological examination is always indicated, to detect evidence of osteomyelitis (see F).

(D) A Gram's stain and culture are indicated only if an antibiotic is required. Most minor paronychias do not require an antibiotic (E) although severe ones, such as this patient had, should be treated with an antibiotic. The Gram's stain showed gram-positive cocci in short chains, and the patient was given erythromycin, 250 mg four times daily for six days, with complete recovery. The culture grew group A beta hemolytic streptococcus. The finding of that organism was somewhat surprising, in that the usual organism is staphylococcus.

(F) In the more advanced paronychia, the matrix of the nail may be destroyed, preventing any regrowth of the nail. The nail bed and the underlying phalangeal tuft may become involved as the infection spreads around the nail and extends deep to the nail bed. Acute osteomyelitis of the phalanx may result, although most patients have such severe pain that they seek relief before that stage is reached.

2. (A, B, D) (A) A felon is an abscess in the distal closed space of the finger. It is usually caused by a puncture wound of the

tip of the finger, with inoculation of organisms from the skin or from the contaminated object causing the puncture wound. Rarely, it occurs as an extension of a paronychia.

The closed space of the fingertip is divided by several fibrous septa, which extend from the phalanx volarward to the skin, where they are anchored. Infection, with its associated swelling and interference with blood flow, causes severe pain, largely because of the distention of the pockets produced by the septa. It is usually that pain, rather than the appearance of the finger, that causes the patient to see a physician.

(B) The causative organism is usually one of the staphylococci, most often coagulase-positive Staphylococcus aureus.

(C) The most common complication is not flexor tenosynovitis, but osteomyelitis of the distal phalanx. The reason seems to be that the cornified skin of the fingertip is so tough that the infection cannot spread in that direction. Therefore, spontaneous drainage is delayed for weeks, or never occurs until after the phalanx is largely destroyed. Although the flexor tendon inserts on the distal phalanx just proximal to the fibrous septa, tenosynovitis does not occur, except in the neglected, advanced felon.

(D) Incision and drainage is almost always necessary; the earlier this is done, the better. Although an antibiotic is indicated in all patients (E), preferably a staphylococcide, treatment with an antibiotic alone should not be depended upon. The definitive therapy is surgical, carried out under digital nerve block or wrist block anesthesia. The incision should be made directly over the area of external pointing, if there is one. If not, the incision should be made longitudinally, a few millimeters from the edge of the nail on one side only and extending across the tip of the finger, with the septa incised just volar to the phalanx. That avoids the digital nerve fibers on both sides of the finger and does not interfere with the finger pad after healing occurs. Extreme care should be used not to contaminate the flexor tendon, since that would lead to pyogenic tenosynovitis with possible permanent dysfunction of the finger.

An alternative site for the incision is along the midline of the volar aspect of the finger, with or without division of the septa to either side. Again, care should be taken not to extend the incision (or the blunt or sharp dissection) proximally as far as the insertion of the tendon.

The traditional mid-lateral hockey-stick or fish-mouth incision is probably too extensive, although one or the other of those is still preferred by many surgeons.

The wound should be held open by a small drain or a piece of nonadherent gauze, such as Xeroform®. Soaking the finger at least three times a day is indicated, and dressing the finger every two to four days is advisable. Immobilization of the finger with a protective splint is also helpful.

Most other infections of the hand require surgical consultation and incision and drainage in the operating room, along with hospitalization for intravenous administration of antibiotics.

CASE 40: SMOKE INHALATION DAMAGE

HISTORY:

A 58-year-old woman was smoking and drinking alcoholic beverages alone in her house when it caught fire. She sustained extensive burns over her face and body. She was treated briefly in her community hospital and arrived at the burn center almost two hours postburn. Her medical history was not remarkable, except for chronic obstructive pulmonary disease, chronic peptic ulcer disease, and arthritis of unknown type.

Approximately 80% of her body surface was burned. Most of the burns were second-degree; some were third-degree, including those of her entire face. She had a great deal of upper airway secretion, and her sputum contained soot particles. Hyperemia, edema, and soot particles were apparent in her mouth and pharynx.

The anterior-posterior diameter of the chest was moderately increased. No basal rales were noted, but there were moderate rhonchi throughout her lower lung fields on both sides. The results of the remainder of the physical examination were normal.

QUESTIONS:

1. The diagnosis of smoke inhalation damage in this patient is based primarily on:
   A. The circumstances that led to the accident
   B. The pulmonary findings
   C. The burns around the mouth
   D. The oropharyngeal findings

2. The proper initial therapeutic measures for this patient are which of the following?
   A. Administer high concentrations of oxygen
   B. Immediate tracheostomy
   C. Corticosteroids in large intravenous doses
   D. Insertion of a nasogastric tube, with suction applied
   E. Penicillin therapy
   F. Morphine intravenously, for pain and anxiety
   G. Admission to the respiratory intensive care unit or burn unit
   H. Add 5% carbon dioxide to the oxygen

- I. The usual management of a patient with a cutaneous thermal burn
- J. All of the above

3. The proper initial laboratory studies to obtain are:
   - A. Blood carboxyhemoglobin determination
   - B. Arterial blood gases and pH
   - C. Portable chest roentgenogram
   - D. Sputum culture
   - E. Electrocardiogram
   - F. Pulmonary radionuclide scan
   - G. All of the above

4. The patterns of respiratory tract injury are:
   - A. Thermal burn of the upper tract
   - B. Lower tract damage due to noxious products of combustion
   - C. A and B

TRUE OR FALSE (Questions 5-7):

5. Pulmonary damage without cutaneous burn is almost unheard of.

6. The longer the exposure to flame or smoke in a closed space, the greater the severity of the pulmonary injury.

7. Patients with an extensive cutaneous burn do not usually develop pulmonary complications unless there is also smoke inhalation present.

8. Which of the following noxious gases that may be present in smoke are direct irritants to lung tissue?
   - A. Carbon monoxide
   - B. Hydrochloric acid fumes
   - C. Sulfuric acid fumes
   - D. Nitric and nitrous oxide fumes
   - E. Sulfur dioxide fumes
   - F. All of the above

9. Which of these statements are true regarding fires with combustion of plastic materials?
   - A. They spread faster than a wood fire.
   - B. They produce more heat than a wood fire.
   - C. Most of the breakdown products are now known.
   - D. Certain plastics used in homes are fire-resistant, but dangerous when they do ignite.
   - E. All of the above

ANSWERS AND COMMENTS:

1. (A, C, D) The diagnosis of cutaneous burn is usually not difficult, although the evaluative diagnostic approach, as outlined in Case 41, is sometimes tricky. On the other hand, even if the clinician is looking for it, smoke inhalation with respiratory tract damage can be very elusive. Occasionally, a patient (a firefighter, for example) is seen in the emergency department with all of the historical and physical clues to this diagnosis, treated with 20 to 30 minutes of oxygen and allowed to go home, or even return to his job. In the case presented here, the possibility that the victim might have been in an alcoholic stupor and thus might have spent more time in the smoke-filled surroundings; the presence of soot in the mouth, pharynx and sputum; the hyperemia, edema and secretions in the upper airway; and the extensive facial burns, all suggested smoke inhalation damage. Since this patient had a history of chronic obstructive pulmonary disease, the pulmonary findings were not informative. In a young healthy patient with no history of pulmonary disease, the presence of rhonchi, so soon after exposure to smoke, would be an ominous finding, especially if rales were also present, since pulmonary changes so manifested are usually delayed in smoke inhalation.

2. (A, D, E, F, G, I) (A) Because carbon monoxide intoxication is always a possibility with exposure to smoke, it is always wise to administer high concentrations of oxygen. Humidification of the inspired oxygen and ambient air mixture is a must, especially in children, in whom a hood or croup tent may be quite satisfactory. The concentration of oxygen may be adjusted on the basis of serial arterial blood gas and pH levels, but the PaO_2 should be kept above 70 mm Hg for most patients. (H) Carbon dioxide should not be added to the oxygen.

(B) Tracheostomy should not be necessary nowadays in most such patients. It is certainly not an emergency procedure, since upper airway obstruction does not usually occur until six to thirty hours postburn. Endotracheal intubation is usually more satisfactory and is safer than tracheostomy in such patients. If possible, the intubation should be nasotracheal, for more patient comfort and for longer use, should several days of intubation become necessary. A tube with a high compliance, low-pressure cuff should be used, thus allowing extended periods of assisted or controlled ventilation and complete control of the airway. Although tracheostomy is still necessary in a few instances, it is more likely than endotracheal intubation to cause pulmonary sepsis in a patient with both cutaneous burns and smoke inhalation injury.

In the face of severe hypoxemia or deteriorating pulmonary function, positive-end expiratory pressure ventilation (PEEP) is indicated. Following nasotracheal intubation, PEEP was established for this patient, with administration of 100% oxygen at first.

(C) The use of steroids in large doses for massive cutaneous burns is controversial, because the benefits are still unproved. For an adult, hydrocortisone sodium succinate, in a dose of 100 to 200 mg, is usually administered intravenously. The dose may need to be repeated after six to twelve hours, and then daily for a few additional days. However, in the patient with predominant thermal burn of the upper air passages, steroids may do more harm than good. There are already breaks in the mucosa, which allow entry of bacteria. Any infection that develops is likely to be more difficult to control in the patient receiving steroids. But the chief deterrent to the use of steroids is the unresolved question of whether they benefit the patient, even a patient who has diffuse pulmonary damage from noxious gases in smoke. Pending accumulation of more controlled data, most clinicians still use steroids in the hope that they will help.

(D) Insertion of a nasogastric tube with suction empties the stomach and helps prevent the adynamic ileus that is so common in patients with burns. Also, nothing is allowed by mouth for the first few days. The tube also prevents regurgitation and aspiration by a patient who is obtunded. Aspiration pneumonitis in a patient with smoke inhalation injury would be a dangerous complication of an already serious injury.

(E) For the patient not allergic to it, penicillin by parenteral administration gives adequate protection against bacterial colonization of the lungs. Changes in antibiotic should be made only on the basis of sputum or blood culture and sensitivity reports. It is not recommended routinely for the patient with a cutaneous burn only, but probably should be given to a patient such as this.

(F) In a patient with such extensive and deep burns, a narcotic is usually required. However, it must be recalled that third-degree burns are frequently painless, at least at first. In the presence of probable pulmonary damage, only small doses (3 to 4 mg) or morphine should be given intravenously, in order to avoid the side effects of respiratory depression. This dose can be cautiously repeated every ten minutes, until pain relief is obtained.

(I) See Case 41 for management of a patient with cutaneous thermal burns.

3. (A, B, C, D, E) These are all studies that are necessary for confirmation of smoke inhalation damage to the respiratory tract and for planning therapy. Routine venous blood studies and urinalysis should also be done to establish baseline levels.

(A) The blood carboxyhemoglobin level is necessary, because early on, there is little objective evidence of the diagnosis, except as given in the case presentation. This test is a measure of the percentage of hemoglobin from which oxygen has been displaced by carbon monoxide. (See Case 44 for a more complete discussion of carbon monoxide intoxication.)

(B) Arterial blood gases and pH are necessary for baseline levels against which serial studies can be judged. In addition, if acute pulmonary changes are present - chiefly indicated by lower than normal PO_2 - the patient requires aggressive treatment for respiratory insufficiency, due to probable smoke inhalation.

(C) Chest roentgenography is also necessary as a baseline study for future comparison, but is not likely to be abnormal in the first hour or two after the patient's exposure to smoke. Another film should be exposed in six to eight hours, another in 16 to 24 hours, and one daily thereafter. The average time for roentgenological abnormalities to develop is 24 to 36 hours after exposure to smoke.

(D) Sputum culture, although not urgent, is valuable for future decisions about antimicrobial therapy. If the sputum is purulent due to pre-existing chronic obstructive pulmonary disease, as in this patient, or due to acute bronchitis or pneumonitis, a Gram's stain may immediately suggest the organism involved.

(E) An electrocardiogram should be obtained in patients of all ages, because of the tendency of cardiac dysrhythmias to develop in patients with smoke inhalation damage. In addition, continuous electrocardiographic monitoring should be done. It is almost always possible to find suitable places for the electrodes on normal skin. Otherwise, they may be placed in burned areas.

(F) A pulmonary radionuclide scan of the lungs is not likely to add useful information and should not be done initially in such a patient.

4. (C) (A) The upper tract thermal burn is an important aspect of respiratory tract damage, although it is less common than the lower tract damage. Its importance lies in the potential for upper airway obstruction, which can occur suddenly. Such obstruction is usually caused by edema and hyperemia, both of which are inflammatory reactions to toxic smoke products, or heat, or both. Therefore, preparation must be made to take care of this eventuality (see answer 2B).

(B) Lower tract injury is usually not caused by direct heat, because the transport of heat by smoke and air is not efficient enough to reach the lower respiratory tract. Rather, such injury is due to chemical irritation by products of combustion within the smoke, in other words, the particulate matter and noxious gases present in smoke. One exception to this occurs when a blast of smoke and burning gases suddenly strikes a person, such as when that person enters a hallway filled with superheated smoke or breaks a window of a burning room in a rescue operation. Another exception occurs when steam is inhaled by the victim, causing a thermal burn in the lower respiratory tract.

5. (False) Although unusual, pulmonary damage can occur when there is no cutaneous burn visible. This usually occurs when the patient is unconscious, under which circumstance, the damage to both the upper and the lower tracts is worse.

6. (True) The air in the room becomes hotter and the smoke becomes more concentrated, thus increasing the damage to the tracheobronchial tree in proportion to the time of exposure. In addition, there is a reflex increase in respiratory rate in response to increased carbon dioxide in the inhaled air; thus, more of the noxious smoke is pulled into the lungs. Even the bronchioles and alveoli are damaged during prolonged exposure in an enclosed space. This damage causes a rapid inflammatory response with hyperemia, edema, and exudation, with frank pulmonary edema as the end result. For severe inhalation injury, the treatment is not entirely satisfactory, even in the best run intensive care units, and many of these patients die.

7. (False) Patients with extensive cutaneous burns may develop pulmonary insufficiency as a delayed, but serious, complication (adult respiratory distress syndrome). The mechanism is not clearly understood, but a postulated mechanism is toxins moving through the blood stream from the burn wound to the lungs.

8. (B, C, D, E) (A) Carbon monoxide is not a direct irritant to

lung tissue, but it enters the body through the lungs and causes serious toxicity, as will be discussed in Case 44. All of the others are frequently found in smoke, and they act as chemical irritants to the mucosa of the respiratory tract.

Smoke, especially from industrial fires, often contains other toxic gases, such as chlorine, ammonia and carbon dioxide. As mentioned in answer 6, the latter stimulates respiration, causing inhalation of larger quantities of smoke than would otherwise be the case. Exertion or emotional stress also has the same result. Finally, since smoke has a reduced oxygen content, the hypoxia it causes also reflexively increases respiratory rate.

9. (A, B, D) (A) A fire involving plastic materials spreads faster (A) and burns hotter (B) than a wood fire does. (C) Of the dozens of possible breakdown products, only a few are known and understood. The pathophysiological effects of those that are known are usually poorly understood or not at all.

(D) The plastic products found in homes, although fire-resistant in many instances, are dangerous when they do ignite, largely because of the noxious gases produced when they burn. One of these substances, polyvinylchloride (PVC) produces anhydrous hydrogen chloride when burning. This gas causes lung irritation, which may lead rapidly to pulmonary edema.

COURSE:

It was unlikely that this patient would survive, because 80% of her body surface was burned. At least half of all patients succumb to 60% third-degree burns and only a few survive 70%, or larger, third-degree burns. However, since her burn was at least half second-degree rather than third-degree, there was every reason to try vigorously to get her through the first few difficult days.

This attempt was thwarted by her pulmonary damage. The most difficult time for a patient with pulmonary damage is also the first three or four days. This patient died 30 hours postburn, after developing progressive respiratory insufficiency and both metabolic and respiratory acidosis. Autopsy showed extensive edema of the tracheobronchial tree and extensive pulmonary edema.

::

CASE 41: EXTENSIVE THERMAL BURNS

HISTORY:

A 36-year-old woman was extensively burned when her house trailer caught fire at 5:00 a. m.

EXAMINATION:

She was brought to the emergency department where the following were found: first- and second-degree burns of the face including the perioral region; first-degree circumferential burns of the neck, burns of the left shoulder, second- and third-degree circumferential burns of the right forearm and hand; second- and third-degree burns of the left hand and forearm; first-degree burns of the entire back and anterior chest; and second- and third-degree burns of the lateral aspect of the right thigh. Her hair was singed; there was erythema of the oral mucosa and soot on the tongue, but no hoarseness. Pulse rate was 110/ min, and regular. Peripheral pulses were strong and equal. The results of the remainder of the examination were normal.

Serial measurements of arterial blood gases and pH, and roentgenograms of the chest, did not suggest significant inhalation injury.

QUESTIONS:

1. Which of the following general statements about burn injuries are true?
   A. Burn injury is the third most common cause of accidental death in the United States.
   B. Thermal burns are the most common cause of serious burn injuries.
   C. In infants and small children, scalding is the most common burn.
   D. High-risk patients are abusers of alcohol and other drugs and those with neurological impairments, such as seizure disorder.
   E. All of the above

2. Which of the following characterize the pathophysiology of the <u>early</u> phase of moderate to severe cutaneous burns?
   A. Hemodynamic changes: altered capillary permeability with extravasation of fluid, hypovolemia, hemoconcen-

tration and edema
B. Diuresis
C. Loss of plasma from the burn area
D. Loss of circulating red blood cells
E. Electrolyte imbalance
F. Disordered fat and vitamin metabolism
G. All of the above

3. The full descriptive evaluation of a burn is based upon:
   A. The age of the patient
   B. The location of the burn
   C. The cause of the burn
   D. The depth of the burn injury
   E. The extent of the burn injury
   F. Associated injuries or pre-existing diseases
   G. All of the above

4. Whether to hospitalize the patient for a burn is a pertinent question for emergency physicians. Which of the following are generally accepted criteria for hospital admission of adults with thermal burns, based solely upon the depth and extent (percentage of total body surface) of the wound?
   A. Partial-thickness burn of less than 10 to 15%
   B. Partial-thickness burn of over 15 to 25%
   C. Full-thickness burn of less than 3%
   D. Full-thickness burn of over 3%

5. Initial management of a patient such as this one should include which of the following?
   A. Perform an immediate tracheostomy.
   B. Apply ice water or ice packs to the burn and cover with a sterile sheet.
   C. Obtain a history of the accident and do a brief physical examination.
   D. Administer intravenous fluid therapy through at least two lines, plus a central venous catheter.
   E. Relieve pain by a narcotic administered orally or subcutaneously.
   F. Insert a Foley catheter.
   G. Administer oxygen and assist ventilation if necessary.

6. Fluid therapy is the mainstay of initial burn care. Which of the following are correct for the first 24 hours?
   A. Electrolyte solution (lactated Ringer's solution) should be given in 1.5 ml/kg of body weight times the percentage of body surface burned.
   B. Colloid should be given in the amount of 0.5 ml/kg of

body weight times the percentage of body surface burned.

C. In adults, an additional 2000 ml of dextrose 5% in water must be given to replace insensible fluid loss.

D. Fluid requirements should be calculated on the basis of a maximum of 50% of body surface burned.

E. One-half of the estimated fluid requirement should be administered in the first four hours following injury.

7. Additional steps that should be taken are:
   A. Cleanse and debride the wounds, preferably in a Hubbard tank.
   B. Apply an ointment to the wound to prevent bacterial infection.
   C. Administer an antibiotic systemically.
   D. Administer a whole blood transfusion.
   E. Monitor vital signs, central venous pressure, and arterial blood gases and pH.
   F. Monitor intake and output.
   G. Administer a diuretic to prevent acute renal failure.
   H. Administer tetanus prophylaxis.

8. If the burn is suitable for outpatient treatment, which of the following are recommended?
   A. Wash the burn with water and bland soap.
   B. Debride and cover the burn with a topical ointment then dress it.
   C. Control pain.
   D. Arrange for frequent follow-up visits.
   E. Start systemic antibiotic therapy.
   F. All of the above

ANSWERS AND COMMENTS:

1. (E) All. Each year in this country, two million persons are burned, of which 200, 000 seek medical attention and 75, 000 are hospitalized. Twelve thousand of these patients die of the burns or their complications.

Fifty per cent of these burns occur in the home, and at least two-thirds of these are preventable.

2. (A, C, D) (A) Even with a relatively small and superficial burn, there are some systemic changes. Although the systemic blood pressure may rise transiently (due to peripheral vasoconstriction) instead of dropping, this is the stage of clinical shock, of which blood pressure is only one indicator. Tissue hypoxia occurs, due to decreased blood flow and decreased oxygen de-

livery to the tissues (see D). Further aggravating this hypoxia is decreased cardiac output, which results from the decreased circulating blood volume.

Fluid resuscitation is designed to correct these derangements; without it, the derangements progress to hypovolemic shock, which becomes irreversible, leading to death. Most moderately to severely burned patients die within 24 to 72 hours if treatment is not available.

(C) Loss of plasma from the burn area, chiefly from second- and third-degree burns, can run as high as 4000 ml per day, per square meter of burn surface. Evaporation of so much water requires expenditure of energy, accounting for the negative nutritional balance for such patients if the extra calories required are not furnished by mouth or by intravenous hyperalimentation.

(D) The number of circulating red blood cells decreases, because many are destroyed in the burn area at the time of the burn. Effective or functional circulation of red blood cells decreases because of the sludge phenomenon, which slows microcirculation as hemoconcentration supervenes. The survival of red blood cells may also be decreased, further contributing to reduction in circulating red cells which are required for oxygen transportation at a time when tissue oxygen requirements are greatly increased.

(B, E, F) Diuresis, electrolyte imbalance and disordered fat and vitamin metabolism are all characteristics of the subacute (after 72 hours) phase of burn pathophysiology. Other characteristics include anemia, accelerated metabolic rate (rarely, the syndrome of burn hypermetabolism occurs), nitrogen disequilibrium, impairment of hepatic and endocrine function, and reduced resistance to infection. This later stage is seldom seen in the emergency department.

3. (G) All. The history and appearance of the patient will, in most instances, establish the diagnosis of thermal burn. Although occasionally an obtunded patient, for example, an alcohol- or drug-intoxicated patient, will present with a skin lesion that is not obviously a burn, the basic diagnosis is not usually a problem. However, determining the type, degree and extent of the injury and determining the clinical characteristics of the patient in whom it is present, are more important in the full evaluation of burn injury than in the evaluation of almost all other types of disease or injury. Greatly simplified, a burn

that is life-threatening, based on a combination of all the listed factors in the question, is called a critical, or severe, burn injury. A minor burn is shallow and small. The burns between these two extremes are called moderate, or noncritical, again, their description being based on all of the listed factors. Since all of these factors are so important, each will be considered separately.

(A) It is impossible to separate the depth and extent of the burn from the other items in the list, especially the age of the patient. It is known that small children and elderly patients tolerate burns very poorly.

(B) The location of the burn is at least as important as the age of the patient in this evaluation. We usually think of a burn as a burn, regardless of where it appears on the body, but where it is located is crucial to both treatment and prognosis. A burn of the face, neck, hands, genitalia, perineum and feet requires a different approach and carries a different prognosis from burns of the trunk and the proximal portions of the extremities. Location is also important in determining whether the patient may be treated as an outpatient or an inpatient, as indicated later.

This patient illustrates the problem of burns around the face, which are frequently associated with smoke inhalation injury (see Case 40). Also, she had an injury of the hand, which required special attention, namely, early escharotomy and grafting.

(C) The cause of the burn is vital in determining the overall management. For example, a flash or flame thermal burn is a far different problem from an electrical burn, as will be discussed in Case 42.

(D) Thermal burns are classified according to depth: (1) A first-degree burn is a painful, erythematous lesion, of which a sunburn is typical. (2) A second-degree or partial-thickness burn is painful, erythematous, and vesiculated. The blebs or vesicles are characteristic, but they may have already ruptured or some may not yet have formed by the time the patient is seen. (3) A third-degree or full-thickness burn has a white or charred, dry appearance and is anesthetic to touch. In the early hours, it is not painful, although the second-degree burn area which frequently surrounds it may be painful.

(E) The extent of the thermal burn is usually readily apparent and is easily approximated by the rule of nines, in which the total body surface is divided into areas of 9% or multiples of nine. Each upper extremity is 9% and each lower extremity 18%, with the head and neck together equalling 9% and the genitalia 1%. The anterior and posterior portions of the trunk are 18% each.

A convenient way to estimate the percentage of total body surface of a small burn is to recall that the palm of one hand represents 1%. A more accurate method makes use of the burn charts developed by Lund and Browder, a copy of which should be posted in every emergency department.

It is often difficult to accurately estimate the degree or depth of burn at the initial examination. This assessment should be tentative, at least until re-examination can be done in a day or two. If, as in this patient, circumferential burns of the neck or extremities are thought to be first-degree, the clinician should be very careful in his follow-up to be certain that the degree of burn has not been underestimated. Contracture from second- or third-degree burns does not begin in the first few hours, but edema does occur early, even in a minor burn, and can cause respiratory embarrassment when the burn is on the neck, or can cause neurovascular impairment when the burn is on an extremity. If there is any evidence of such impairment in an extremity, a fasciotomy must be done at once if gangrenous changes of the extremities are to be avoided. This was not required in this patient, since her neck wound, although circumferential, proved to be first-degree, as originally thought. At no time was there vascular embarrassment to any of the involved extremities.

(F) Associated injuries or pre-existing diseases are also an important aspect of this initial evaluation. They must be determined by a careful history and physical examination, as well as routine laboratory and other special studies. A small cutaneous burn in a healthy young adult may be a minor burn, whereas in an elderly patient with diabetes, it may represent a critical, even life-threatening injury. The reason is that fluid and electrolyte derangements are poorly tolerated by the patient with pre-existing disease, such as diabetes, and healing is defective, with infection almost a certainty.

4. (B, D) The patient with a first-degree burn can almost always be managed by home treatment, with careful follow-up in a physician's office or clinic. Most of these burns will heal without significiant infection and with almost no scarring, no matter what treatment is used.

(A, C) In most adults, minor burns are those partial-thickness thermal burns of less than 10 to 15% and full-thickness burns of less than 3%. Patients with burns of these magnitudes can usually be treated on an outpatient basis.

Moderate burns are partial-thickness burns of 15 to 30% or full-thickness burns of 3 to 10%. These usually require hospitalization.

In children, even smaller burns require hospitalization. The same can be said of burns in the elderly, especially if there is an associated disease or if the home setting is not satisfactory for the patient's care.

Severe or critical burns are all partial-thickness burns greater than 30% and all full-thickness burns greater than 10%. All patients with severe burns should be hospitalized. Patients with severe or special types of burns should almost always be transferred to a hospital or burn center where special care is available.

As implied in answer 3, the decision to admit a burned patient to the hospital is, in actuality, based on far more than just the depth and extent of the wound. Other relevant factors include the location of the burn, the age of the patient, the presence of associated injuries, and the presence of pre-existing diseases, as well as the type of burn. Patients with electrical burns should always be hospitalized. Patients with respiratory tract burns require admission, as do patients with almost any burn associated with other injuries, such as fractures. If a patient has no one available to take care of him at home, this may influence the decision to bring him into the hospital for at least the initial care. All burns in infants under 18 months of age, and in patients over 60 years of age, are legitimate reasons for hospitalization.

There is a tendency to underestimate the severity of burns in certain locations. These include the face, hands, perineum, genitalia, and feet. For this reason, patients with burns in these areas should be hospitalized, at least initially. The patients with burns of the feet who are allowed to go home for outpatient care are the ones who most often require hospitalization later, when it is found that the arrangement for home care is unsatisfactory.

Ideally, the decision about admission should be made after consultation with the physician who will provide definitive care.

5. (B, C, D, F, G) (A) Tracheostomy is rarely performed, since it creates a portal of invasion of bacteria or fungi. However, maintaining an airway is of vital importance, especially for the patient with possible smoke inhalation injury. If required, endotracheal intubation may be carried out and the oxygen administration and assisted ventilation (G) accomplished in this manner. If a significant degree of inhalation injury is judged to be present, tracheostomy may be required later as an elective procedure.

(B) Application of ice water or ice packs can be very helpful immediately following the burn for stopping the burning process and for relief of pain. It can often be advised by telephone or radio before the patient leaves for the hospital. However, an hour or so after the injury, it is not likely to be helpful. Its chief use is to relieve the early pain of smaller burns.

(C) At the minimum, the clinician needs to know how and when the burn occurred, by what agent, and whether there were other injuries sustained, as well as personal medical information, such as age, previous illnesses, medications being used, and any allergies, especially to medications.

The brief physical examination should indicate depth and extent of the burn, with the percentage of total body surface of each burned area by degree (disregarding first-degree burns), the status of the central nervous system and cardiopulmonary system and the presence of any associated injuries or illnesses.

(D) Fluid therapy for a burn patient is the most important aspect of early care. At least two intravenous lines should be opened as soon as possible, plus a central venous line. These should be placed in nonburned areas, if possible. See answer 6 for additional discussion of fluid therapy.

(E) Narcotics should never be administered by the subcutaneous or intramuscular route during the first 48 hours following a moderate to severe burn, because the edema that invariably develops prevents absorption of the drug. Later, when the edema subsides, the drug will be absorbed into the blood stream, and the patient may suffer the lethal effects of an overdose. The oral route is not satisfactory either, because the patient is likely to develop paralytic ileus, and the medication will not be absorbed fully, if at all. (For the same reason, the patient should be denied oral liquids and food.)

Morphine is the narcotic of choice in most patients. An intravenous dose of 3 to 5 mg is usually satisfactory for adults, the dose to be repeated every 5 to 10 minutes as necessary for initial pain relief.

(F) As in most cases of severe trauma, an indwelling Foley catheter should be placed in the bladder. This will allow much finer adjustments in fluid therapy by allowing easy and frequent measurement of the urinary output.

6. (A, B, C, D) (A, B, C) For calculating the extent of burn, first-degree burned areas are disregarded and the calculation is made only on the basis of second- and third-degree burned areas (see D). It is very important to know the patient's weight (and height), especially if a child, in order to calculate fluid requirements and medication dosages. For all ages, a baseline weight is useful in determining fluid retention, as well as nutrition.

The formula as outlined in A, B, and C is called the Brooke formula, and it is widely used in this country and many other parts of the world. Most of the colloid should be given early, and children require a larger proportion of colloid than adults. However, it is possible to limit initial fluid replacement to lactated Ringer's solution, in the amount of 3 to 4 ml/kg times the percentage of burned area. This is called the Parkland Hospital or Dallas formula and is based on the premise that colloid is not required in the first 24 hours for most patients.

This latter formula is not listed in the question, but it is becoming popular in more and more burn centers.

Whichever formula is used, approximately one-half of this calculated amount should be given in the first eight hours - not four hours (E) - after injury. The start of the eight-hour period should be the time of injury, not the time the patient was first seen. One-fourth of the calculated amount of fluid is then given in each of the second and third eight-hour periods.

Formulas are only guidelines for initial therapy and must be flexible. After 8 to 12 hours, re-evaluation of the patient will determine the type of fluid and the optimal amount needed. This re-evaluation includes hourly measurement and recording of the urinary output (the desired amount being 0. 5 to 1. 5 ml/kg/hr), pulse, blood pressure, and central venous pressure, as well as assessment of the patient's general condition.

(D) There is no basis for calculating the fluid requirement on more than 50% of total body surface burned. The fluid requirement parallels the extent of the burn up to 50%, but above that level, the requirements are variable. To use a higher figure would increase the risk of producing fluid overload and pulmonary edema. When using the Brooke formula for burns above 40% of body surface, it is wise to increase the colloid estimate at the expense of the electrolyte requirement.

In the second 24 hours, about one-half of the electrolyte and colloid fluid used in the first 24 hours is needed.

7. (A, B, E, F, H) (A) For moderate to severe burns, gentle washing and debridement are best done in the Hubbard tank. This should be deferred until the patient's condition has stabilized, usually at least one to three hours after arrival if the burn is the only injury found.

(B) One of the several ointments available is then applied, the purpose of which is to prevent or minimize bacterial colonization of the wound. Although some of these agents do not penetrate the eschar to the interface between the living and devitalized tissue, they do lessen or prevent cellulitis and septicemia, which are the major complications of burns. One of the creams that does penetrate the eschar is 10% mafenide, used in the acetate form to reduce or prevent problems of metabolic acidosis. It should be applied to a depth of approximately 5 millimeters. It exerts a bacteriostatic effect, although it does not sterilize the wound. It is nonstaining, but it does cause pain on application. For this reason, the patient may require a narcotic before the ointment is applied.

Silver sulfadiazine is another preparation that is suitable for this purpose, since it also penetrates the eschar well and is nonstaining. It has an advantage over mafenide acetate in that it is less painful on application; and there have been no reports of metabolic acidosis resulting from its use.

Both of these preparations interfere with spontaneous separation of the eschar; therefore, daily hydrotherapy and debridement are required.

(C) Prophylactic administration of antibiotics for patients with moderate to severe burns is still controversial. The matter revolves around whether such antibiotics actually reach the burn area, in view of the compromised circulation in that area. Also, there is the question of whether they are needed in the first 24 hours before actual colonization takes place. It is not certain that antibiotics administered early actually prevent infection in the burn wound.

(D) Whole blood transfusion will not be indicated in the emergency department, unless whole blood loss can be demonstrated or is at least strongly suspected. However, as for any seriously injured patient, whole blood should be cross-matched for the burn patient and made available for possible bleeding from associated injuries. Also, if the patient develops hypovolemic shock of uncertain cause, blood will probably be required. Only plasma will be needed if the drop in blood pressure proves to be due to the loss of fluid from the burn itself. If whole blood is given, it should, of course, be counted as colloid in calculating fluid needs.

(E, F) Monitoring these variables is routine for special care units, such as the emergency department and the intensive care unit. All levels or readings should be recorded on a flow chart for easy detection of any deleterious trends.

(G) A diuretic is not indicated routinely for any reason. The best assurance against acute renal failure is adequate fluid administration.

(H) Tetanus prophylaxis in the form of a booster injection of tetanus toxoid or 250 to 500 units of tetanus immune globulin, is particularly needed for third-degree burns, not as much for second-degree burns, and not at all for first-degree burns. However, one may reasonably give the injection if the usual criteria for a booster are met.

8. (A, B, C, D) Although the initial treatment depends somewhat upon the type of burn sustained, certain general rules apply to all burns that are to be treated on an outpatient basis.

All patients require review of their tetanus immunization and prophylactic injection if necessary, as mentioned previously.

(A) Gentle washing with a bland soap and water is indicated to remove as much debris and as many contaminating bacteria as possible. This should reduce the massive bacterial colonization that is sometimes present after 24 hours and that leads quickly to actual infection.

(B) Debridement in the initial phase of care involves removing the loose ends of tissue, such as the ruptured vesicles. Generally, unruptured vesicles may be left intact at the initial treatment. In third-degree burns, debridement involves removing charred tissue and any dirt and debris that was not washed off. These procedures should cause little or no pain. Although burns treated in the hospital are usually left exposed, burns in ambulatory patients treated on an outpatient basis are best covered by a light, nonadhering dressing. The initial dressing must be changed one or two days later, and subsequent dressings must be changed every two to three days in the physician's office or clinic. Thus, frequent follow-up visits are necessary (D).

(C) The use of ice water or ice packs as soon as possible after a minor burn occurs is often useful in stopping the burning process and for relief of pain. For more severe burns, pain and anxiety should be relieved immediately by the use of a narcotic, and arrangements should be made for control of pain after the patient leaves the emergency department. Meperidine, codeine, or pentazocine is suitable for this purpose, often combined with another analgesic if an additive effect is needed for more severe pain. A sedative may be indicated for the first week or two. Narcotics, analgesics, and sedative-hypnotic drugs should be reduced as soon as possible to decrease the chance of addiction or habituation.

(E) Systemic antibiotic therapy is rarely, if ever, indicated for such burns. In fact, an antibiotic ointment is usually not indicated, although the patient and the physician may prefer the use of some mild ointment, not necessarily an antibiotic type, before the dressing of minor burns.

COURSE:

This patient was admitted to the hospital, and her burns were treated with mafenide acetate. She had no respiratory insufficiency at any time. On the ninth hospital day, the eschar of the right hand and forearm was excised; six days later, split-thickness grafts were applied to these wounds and "took" successfully. The other wounds healed well without grafting. On the twenty-fourth hospital day, she was discharged home to continue physical therapy and to be followed up by a plastic surgeon.

::

CASE 42: ELECTRICAL BURN

HISTORY:

A 34-year-old man had tried to free a fishing line from a power pole by climbing the pole. He touched a live high-voltage electrical wire with his right hand and was thrown from the pole. The voltage involved and the height from which he fell were not known. He was unconscious for an undetermined period of time, and had amnesia for the incident.

When he arrived at the emergency department, he was alert and oriented. His blood pressure was 110/80 mm Hg; pulse, 90/min, and regular; and respirations, 16/min and regular.

There were third-degree burns of the entire right hand with deeper burns of the volar aspect of the index and middle fingers. He had a circumferential burn of the right wrist 6 cm wide, with thrombosed veins in the burn area. The radial pulse was not palpable. The wrist was fixed in 80 degrees of flexion, with only 20 degrees of motion possible. The fingers were in fixed flexion contracture. Several small burns were noted in the right elbow area, including a third-degree burn in the antecubital space, measuring 3 x 6 cm. The volar aspect of the left wrist had a 2 x 3-cm third-degree burn. The penis had a third-degree circumferential burn, 3 cm wide in the midportion of the shaft. A deep burn, 3 x 4 cm, was noted over the left side of the anterior aspect of the scrotum; the testicle was exposed. The right side of the scrotum had a 2 x 2-cm third-degree burn of the anterior surface. Both thighs had multiple small areas of third-degree burns, some of them deep.

The results of the remainder of the general and neurological examination were normal. There was no evidence of associated injuries.

QUESTIONS:

1. Which of the following are true regarding the injury potential of electricity?
   - A. Direct current is more dangerous than alternating current.
   - B. The tissue damage results from the conversion of electrical energy to thermal energy, with heat production.
   - C. The risk of thermal injury is directly proportional to the voltage.

D. Low-tension (voltage) injuries (below 500 volts) usually produce only local thermal damage.
E. High-tension injuries (above 500 volts) are often associated with arcing, with the production of intense heat.
F. Electrical current flows preferentially along blood vessels and nerves.
G. Fractures can occur from severe muscle contraction.

2. Which of these statements about electrical injuries or burns are true?
   A. Most severe electrical burns are job-related.
   B. Electrical burns constitute approximately 3% of all burns.
   C. Mortality rate is 18 to 20%.
   D. There is always a single wound of entry of the current and a single point of exit.
   E. The smaller the area of contact, the more severe the burn.
   F. Twenty per cent of patients require at least one major amputation.
   G. Thermal damage to internal organs is usual.
   H. The extent of the burn should be apparent at the initial examination if one checks carefully.

3. Immediate treatment of patients with electrical burns consists of which of the following?
   A. Removal of the patient from contact with the source of electricity.
   B. Cardiopulmonary resuscitation, if required
   C. Application of ice directly to the burn wound
   D. Careful search for associated injuries
   E. Large amounts of fluid intravenously
   F. Debridement of the burn with application of antibacterial ointment, using the exposure method of care
   G. Tetanus prophylaxis
   H. Gas gangrene prophylaxis
   I. Antibiotic therapy

4. Additional treatment of patients with electrical burns consists of which of the following?
   A. Blood transfusion
   B. Escharotomy, fasciotomy, or excision of nonviable tissue as soon as feasible
   C. Enzymatic debridement
   D. Nasogastric suction
   E. Monitoring of central venous pressure and urinary output
   F. Hospitalization

5. Which of the following are potential complications of electrical burns?
   A. Cardiac dysrhythmias and cardiovascular collapse
   B. Vascular obstruction requiring major amputation
   C. Contracture of tendons, which may cause permanent deformities
   D. Visceral injury
   E. Renal failure
   F. Sepsis
   G. Hemorrhage
   H. Permanent nerve damage
   I. False aneurysm
   J. Cataracts
   K. All of the above

ANSWERS AND COMMENTS:

1. (B, C, E, F, G) Alternating current at any voltage is much more dangerous than direct current (A). Low-tension injuries by alternating current frequently cause ventricular fibrillation, instead of thermal burn, or they may cause both (D). The most dangerous current to the heart is alternating current at 40 to 60 hertz.

(B, C) The mechanism by which damage is produced from electrical current is very complex. It relates to several variables: the voltage, the duration of the contact, the resistance of the tissues, and the variability in individual response to electrical current. Damage is produced by the conversion of electrical energy to thermal energy, and this is directly related to voltage differences (E). When the voltage is high, the electrical flow and the heat produced will be great, causing coagulation necrosis, especially at points of entry and exit of the current. Locking to the electrical source is much less likely to occur with high-voltage than with low-voltage contact.

Arcing is a special problem with high-tension current, in that the current jumps from the contact source to the body producing incredible heat, from 3000° C to $20,000^{\circ}$ C, which burns deeply into tissues and organs beneath the skin.

(F) Body tissues vary greatly in their resistance to electrical current. Nerve tissue offers the least resistance, blood and blood vessels, muscle, skin, tendon, fat, and bone offer, in increasing order, more resistance. Blood coagulates, due to the heat, especially in the veins, and the arteries sustain medial necrosis. Arterial thrombosis is spotty, probably because the blood moves more rapidly through the arteries than through the veins.

(G) Fractures occur from tetanic contractions in the victim who remains in contact with the source of electricity. It is usually the vertebral bodies that fracture, although long bones may fracture in a fall such as this patient sustained.

2. (A, B, C, E, F) Electrical burns differ from thermal burns, in that the damage is almost always more severe and deeper. Therefore, electrical burns are less obvious at times, with normal skin hiding necrosis of the underlying muscle. In fact, the differences are so great that (1) many authorities consider electrical injury as not being primarily a burn and (2) confusing the two is likely to cause one to underestimate the severity of the injury and to administer inadequate fluids for resuscitation. This can cause an early or late death and represents one reason emergency department physicians need to be aware of the implications of electrical injury.

A related problem is that a thermal cutaneous burn, as from ignition of clothing, may mask even further the extent of the tissue damage from the electrical current.

(A) Most severe electrical injuries are job-related, and occur in men rather than women. However, many of the injuries are caused during do-it-yourself home repairs or installations, such as of television antennas.

Children sustain electrical burns from chewing through electrical cords. These are usually not severe, although a few deaths have occurred. The burn is usually confined to the mouth, and reconstructive surgery may be required several months later.

(B) Three per cent of all major burns are electrical and three to five per cent of all admissions to major burn centers are for this type of injury. The number of electrical injuries is gradually increasing, despite safety warnings and precautions, such as better shielding of high-tension sources from contact with workers. Electrical linemen make up the largest single group injured.

(C) In the United States each year, there are over one thousand deaths from contact with electricity, plus an additional 200 deaths caused by lightning. Most of the immediate deaths are due to ventricular fibrillation in the case of low-voltage injury, and to asystole or respiratory arrest in the case of high-voltage injury. Of those victims who survive long enough to reach the emergency department, the mortality rate is 18 to 20% with at least 20% requiring one or more major amputations (F).

(D) There is frequently a single entrance wound - as in this patient, whose entry wound was on his right hand - but there are usually multiple exit wounds. These may be the only cutaneous burns. In this patient, the left hand possibly, and the thighs, scrotum and penis certainly, were sites of exit wounds. The number of entry and exit wounds varies widely, depending upon how the initial contact was made, the degree of arcing that occurred, and the voltage involved. Severe arcing occurred in the region of this patient's hand, in addition to the direct contact of his hand against the wire, causing the contracture of the fingers and wrist.

(E) One of the greatest pitfalls in evaluation of a patient with possible high-tension electrical injury is that the smaller the area of contact, the more severe the damage. The mechanism of such damage is a concentration of the current into that small area, which may be either the site of entry or a site of exit. Lightning injuries often present the smallest cutaneous wounds and often no external wound at all, even when the victim has sustained severe internal injury. This is occasionally true for a victim killed outright.

(G) Thermal damage to internal organs is unusual. The reason is not entirely clear, but the skin of the trunk reduces the amount of heat released and protects the organs in the thoracic, abdominal, and pelvic cavities. When the current enters or exits through the head, it is the scalp (and occasionally the skull) that sustains the burn. If cerebral damage occurs, it does so by way of the diploic veins. This patient's presumed unconsciousness was probably due to the effect on the brain of the sudden, severe high-tension shock, although a dysrhythmia, such as ventricular tachycardia with hypotension, or a head injury sustained in the fall, cannot be ruled out as the cause.

(H) The extent of electrical burns is almost never fully apparent at the initial examination; in fact, several days may pass before the damage can be fully assessed. It is true that third-degree burns are usually apparent at the electrical contact points, but the extensive coagulation necrosis of the vessels, nerves and musculotendinous structures is hidden at first and may not become apparent until dysfunction occurs, due to swelling or necrosis.

3. (A, B, D, E, F, G, I) (A, B) Care at the scene of the accident is critical, particularly if the victim is locked to the wire or other contact object. It is also critical if cardiac arrest has occurred. Unless the electrical circuit is broken and the heart restarted if necessary, the victim will obviously not arrive at the emergency department alive. An electrocardiogram should always be done as soon as possible, since the patient may have, or may subsequently develop, serious dysrhythmias, especially ventricular fibrillation.

(C) The purpose of applying ice water to a burn is to stop the burning process and to relieve pain. It is reserved for thermal burns not larger, say, than 10% of body surface. To be effective, it must be used early after the injury. Ice should never be applied directly to a wound, since the consequent development of frostbite would only increase the extent of injury.

(D) Associated injuries are usually of secondary importance to the shock and burns, unless they are serious head injury, spinal cord damage, tension pneumothorax, or bleeding into the chest or abdomen. A brief preliminary examination, plus appropriate ancillary studies, will usually reveal any associated injuries.

(E) The amount of fluid required for resuscitation is frequently quite high because of the extensive damage, especially to the tissues deep beneath the skin. Since the formula method used for initial fluid replacement in patients with cutaneous burns is not appropriate for electrical burns, determination of functional blood volume and measurement of urinary output are the best methods of determining fluid requirements. However, the urinary flow should be kept at a rate approximately twice that sought in patients with only cutaneous burns, in an attempt to avoid renal failure from pigmenturia. In an adult, this usually means a urinary output of at least 75 to 100 ml/hr.

(F) Initial, preliminary debridement may be done in the Hubbard tank or in the operating room, provided the patient's condition is stable. Debridement is one of the best methods of determining the extent of the underlying tissue damage and of removing obviously necrotic tissue. Initially, the excision of tissue should be conservative, since the viability of tissue is impossible to determine by inspection. Daily removal of obviously nonviable tissue is indicated, preferably with the patient in the Hubbard tank. For the most severe burns, extensive exploration of the burned area is indicated within the first few hours or days, with removal of all nonviable tissue, regardless of the depth and the type of tissue.

There is no doubt that the exposure method for local wounds is preferable to the closed method. This allows frequent inspection of the wounds, and the area between the entrance and exit wounds, for possible necrosis. Either silver sulfadiazine or mafenide acetate should be applied topically, the latter being preferred because of its ability to penetrate more deeply into the burned tissue.

(G, H) Prophylaxis against tetanus is especially important in patients who have electrical burns because of the deep tissue damage that is usually present. If there is any doubt about the patient's protection, tetanus immune globulin should be given. There is considerable controversy over the effectiveness of the gas gangrene antitoxin for prophylaxis, as well as for treatment. In any case, this prophylactic treatment for both tetanus and gas gangrene must be combined with adequate debridement, including amputation when necessary, if extensive necrotic tissue is involved. Massive necrosis of muscle tissue especially is likely to result in sepsis, such tissue becoming secondarily infected with both aerobic and anaerobic bacteria. This frequently clears after early, adequate debridement, repeated as necessary, plus adequate doses of appropriate antibiotics.

(I) Antibiotic therapy, such as penicillin, ten million units daily, intravenously, is recommended for the first ten days or so.

4. (A, B, D, E, F) (A) Often large amounts of blood are required in the first few days to maintain adequate blood volume and support debridement. The extensive debridement required with electrical burns often leads to hemorrhage from friable vessels, as well as to rupture of major vessels, either during or after the procedure.

(B) Fasciotomies, deeper than escharotomies, play a definite role in the management of electrical injuries. The deeper the muscle injury present in any extremity, the more the edema and the more the likelihood of vascular insufficiency, both arterial and venous.

(C) Many preparations have been used for enzymatic debridement, but none are capable of cleansing a wound sufficiently for grafting within a few days. Some burn centers do not use them at all, but prefer to use antibacterial ointment, saline soaks, and daily sharp debridement, preferably in the Hubbard tank.

(D) Most of the patients have adynamic ileus following the injury and require nasogastric suction for several days. Although damage to abdominal organs is unusual, necrosis of retroperitoneal muscle is not unusual and contributes to the ileus.

(E) Monitoring the central venous pressure is necessary even in a patient with normal cardiovascular dynamics. In those with cardiac disease or with massive necrosis, more sophisticated monitoring is probably indicated. As mentioned earlier, the urinary output is the major factor in determining whether fluid resuscitation is adequate or not.

(F) It is essential to admit to the hospital any patient who has sustained a significant electrical burn. Significant means almost any cutaneous burn, since the extent of the damage to underlying or remote tissue bears little correlation to the size and depth of the cutaneous damage. It is also impossible to predict, on the basis of the history and extent of cutaneous burn, how much swelling with secondary vascular insufficiency will occur and how soon. If the patient is allowed to return home he may, within a few hours, develop irreparable damage to any extremity involved either in the entry or the exit of the current. As in this patient, the male genitalia can also be involved and require extensive grafting or radical surgery.

5. (K) All of the answers represent potential complications, A through G occurring within the first week or so, and H and I being delayed, usually for weeks or months. Some have already been discussed or are obvious from the case report.

(B) Vascular obstruction is due to damage to the walls of the vessels, as well as to clotting within the lumen of both veins and arteries. This causes ischemia and necrosis of the part, usually an extremity, supplied by the arteries involved. Such damage can lead to early or late rupture of a vessel with bleeding (G), or the escaping blood may be contained by a sac composed of the surrounding tissues - a false aneurysm (I). The Doppler flowmeter can be helpful in assessing blood flow, and this information can be used in determining the need for fasciotomy. Testing for loss of sensation is useful for the same purpose.

(E) Renal failure occurs in major electrical burns due to hematuria, proteinuria, and myoglobinuria. It is the most common cause of early hospital death following major electrical burn.

Urinary flow should be maintained at a minimum level of 75 to 100 ml/hr as a preventive measure. An osmotic diuretic, such as mannitol, may be helpful.

(F) Sepsis comes from secondary infection of necrotic tissue, especially muscle. Infection may be with aerobic bacteria, anaerobic bacteria, or both. Sepsis is one of the major causes of early hospital deaths from electrical burns. On the other hand, it frequently clears without sequelae after early, adequate debridement, plus adequate doses of appropriate antibiotics.

(H) Nerve damage, which may be impossible to detect at early operations, may manifest itself later and be permanent. Both sensory and motor nerves may be affected. The mechanisms seem to be the traversing of the nerve by the electrical current, the ischemia that usually develops, and the local infection which may develop with secondary perineural fibrosis.

(J) Cataracts may occur months or years later and must be remembered when discussing prognosis with the patient and his family.

COURSE:

Escharotomy of the right upper extremity, dorsal slitting of the prepuce, and debridement of the wounds of the scrotum and both thighs were done in the operating room soon after this patient's arrival in the emergency department. Twelve days after admission, his right upper extremity was amputated above the elbow because of the extensive wrist and hand deformity and because of gangrenous changes of the distal portion of the triceps muscle. The stump was left open and was later closed satisfactorily. A suprapubic catheter was required for several weeks. The left testicle became necrotic, and was removed. Several grafting procedures were required to cover all residual wounds, including the penis. At 18 months' follow-up, he was doing quite well. There had been no clinical or other evidence of injury to the head, heart or abdominal viscera at any time.

::

CASE 43: DRUG OVERDOSE IN A 21-YEAR-OLD WOMAN

HISTORY:

A 21-year-old woman took 10 to 15 five-milligram tablets of diazepam because her "husband is not spending enough time at home." She immediately told a friend what she had done and was promptly brought to the emergency department. She denied alcohol intake and use and abuse of other drugs. The diazepam had been prescribed for nervous tension the week before. There were no known previous attempts to commit suicide.

She was alert and cooperative. The results of the general physical examination were normal. Her affect was flat, but she was of average intelligence and was oriented. She repeated her determination to kill herself.

Thirty minutes after ingestion of the diazepam, repeated vomiting was induced with 60 ml of syrup of ipecac. Gastric lavage was not done.

She was admitted to the psychiatric ward for both her protection and supportive therapy. She had not seemed drowsy at any time during her stay in the emergency department.

QUESTIONS:

1. Which of the following are true regarding suicide?
   - A. At least 22, 000 deaths from suicide occur each year in the United States, making suicide the tenth leading cause of death.
   - B. Suicidal attempts are either manipulative gestures or serious attempts to end life.
   - C. Suicidal attempts are made only by patients who are obviously and seriously depressed.
   - D. Suicidal attempts are twice as common in women as in men.
   - E. Completed suicide, i. e., death, is several times more frequent in women than in men.
   - F. A family history of suicide decreases, rather than increases, the risk.
   - G. In the emergency department, most patients who have attempted suicide require emergency psychiatric evaluation.
   - H. All of the above

2. TRUE OR FALSE: This patient's suicidal attempt was probably a serious one, not just a gesture.

3. Which of the following statements about depression are true?
   A. It may be either psychotic or nonpsychotic.
   B. Most patients who are depressed are receiving adequate treatment.
   C. Approximately 70% of depressed patients respond favorably to tricyclic medication given in adequate doses.
   D. Monoamine oxidase inhibitors are the first-line drugs for nonpsychotic depression.
   E. A depressed mood is never normal and always deserves treatment.
   F. Most severely depressed patients should be hospitalized.
   G. Depression afflicts only middle-aged and elderly persons.
   H. All of the above

TRUE OR FALSE (Questions 4 and 5):

4. The risk of suicide is almost nil in the depressed patient who begins to show signs of clinical improvement.

5. Questioning a depressed patient about suicidal thoughts will cause him to attempt suicide.

6. Depression is characterized by which of the following?
   A. Somatic complaints
   B. Suicidal thoughts or behavior
   C. Psychomotor retardation
   D. Flat affect
   E. Loss of interest, motivation, decisiveness
   F. All of the above

7. TRUE OR FALSE: The management of grief has no place in the emergency department.

ANSWERS AND COMMENTS:

1. (A, B, D, G) (A) The number of completed suicides in the United States each year is at least 22, 000, making suicide the tenth leading cause of death. If accidents that may have been suicides were included, the number would probably be ten times that. The number of attempted suicides is several hundred thousand, many patients attempting to kill themselves multiple times.

(B) Suicidal attempts are either serious attempts to end life or attempts to convey a message, a cry for help. The problem is to decide which; in other words, to assess the risk of the patient's repeating the attempt for whatever reason.

(C) In all depressive reactions, the chief risk is suicide. However, not all persons attempting suicide are depressed. It is estimated that only a little over half of completed suicides are in persons having suffered from depression, although depression is the most common single precursor state of suicidal behavior. Patients with agitated depression are particularly prone to suicide. Therefore, it is necessary to differentiate between that and retarded (nonagitated) depression. Many patients with agitated depression may only seem "nervous and upset" on superficial examination.

(D, E) Suicide attempts are twice as common in women, but completed suicides are much more common in men. That probably has much to do with the method used, men tending to use methods that are more apt to be lethal.

(F) Since the patient has often been affected by a previous family suicide and knows the effect it had on the family, one might expect the patient to hesitate before putting the family through such an experience again. However, that is not true, and a family history of suicide increases, rather than decreases, the risk of suicide.

(G) Not only do such patients require emergency psychiatric evaluation, but they also require hospitalization - involuntary commitment, if necessary.

Hospitalization is not, in itself, an invariable preventive of suicide, since, until circumstances have changed and hope has been re-established, the patient is not safe anywhere. Such a change in circumstances can result from intervention by the clinician and the patient's family and friends, that intervention including whatever changes in the patient's environment are required.

2. (False) Although one cannot be certain, it is very likely that this patient's attempt was only a manipulative gesture. However, her repeated threats of suicide had to be taken seriously, for the reason that she might miscalculate and die the next time. That risk was present, even though she probably did not wish to die and would be making an additional attempt only to make her husband more attentive.

In other words, some persons who attempt suicide do not want to die but are unable to get the attention of persons in a position to help them by any other means. Other persons see no other way out of their hopeless, helpless situation except to die, and they are trying to do so.

Persons at high risk of suicide are lonely, elderly persons (especially male), alcoholic persons or others who are drug abusers, and chronically or terminally ill persons, as well as persons who have previously attempted suicide or who have had a recent significant loss, such as the loss of a loved one or a job. At least 60% of completed-suicide victims had a history of previous suicide attempts, and 75% had given clear warning that they would try to commit suicide. For most patients attempting suicide more than once, the attempts increase in severity until one is successful. Other patients use a stereotyped, usually feeble attempt, which may be tried dozens of times (such as lightly slashing the wrist or forearm).

Ten per cent of attempted-suicide patients will eventually kill themselves, regardless of the amount of attention and treatment they receive. This figure would be much higher, except for the relatively large proportion of those who use mild attempts as suicidal gestures.

3. (A, C, F) The differentiation between nonpsychotic depression and psychotic depression is based on a history of hallucinations and delusions in the latter, those being the usual criteria for diagnosis of psychosis.

(B) Depression is one of the most underdiagnosed and undertreated conditions in our society. It represents approximately half of the total of all major psychiatric illnesses in the United States and is widespread in other countries. Even in this country, probably not more than 20 to 25% of depressed patients are receiving any form of treatment. The failure is partly due to patients who do not seek treatment, but also partly due to physicians who fail to recognize depression.

Clinically, the patient is frequently not obviously depressed or crying. Even if depressed to the point that he is contemplating suicide, a patient will almost never say so. Instead, he will usually complain about vague physical symptoms that may be exasperating to the busy physician and hard to interpret, unless the physician maintains a high index of suspicion. Acute depression is usually a self-limited condition, although treatment can make it more tolerable. From the standpoint of the risk of suicide, acute depression is much safer for the patient than chronic depression. However, acute depression frequently becomes a chronic state, and then the lifetime risk of suicide increases.

(C) Approximately 70% of depressed patients respond favorably to treatment with adequate doses of one or the other of the tricyclic drugs. The prototype drug for depression is imipramine, which, by itself, works in approximately 50% of patients, provided two to three weeks are allowed for its full effect and provided it is given in optimal doses. That titration or individualization of the dose is required because of marked variation in its effect from one patient to another.

Imipramine is indicated in depression with psychomotor retardation, whereas amitriptyline (which is somewhat more sedating) is indicated in agitated depression, which may require a combination of an anti-anxiety drug, as well as an antidepressant agent. The antidepressant chosen must be given in adequate amounts. It is not uncommon to see a patient who is taking the proper medicine, but taking it in subtherapeutic doses, as indicated by lack of improvement over a period of weeks. The dose should be started at a low daily level and increased weekly until a clinical response is noted. For imipramine, that means up to 300 mg daily.

(D) Monoamine oxidase inhibitors are not the first-choice drugs for depression. They should be considered if the tricyclic antidepressants fail to relieve the patient's symptoms, but should never be given in conjunction with the tricyclic drugs.

For the patient with manic-depressive psychosis, lithium carbonate is the drug of choice, for both treatment of the current episode and prevention of future attacks.

(E) A depressed mood is normal after a family death, a long illness, loss of a job, or loss of a part of the body, such as the breast or an extremity. That is not the type of depression that requires treatment.

Even without a loss, many so-called normal persons feel depressed at times. That feeling is usually mild and transient and requires no treatment, although treatment may be sought by persons who believe that there should be no discomfort of any sort in life.

As to diagnosis, one of the most important points to remember is that, with normal grief or depression, the patient does not have the multitude of complaints that the moderately or severely depressed patient has.

(F) Most severely depressed patients should be admitted to the hospital for observation and treatment. In many emergency department settings, that can be arranged even if psychiatric consultation is not immediately available.

Deciding whether a patient such as this one with nonpsychotic depression should be hospitalized or not is often based upon the patient's social setting and emotional support, especially the support from the family or another group.

Even a patient who is psychotically depressed may not require hospitalization, provided his social supports are strong. This means a family or group setting that has adequately served the patient's needs in the past. Also, the patient's ego strength must be evaluated as to whether, with therapy, he can manage without excessive risk of suicide in the same setting from which he came. In most instances, that question should be discussed with his family or other responsible persons.

Another factor that determines the need for hospitalization is a previous history of a long psychotic depression with a lack of response to outpatient therapy.

The procedure for involuntary commitment (a judicial process) of an emotionally disturbed patient varies from state to state. The process is legal in every state, and is controlled by laws designed to protect both the patient and those around him. However, involuntary commitment is legal only if the patient is a threat to himself or to others. Thus, a psychiatric emergency that would require such intervention can be defined as any serious disorder of thinking, feeling, or behavior. It is usually manifested by bizarre, disruptive, or alarming behavior, but may rather be manifested by acute, intense mental or emotional suffering.

There is more legal risk for the physician who fails to recommend involuntary commitment than for the one who does so. The laws in most states have an immunity clause that prevents successful legal action against a physician who acts in good faith and follows the guidelines for involuntary commitment established by each state.

Although involuntary commitment is occasionally necessary for suicidal patients, it is much more often necessary for psychotic patients.

Ordinarily, treatment for depression is usually not started in emergency departments, except under the direct supervision of the psychiatrist who arranges appropriate follow-up care for the patient. That is not to say, however, that nothing should be done in the emergency department for the depressed patient who is not to be hospitalized. If the patient has insomnia, for example, that symptom should be relieved, provided it can be done safely, with the medication being dispensed by a family member or other responsible person.

(G) Depression has been thought of as a condition of middle-aged and elderly persons, and the incidence in those age groups is still quite high. However, it is not as apparent that adolescent and young-adult persons are depressed, and the number of depressed patients in those age groups is increasing rapidly, as is the incidence of suicide.

4. (False) The depressed patient who begins to show clinical improvement may be at an increased risk of suicide. If he has a well-thought-out suicide plan, his improvement may enable him to carry it out successfully.

5. (False) A myth that has been largely dispelled, to the good of both the patient and the physician, is that asking about suicidal thoughts encourages attempts at suicide. Just the reverse is true. The patient appreciates the physician's interest in his well-being and usually responds with an honest answer, even a voluble discussion of his intentions. In fact, discussion of suicidal feelings is the one most helpful thing in the prevention of suicide. That is true in adolescents, as well as in adults. It sets the stage for the physician to offer his support if the thoughts of suicide recur, particularly during the interim before the medication, if any, has taken effect. On the other hand, the physician who gives the impression that he does not care about the patient's problem is probably increasing the risk of suicide.

For a patient who has just attempted suicide, the most important thing is to prevent his repeating the attempt. The primary physician's attitude during the patient's stay in the emergency department may be of as much benefit as the visit of the consulting psychiatrist. It is obvious that the emergency department physician cannot abrogate - or even transfer - his responsibility in that regard. As a rule of thumb, he should consider a suicidal gesture to be as lethal as a serious suicidal attempt. To consider it in any other light is to run the risk of sending the patient away to repeat the attempt, possibly with more successful, albeit disastrous, results.

6. (F) All. In addition to somatic symptoms (loss of appetite and weight, constipation, insomnia, loss of libido, amenorrhea), there are abnormalities of mood, thought, appearance, and behavior, and suicidal thoughts and actions (as in this patient). In the presence of any of those symptoms, it is vital that the clinician maintain a high index of suspicion of depression. The 20-item Zung self-rating depression scale is based upon the previously mentioned symptoms, although some of the questions are arranged to prevent the patient from anticipating the "correct" answer. That rating chart is useful in any setting for screening purposes.

Impotence is a characteristic symptom of depression in middle-aged men. For that reason, all men with impotence should be screened for possible depressive symptoms and signs. However, not all will be found to be depressed, since there are other causes of impotence.

Assessing the risk of suicide in a depressed or disturbed patient is one of the most important tasks a physician will ever undertake. Often, a clue to a patient's real intentions is found in his answer to the general question, "Well, how are things going with you?" If the physician suspects paranoid ideas, he should ask a general question such as, "Do you think your family (or your boss or other key person) is treating you fairly?" Frequently, that will produce a series of comments yielding information on the real problem, as well as anxiety features. The presence of anxiety can cause the hurried, unwary clinician to miss the diagnosis of depression and to treat the patient with anti-anxiety medication, which may make him worse, or at least will not make him any better. Thus, where possible, treatment of an emotional disorder should be started only after an examination of mental status has been done.

7. (False) Normal grief is encountered in an emergency department when a patient is brought in dead on arrival (DOA) or when a patient under treatment dies. Following the loss of a loved one, a depressed mood is normal; in fact, its absence would raise the question of a more serious underlying psychiatric disorder.

The clinician must ask himself whether the degree of grief or depression is normal, excessive, or unduly prolonged for the circumstances.

Pathological grief results when there is an arrest in the normal process of grieving, such as when a patient has a delayed grief reaction, or a distorted reaction, or becomes hyperactive and acts as if the loss has not occurred. Pathological grief may also be present when grief persists for months or years. Even more serious is the precipitation of a psychiatric disease, such as a schizophrenic reaction or a severe depression, or the exacerbation of depression in a person under treatment. If possible, psychiatric consultation is advisable immediately. Failing that, the patient may be treated with sedatives at bedtime until he is able to see a psychiatrist. Such medication should be administered by a responsible family member, since the risk of suicide may be high.

An unresolved grief reaction in children and adolescents can cause irreparable harm. The child should be given special attention in the emergency department and afterwards, and should be encouraged to talk about his feelings of loss, particularly any hostile feelings toward God or any family member. Careful follow-up care should be arranged, especially if the death was sudden and unexpected.

::

CASE 44: CARBON MONOXIDE POISONING

HISTORY:

After leaving a note saying, "I am going to kill myself because I have nothing to live for," a 43-year-old white man connected a hose from the exhaust pipe to the inside of his car through a slightly lowered window, closed himself in the car, and started the engine. He was found unconscious a short time later and a rescue squad was called. The paramedic team found his respirations to be 3/min; pulse, 150/min and weak; blood pressure, 110/50 mm Hg; and his skin "splotchy pink," but also dusky.

His upper airway was cleared; there was no evidence of vomiting. Oxygen in 100% concentration was started by bag-valve-mask administration, and 5% dextrose in water was administered intravenously.

He had exhibited bizarre behavior for three to six months, threatening on at least one occasion to kill his girl friend with a gun.

When he arrived in the emergency department, his blood pressure was 155/88 mm Hg; respirations 12/min; temperature, 99°F (37.2°C); and pulse, 90/min and strong. He was comatose, responding only slightly to painful stimuli. His conjunctivae were rosy-red and his skin was pink. The general examination was negative and neurological examination was otherwise not remarkable.

Intubation was done immediately and oxygen in high concentration given. Naloxone, 0.4 mg, and dexamethasone, 10 mg, were administered intravenously, along with 5% dextrose in 0.5 normal saline. He was then admitted to the intensive care unit.

QUESTIONS:

1. Which of the following statements about carbon monoxide are true?
   A. Next to carbon dioxide, it is the second most common pollutant of the lower atmosphere.
   B. It is formed by incomplete combustion of carbonaceous material.
   C. It is responsible for about half of the fatal poisonings in the United States.

D. It has a characteristic pungent odor.
E. Natural gas contains large amounts of it.
F. Intoxication occurs only when the atmospheric level of carbon monoxide is high.
G. The affinity of hemoglobin for carbon monoxide is over 200 times greater than that for oxygen.
H. It is a severe lung irritant.
I. All of the above

2. Which of the following are particularly susceptible to the toxic effects of carbon monoxide?
   A. Children
   B. The elderly
   C. Anemic persons
   D. Individuals engaged in strenuous exercise or under emotional stress
   E. Heavy cigarette smokers
   F. All of the above

3. **TRUE OR FALSE**: Another common source of carbon monoxide toxicity is smoke.

4. With a history such as this, the diagnosis is relatively easy. When the history is not so clear-cut, which one of the following is the <u>most</u> suggestive of carbon monoxide intoxication?
   A. History of exposure to smoke, fire or "gas" in an enclosed space
   B. History of drowsiness, blurred or reduced vision, decreased mentation
   C. Cherry red skin and mucous membranes
   D. Elevated levels of carboxyhemoglobin in the blood
   E. Arterial blood gases and pH levels, indicating oxygen desaturation and metabolic acidosis

5. The treatment for acute carbon monoxide intoxication is which of the following?
   A. Removal of the patient from the carbon monoxide environment
   B. One hundred per cent oxygen therapy
   C. Methylene blue given intravenously
   D. Hypothermia
   E. Hyperbaric oxygen chamber
   F. All of the above

ANSWERS AND COMMENTS:

1. (A, B, C, G) (D) Carbon monoxide has no odor, making it all

the more dangerous. It is also colorless and tasteless, the truly "silent" killer. It is responsible for more deaths due to poison than any other single substance - the latest report being 3, 500 accidental or suicidal deaths in the United States per year.

(E) Natural gas contains no carbon monoxide, although it may produce a poisonous gas if burned without adequate oxygen. Illuminating gas of a former era and some gas used for heating have appreciable amounts of carbon monoxide. However, any carbonaceous material that burns incompletely can be the source of carbon monoxide.

(F) Intoxication can occur even when very small amounts of carbon monoxide are present in the atmosphere. In an atmosphere of 1% carbon monoxide (10, 000 parts per million) and 20% oxygen, a lethal concentration of carboxyhemoglobin can occur in the blood in as short a time as ten minutes. Symptomatic levels are reached in one to two minutes. The reason is that hemoglobin has an affinity for carbon monoxide that is greater than 200 times its affinity for oxygen (G). So long as there is a significant level of carbon monoxide in the ambient air, the concentration of carboxyhemoglobin will continue to build up in the body, with symptoms increasing proportionately. This is particularly true if the air being breathed has a reduced level of oxygen for any reason, as in the case of a fire with large amounts of smoke present in the immediate vicinity of the patient.

Another way in which carbon monoxide is harmful is that it prevents the release of oxygen from the hemoglobin not yet displaced by carboxyhemoglobin. It does this by shifting the oxyhemoglobin dissociation curve to the left, resulting in greater affinity of hemoglobin for oxygen, thus preventing release of oxygen to the tissues. This produces profound hypoxia, which leads to death if not corrected. The dysfunction caused by a carboxyhemoglobin concentration of 50% is much greater than the effect of reducing the hemoglobin concentration 50%, as in ordinary anemia.

There may also be a direct toxic effect of carbon monoxide on the myocardium, constituting a third threat to the person who inhales it. However, this patient's electrocardiogram showed only mild, nonspecific changes, and he had no cardiac dysrhythmia at any time after his arrival in the emergency department.

(H) Carbon monoxide causes no lung irritation, thus adding to the hazard of exposure, since it causes no coughing or other warning symptoms. Unless the patient has pre-existing changes or has vomited or aspirated, there should be no abnormalities on a chest roentgenogram.

2. (F) All. For little understood reasons, there is marked variation in susceptibility to carbon monoxide among persons in whom these variables are the same. However, overall, the relatively increased metabolic rate in children causes them to build up higher percentages of hemoglobin occupied by the carbon monoxide than adults exposed for the same duration. The elderly are more susceptible than young adults because of associated illnesses, especially cardiac problems. The person who has anemia is especially sensitive to the toxic effects of carbon monoxide. Rapid or deep breathing, as occurs with physical exertion or emotional stress, allows larger amounts of carbon monoxide to accumulate in the blood more rapidly. Many heavy cigarette smokers already have carboxyhemoglobin levels as high as 8 to 15%. The additional amount from acute exposure to carbon monoxide causes the carboxyhemoglobin level to reach toxic proportions earlier than in nonsmokers.

3. (True) Smoke contains carbon monoxide in concentrations of 0.1 to 10%. Even a few deep breaths of smoke containing the higher concentration can cause toxic symptoms; and 30 seconds of heavy exertion in ambient air that contains 10% carbon monoxide produces dangerously high levels of carboxyhemoglobin in the blood.

4. (D) (A) It is seldom that a confirmed history of exposure is available at the time the patient is first seen. Exceptions are when the patient is found unconscious under the circumstances described for this patient, and when the patient is rescued from a burning building. In the latter instance, exposure to carbon monoxide and other harmful gases found in smoke must be assumed and the patient treated accordingly.

Even in the absence of such clues, a patient must be suspected of having been exposed to carbon monoxide if the diagnosis is obscure and if the circumstances are uncertain. This is especially true if there are physical findings suggestive of this entity.

(B) Unfortunately, the symptoms of carbon monoxide intoxication are nonspecific. Therefore, it is very important that the clinician maintain a high index of suspicion, and that he search for any clues to this type of poisoning. The patient who has been accidentally exposed to carbon monoxide has no reason to suspect that anything is amiss, except that he is drowsy and has headache, weakness and blurred vision. His higher centers of judgment are likely to be affected early, and he may not recognize these or other warning symptoms until it is too late. In fact, the longer the exposure and the higher the carboxyhemoglobin level, the more likely neurological symptoms are to develop. These include mental deterioration, tremors, and psychotic behavior. The reason for this is that the central nervous system is the body tissue most vulnerable to tissue hypoxia, which is the crux of the problem in acute carbon monoxide intoxication. Even with early and intensive treatment, the neurological symptoms may persist for hours to days, and are occasionally permanent.

The symptoms depend almost entirely on the concentration of carboxyhemoglobin in the blood (D). In general, at levels of zero to 10% of blood saturation, there are usually no symptoms. Many persons, especially cigarette smokers, fall in this range or higher, developing some tolerance to elevated carboxyhemoglobin levels. At concentrations of 10 to 20%, tightness across the forehead or headache develops, becoming much more severe when the concentration rises toward 30%. It should be noted that these "stages" are passed through in a matter of minutes if the exposure is intense. At concentrations of 30 to 40%, severe headache, weakness, blurring of vision, nausea and vomiting occur. Tachypnea, tachycardia and collapse occur as the concentration rises toward 50%; and above 50 to 60%, seizures, coma, depressed cardiac and respiratory function, and death occur.

The diagnosis is confirmed by the finding of elevated carboxyhemoglobin in the blood. However, this test is not universally available, especially at night and on weekends when it is most likely to be needed. In this patient, the test could not be run for 12 hours after his arrival, and it was then invalidated for technical reasons. Since the concentration of carboxyhemoglobin drops at a variable rate after the patient is removed from the contaminated environment, extrapolation of results is impossible. The variability depends largely upon the rate of administration of oxygen.

It is possible to obtain circumstantial evidence for the diagnosis by finding an elevated concentration of carbon monoxide in the atmosphere at the scene of the exposure, provided, of course, that conditions have not changed markedly since the exposure is thought to have occurred.

There are relatively simple blood tests that give a fair estimate of whether carboxyhemoglobin is present in an amount sufficient to cause symptoms (even normal blood contains small amounts of it). One such test is to boil the blood. If more than 40% of carboxyhemoglobin is present, the blood will turn brick red, whereas normal blood will turn brownish black. The details of other qualitative tests can be found in any poison handbook or text, some of which are found in the suggested reading list in the back of this book.

Unfortunately, the physical findings are also nonspecific, suggesting drug abuse or overdose or several different types of toxic exposure. The cherry red color of the skin and mucous membranes that is considered a classic sign of carbon monoxide poisoning is actually rarely seen in patients who are alive when they reach the emergency department. It may also be obscured by the cyanosis of oxygen insufficiency. This patient had skin described as "splotchy pink" and dusky, and had a markedly slow respiratory rate (three per minute). He was in a preterminal stage when found, suggesting that his carboxyhemoglobin concentration was well above 60%. The reason for the pink or red color, when it is seen, is that carboxyhemoglobin is red. However, the physician should not plan to base his diagnosis on this coloration, since it is so rarely found, even with significant toxicity.

It is always wise to obtain blood, urine, and possibly vomitus for toxicological examination. Not infrequently, the patient who attempts suicide will have taken various substances in preparation for the event or in order to ensure his death. Such substances can complicate the patient's recovery. Treatment can be altered if it is known or suspected that other toxic preparations, or medications in toxic amounts, are present.

This patient, according to history obtained later, had taken one 5-mg diazepam tablet and some alcohol shortly before his attempted suicide. His "drug screen" had shown that neither was present in significant amounts.

(E) Metabolic acidosis is not specific for this condition, but, taken with all other findings, would help suggest the diagnosis. In some patients, arterial blood gases and pH can actually be confusing. Oxygen tension can be near normal, although the oxygen saturation before therapy will be low.

In this patient, oxygen saturation was greater than 99% when he arrived, his having received oxygen en route. His PaO_2 was 479 mm Hg; $PaCO_2$, 23 mm Hg; pH, 7.33; and HCO_3^-, 11.8 mEq/l. These levels represented a significant degree of metabolic acidosis, but it was rapidly corrected with adequate ventilation and oxygenation, and sodium bicarbonate was not administered. The mechanism of such correction is that anaerobic metabolism is stopped, and aerobic metabolism substituted, in the presence of high-oxygen tension in the blood and tissues as carboxyhemoglobin is displaced.

5. (A, B, D, E) The patient must be removed from the carbon monoxide environment as quickly as possible. As long as he is being exposed to even small amounts of carbon monoxide, he will not be able to reverse the toxic process to allow significant oxyhemoglobin to replace carboxyhemoglobin.

The half-life of carbon monoxide is two to four hours, with the victim breathing room air. Unfortunately, carboxyhemoglobin is eliminated at a much slower rate than it is formed. It is solely eliminated through the lungs, meaning that, with impaired ventilation from any cause, it is likely to be eliminated very slowly. Thus, acute injury to respiratory tissue by irritating gases must be corrected as rapidly as possible.

The half-life of carbon monoxide is only 15 to 30 minutes, with the victim breathing 100% oxygen. This fact dramatically highlights the importance of administering 100% oxygen at the earliest possible moment after the victim is found and the diagnosis is suspected. Since a short period of administration of 100% oxygen is not harmful to the vast majority of patients, one should not wait for confirmation of the diagnosis to start oxygen therapy. In most patients, it should be continued until the carboxyhemoglobin blood level is below 5%, if this measurement is available.

(C) Although it gained some popularity for this purpose, methylene blue has <u>no</u> place in the treatment of carbon monoxide intoxication, since it may further reduce oxyhemoglobin by causing the formation of methemoglobin.

(D, E) Both hypothermia (30-31°C reduces oxygen requirement by approximately 50%) and hyperbaric oxygenation (at two to three atmospheres of pressure) are helpful in patients with carbon monoxide poisoning. Unfortunately, these modalities are frequently not available early enough to influence the outcome in such patients.

COURSE:

This patient was maintained on a ventilator with 100% oxygen, gradually reduced to 25%. He was then noted to be breathing spontaneously. Two units of whole blood were given in an effort to increase his oxygen-carrying capacity. Extubation was possible 20 hours postinjury.

Dexamethasone was continued at 4 mg every six hours intravenously for a total of six doses in an attempt to decrease cerebral edema.

Psychotic organic brain syndrome was diagnosed on later consultation, presumably due to the carbon monoxide toxicity, and the patient was transferred to a long-term facility. It was considered likely that he had a pre-existing functional psychosis.

::

CASE 45: DRUG OVERDOSE IN A 35-YEAR-OLD HOUSEWIFE

HISTORY:

A 35-year-old housewife was found unconscious at her home. She had vomited at least once. An empty bottle labelled imipramine was found nearby. The patient also had containers labelled diazepam and flurazepam; some of the contents were thought to be missing. She was cyanotic and her respirations were shallow. Her pupils were widely dilated and did not respond to light. She was treated in a community hospital with orotracheal intubation with cuffed tube, assisted ventilation, and gastric lavage with a #18 French nasogastric tube, and then referred to a larger hospital for further care. She had been depressed for six months.

EXAMINATION:

Examination at the second hospital revealed a stuporous woman, with pupils in mid-position of dilation and reacting sluggishly to light. She was able to move all four extremities. Her pulse was 106 per minute; all other vital signs were within normal limits. No needle marks were found. General examination and neurological examination were otherwise within normal limits.

LABORATORY DATA:

Hemoglobin: 13.7 gm/dl
White blood cell count: 17,600 with normal differential
Urinalysis: negative except for 5 to 10 white blood cells per high-powered field; urine specific gravity, 1.008
Arterial blood gas analysis:
- pH: 7.45
- PCO_2: 27 torr
- PO_2: 119 torr
- HCO_3^-: 18.2 mEq/l

OTHER STUDIES:

Electrocardiogram: negative, except for sinus tachycardia of 110 per minute.
Chest roentgenogram: not remarkable; the endotracheal tube was in good position, and there was no evidence of pulmonary aspiration.

All other initial studies were within normal limits.

QUESTIONS:

1. Which of the following statements about excessive multiple-drug ingestion are true:
   A. Often, signs and symptoms of multiple drugs partly, or completely, cancel each other out.
   B. A history of multiple-drug ingestion is usually available and reliable.
   C. Multiple-drug ingestion should be suspected in any comatose patient whose diagnosis is not immediately apparent.
   D. All of the above

2. Initial management of an obtunded patient believed to have taken an excessive amount of multiple drugs consists of which of the following?
   A. Opening and maintaining of the airway
   B. Assisted or controlled ventilation
   C. Prevention of aspiration by cuffed endotracheal tube
   D. Identification of the drug or drugs ingested
   E. Administration of a specific antidote, if available
   F. Decrease or elimination of further drug effects by emptying the stomach
   G. Electrocardiographic monitoring
   H. All of the above

TRUE OR FALSE (Questions 3-5):

3. Emptying the stomach by gastric lavage or administration of emetic drugs is mandatory for all cases of oral poisoning or drug overdose.

4. In an adult, the use of a #16 or #18 French nasogastric tube for gastric lavage is quite satisfactory.

5. Specific antidotes are available for most drugs and poisons ingested.

6. When anticholinergic drugs are taken in excessive amounts, which of the following will <u>not</u> occur?
   A. Hallucinations, delirium, seizures
   B. Lethargy, stupor, coma
   C. Hypothermia
   D. Hypertension, tachycardia, arrhythmias with possible cardiac arrest

E. Dry mucous membranes, abdominal distention with ileus, dilated pupils

7. TRUE OR FALSE: Phenothiazines may be used for control of toxicity due to tricyclic antidepressants (imipramine), such as this patient took.

8. In recent years, physostigmine salicylate (Antilirium) has been found to be a specific antidote for poisoning by most anticholinergic agents. The following are true of this drug in the treatment of anticholinergic poisoning except:
   A. It is a cholinesterase inhibitor.
   B. The intravenous dose in adults is 2 mg given over 2 minutes (1 to 4 mg).
   C. The intravenous dose in children is 0.5 mg, repeated at 5-minute intervals until toxic effects have been reversed or a maximum of 2 mg has been given.
   D. It is destroyed in the body within 60 to 120 minutes and may need to be repeated cautiously for hours or days.
   E. It is contraindicated in the presence of asthma, gangrene, diabetes, cardiovascular disease and certain other conditions.
   F. It can cause cholinergic crisis, if used in excess.
   G. Atropine can be used to counteract the cholinergic crisis.
   H. It can safely be used as a trial in any delirious or comatose patient.

ANSWERS AND COMMENTS:

1. (A, C) Since it is true that suicidal patients are prone to take any and all drugs in sight, multiple-drug ingestion must be assumed until ruled out (C). Unfortunately, which drugs were taken and how much of each (B) is usually not known, at least at first, and signs and symptoms may be confusing (A). Friends and relatives may bring in empty bottles or other containers or may be willing to return to the scene to look for such items. But at the time when it is needed most, that is, at the beginning of emergency medical care, information about the drugs themselves and the number taken is usually not available. Therefore, the patient must be treated on the basis of probabilities derived from what little history is available; clues provided by physical examination; phone calls to physicians and pharmacies; and search of hospital records to determine which medications have been prescribed for the patient and which might, therefore, have been available.

2. (H) All. In fact, these steps epitomize the best approach to

any patient who may have taken an excessive amount of medication, or have ingested a material that can cause serious injury or death. Arena has stated that such incidents are so often mismanaged, in that the wrong thing is done or too much of the correct thing is done, that it is often impossible to determine whether recovery occurred because of, or in spite of, the treatment.[1]

In this patient, A and B were taken care of at the first hospital, and arterial blood pH and gases measured at the second hospital indicated satisfactory oxygenation and slightly more ventilation than was necessary. This was corrected, and her arterial blood pH and blood gases remained normal after that. There was never any indication that the patient had aspirated gastric contents (C), although she had vomited at least once at her home, presumably before she became unconscious. The only leads to the identification of the drug(s) ingested (D) were the history of depression, and the finding of the empty bottle of imipramine, as well as partly emptied bottles of diazepam and flurazepam. This is considerably more information than one usually has in the first few minutes or hours in such cases. (E) The history of imipramine use led us to give this patient physostigmine salicylate intravenously, in a dose of 2 mg over 60 seconds. She almost immediately became more alert and tried to remove the orotracheal tube and the orogastric tube being used to evacuate her stomach. In fact, she improved so much that the orotracheal tube could be removed four hours after she had been admitted to the intensive care unit. Had this patient not responded so promptly, naloxone, 0.4 mg, would have been given intravenously, in the hope of reversing any respiratory and cerebral depressant effects produced by any narcotics taken. The dose for children is 0.01 mg/kg given intravenously or intramuscularly. Naloxone is specific for narcosis, but may need to be repeated once or twice at two- to three-minute intervals. Answer F will be discussed in the answer to the next question; answer G in the answer to question 6.

3. (False) The exceptions are patients who have ingested caustic alkalis, since the mucous membranes are probably damaged and further trauma will lead to perforation or hemorrhage. Previously, it was thought that gastric emptying was also contraindicated after ingestion of petroleum products, specifically kerosene, but now many believe that careful induction of emesis is reasonably safe, provided of course, that the patient having ingested these products is not comatose. Gastric emptying is probably safer if such a patient is sitting or semi-erect during the procedure.

The trend in poison management is to induce emesis instead of using gastric lavage, partly because emesis is more effective and partly because it will help empty the upper small intestine, as well. Emesis is best induced with syrup of ipecac (never with the fluid extract, which is more toxic), 15-30 ml given orally for an adult (10 to 15 ml for children), followed by one to three glasses of clear liquid. The additional fluid is essential, since emesis may not take place unless the stomach has some bulk in it. The syrup of ipecac may be repeated only one time after 20 minutes if vomiting has not occurred. If vomiting still does not occur, the stomach must be emptied by lavage because of the cardiotoxic effects of ipecac.

Apomorphine works much more rapidly than syrup of ipecac in most instances; but it is not without risk, in view of the central nervous system depression that it may produce. Some children continue to vomit during the depression, making the situation dangerous. Apomorphine also makes it difficult to monitor a systemically depressed patient for later signs of toxicity. Naloxone must be administered to correct the depressant effect of apomorphine.

It should be added that inducing emesis by any method usually fails if the patient has ingested antiemetic drugs, such as antihistamines or phenothiazines. If the patient is comatose, the stomach may be emptied by means of gastric lavage, provided a cuffed endotracheal tube is in place to prevent aspiration. However, insertion of a cuffed endotracheal tube is not recommended in children under seven to nine years of age, because the trachea is small and the risk of tracheal stenosis is greater than in adults. In such children, a snug-fitting, uncuffed tube is preferred for the obtunded patient who requires gastric lavage.

Emptying the stomach may not be indicated if several hours have passed since the ingestion of the drug or poison. However, many authorities believe that the stomach should be emptied in all cases, since certain drugs (such as methyl salicylate) remain in the stomach for six or more hours after ingestion and continue to release their contents into the system until they are removed.

Following gastric emptying, activated charcoal should be given by mouth to bind the remainder of the poison, thus preventing absorption during its passage through the intestine. A cathartic is also helpful in elimination of the offending substance. The activated charcoal should <u>not</u> be given at the same time as syrup of ipecac, since it binds ipecac and prevents the desired systemic and local emetic effect. However, activated charcoal may be given orally, simultaneously with parenteral administration of apomorphine.

4. (False) Unless contraindicated (see answer 3), and if chosen as the means of emptying the stomach, gastric lavage should be done as early as possible, but not with so small a tube. An Ewald orogastric tube, #28 to #34, is more apt to allow recovery of solid material from the stomach, including portions of tablets and capsules. The larger tube was used in this patient at the second hospital, with pieces of both flurazepam and imipramine being recovered. In children, a smaller tube should be used.

The return from the first washing, or gastric contents aspirated before the start of lavage, should be kept separate and sent to the laboratory for analysis. Thereafter, in the adult, lavage is done in cycles of 300 to 500 ml of fluid (tap water or normal saline) instilled over one to two minutes, left in place for one minute, and drained by gravity or suction over three to four minutes. Once the return fluid is clear, an additional 3000 ml should be washed through on the same schedule.

5. (False) There are only a few specific antidotes available for the hundreds of drugs and other substances that can cause poisoning. Thus, it is vital to identify the poison, so that the antidote, if there is one, can be started as rapidly as possible, and so that, if there is no antidote, less specific counteracting steps can be initiated immediately. The patient's life may depend upon the type of sleuthing one does when the patient first arrives in the emergency department.

The nearest Poison Control (or Information) Center should be contacted for any assistance needed, such as identification of an unknown drug or other substance, and management of the problem. Any information or advice obtained by such a call should be recorded in the record promptly (1) for medicolegal reasons; and (2) as a guide to other physicians who may assist in the patient's later management.

6. (C) Many of these patients have hyperpyrexia due, in part, to their inability to perspire. The skin will often be flushed, especially in children, who are particularly susceptible to anticholinergic poisoning. The central nervous system effects may be either excitation (A) or depression (B). Aspects of both can be present at the same time, and fluctuation from one to the other is frequent. The excitement phase seems to be due to central cholinergic blockade, which accompanies smaller over-

doses. The larger the overdose, the greater the central nervous system depression. Among the peripheral effects, the ones that affect the heart (D) are by far more dangerous than the ones listed in E. Anticholinergic drugs sensitize the myocardium to catecholamines, such as endogenous epinephrine and norepinephrine, which sets the stage for supraventricular tachycardia, ventricular tachycardia and fibrillation, as well as both atrioventricular and intraventricular blocks. These require careful electrocardiographic monitoring (see question 2) for at least three days, during which time the patient should be treated in an intensive care unit. This patient did not develop any arrhythmias and was discharged from the hospital on the fourth day after psychiatric consultation and arrangements for psychiatric care as an outpatient had been made.

7. (False) Phenothiazines should not be used in anticholinergic poisoning (which includes tricyclic antidepressants), as they may intensify the toxicity and plunge the patient into coma. However, phenothiazines, such as chlorpromazine, are useful in controlling toxicity due to amphetamines. It is possible for the two conditions to be confused, since dilated pupils are present in both. Therefore, a fairly accurate differential diagnosis should be made before phenothiazines are given to patients with drug toxicity.

8. (H) All of the other items are true, but physostigmine salicylate must never be used in a cavalier fashion "just to see if the patient will wake up." The cholinergic crisis (F) is potentially fatal, causing severe bronchospasm and respiratory failure, bradycardia and hypotension, or tachycardia and hypertension, depending on the predominance of ganglionic or postganglionic action. Atropine should always be available for immediate use, in one-half the physostigmine dose, to counteract such a crisis. In spite of all of these limitations, physostigmine is a life-saving drug when used with the proper indications and precautions.

REFERENCE

Arena, J. M.: Poisoning. Emerg. Med. 8(4):171-198, 1976

::

CASE 46: BLINDNESS IN A 30-YEAR-OLD MAN AFTER HEAD INJURY

HISTORY:

A 30-year-old man had sustained several blows to his head five days earlier, when he was "attacked by five or six men" on his way home from the night shift at work. Skull roentgenograms taken in another emergency department showed no evidence of fracture. He was released from that emergency department with no follow-up instructions.

Over the next three days, he had short periods of total blindness, described as a "coming and going" of his vision. Then, for two days, he had noted gradual dimming of his vision to the point that he could barely detect light, and he had had to be fed, dressed, and led by the hand.

He had no other complaints, except for generalized headaches since the injury and dizziness for the last three days. For several weeks, he had had early-morning insomnia. He had no history of mental disease.

There were bluish areas around the left temporal area; otherwise, the results of the general physical and neurological examination were normal. He was not able to see hand movements with either eye, but he obviously fixed his gaze on objects at a distance. His pupils reacted to light and accommodation, including both direct and consensual reaction.

QUESTIONS:

1. The probable diagnosis is:
   A. A "blowout" fracture of the left orbit
   B. Subdural hematoma in the left parietotemporal region
   C. Acute schizophrenic reaction
   D. Hysterical conversion reaction
   E. Malingering

TRUE OR FALSE (Questions 2-11):

2. Neuroses are the most prevalent of the mental disorders.

3. Neuroses are rare in childhood.

4. Obsessive-compulsive neurosis and hysterical neurosis constitute 80% of all neuroses.

5. A neurosis is a reaction to stress that is usually identifiable by the patient.

6. Most neuroses are self-limited.

7. Anxiety is, by far, the most common symptom in all of the neuroses.

8. Neuroses are usually distinguishable from psychoses by the absence of delusions, hallucinations, and bizarre affect in the former.

9. Neuroses frequently evolve into psychoses.

10. The types of hysterical neuroses are dissociative type and conversion type.

11. Malingering has almost disappeared as a problem in emergency departments.

12. The characteristic features of personality disorders (also called character disorders) are which of the following?
    A. Onset early in life
    B. Males are predominantly affected
    C. The presence of personality features suggesting immaturity
    D. Maladjustment to one's environment
    E. Resistance to all known treatment modalities
    F. All of the above

13. TRUE OR FALSE: A patient rarely has a personality disorder and another type of mental illness.

ANSWERS AND COMMENTS:

1. (D) Hysterical conversion reaction. There is nothing to suggest a "blowout" fracture of either orbit (A), and a subdural hematoma (B) seems highly improbable. They were ruled out by appropriate studies.

Acute schizophrenic reaction (C) can be precipitated by a stressful experience, such as the attack on this patient, but the absence of other personality disturbances tends to rule out that diagnosis.

Malingering (E) was considered, but since there was no monetary benefit to be gained from the patient's continued illness, it was the opinion of the emergency department physician and the neurology consultant that the patient had hysterical conversion reaction, or "functional" blindness. That was borne out by his gradual improvement under outpatient psychiatric care, with restoration of normal sight.

2. (True) Neuroses are the most prevalent of the mental disorders, accounting for at least 50% of the psychiatric patients seen in outpatient clinics and in family practice. Neuroses are, by far, the most common mental disorders for which patients are treated in emergency departments. Although females are more susceptible to hysterical neuroses and depressive neuroses, there is no significant difference in the overall incidence of neuroses between the sexes.

3. (True) Symptomatic neuroses are rare in childhood. However, personality traits associated with adult neuroses are present before puberty in many patients. Even that early, the pattern of neurotic symptoms and behavior seems to be set, and neuroses tend to take the same form throughout the patient's life.

4. (False) Obsessive-compulsive neurosis and hysterical neurosis together constitute a relatively small per cent of the total. It is anxiety neurosis and depressive neurosis that, together, constitute more than 80% of all neuroses seen in practice. Other types include phobic neurosis, neurasthenic neurosis, depersonalization neurosis, and hypochondriacal neurosis.

5. (False) Although it is true that neurosis is a decompensation in the patient's level of adaptation to life's stresses, the specific stress to which a neurosis is the abnormal response is seldom identifiable by the patient and is usually beyond his conscious awareness. When the source of stress is identified, with the help of a therapist, it is often "disappointing" to the patient, because it seems such an insignificant cause of so much mental distress and such associated behavioral abnormalities. That is especially likely to be true if the reaction to the stress has incapacitated the patient. Characteristically, although he may gain some insight into the origin of his symptoms, the patient is powerless to overcome or change them. They are not under conscious control. Such incapacitation (functional) may be manifested by an apathetic attitude toward work, an inability to concentrate or to complete tasks, or an inability to relax and enjoy experiences, no matter how pleasurable. There are also

physical symptoms, such as tremulousness, tachycardia, urinary frequency, or diarrhea. Secondary guilt feelings, with depressed moods, are also common. Even though the stress that causes a neurosis may become known, why only some persons react to stress with a neurosis is not known. Certainly, there is no known organic basis for any neurosis. It seems reasonable to consider the neurotic symptoms to be unresolved intrapsychic conflicts, possibly drives of either the aggressive or sexual type.

6. (True) Most neuroses are self-limited and may be managed without psychiatric referral or hospitalization. The overall prognosis is good. Neurotic patterns of behavior that do become chronic probably do so because of the persistence or frequent recurrence of the type of stress that is capable of producing them. That development of chronicity applies especially to anxiety neurosis, obsessive-compulsive neurosis and phobic neurosis.

Obviously, if the discomfort or functional disability of neurosis is severe enough or long-standing enough to require relief, the patient should be treated.

7. (True) Anxiety is the most widespread of all of the symptoms of neurosis, with depression and various physical symptoms being the next most common symptoms.

8. (True) In most instances of neurosis, there is an absence of the delusions, hallucinations, and bizarre affect that characterize psychosis, schizophrenia in particular. In other words, the neurotic patient usually retains his grasp on reality, and that is the essence of the differential diagnosis. However, in some neurotic patients, the symptoms are bizarre enough that differentiation from psychosis may be difficult without a period of observation, preferably in the hospital.

The diagnosis of neurosis in any of its forms is based largely on the exclusion of a physical (organic) cause of the symptoms and a positive finding of the features of neurosis by history, physical examination and mental-status examination. Some of the organic diseases that can be mimicked by the various neuroses are multiple sclerosis, drug abuse (especially of amphetamines and marijuana), thyrotoxicosis, weakness due to a malignancy, temporal lobe epilepsy, and general fatigue from any cause.

A differentiation must also be made among neurosis, psychosis, and personality disorders (see question and answer 13 and Case

47). Tests that can be used for confirmation of the diagnosis of neurosis are the psychological tests for intelligence, perception and personality, and, in particular, the projective tests, such as the Rorschach test. The Rorschach test is particularly helpful in differentiating neurosis from both functional and organic psychosis. However, those tests have limited usefulness in the emergency department.

9. (False) There is no evidence that neuroses evolve into psychoses, although being neurotic probably does not protect one from becoming psychotic. Psychosis may be manifested by neurotic symptoms, which can deceive the unwary clinician.

10. (True) Those two types of hysterical neurosis are related but distinct. The dissociative type is manifested by disorders of consciousness; the conversion type is manifested by disorders of the neuromuscular and sensory systems, as in this patient.

In both types, there is an ability to comprehend reality, although, as mentioned earlier, the symptoms are on an unconscious level. That combination confirms hysterical neurosis, provided the physical disease it simulates, however remotely, can be ruled out.

Hysterical dissociative neurosis is not common, but is seen equally between the sexes. The symptoms include amnesia, fugue states (amnesia for long periods of time), and somnambulism. Those states may be brought on by the sudden emergence into consciousness of unacceptable impulses, such as to harm someone. On the other hand, they may occur after the patient has committed a violent act.

Hysterical conversion neuroses occur predominantly in women and often arise following industrial or vehicular accidents or injuries, especially if an insurance settlement or litigation is pending. The symptoms are varied but are usually suggestive of disorders of the nervous system, such as localized paralysis, paresthesias, gait disturbances, blindness (as in this patient) and bizarre seizure-like states. The neurosis is on an unconscious level, even though the patient appears to be seeking secondary gain. That causes some confusion with malingering (see question and answer 11). Often, settlement of the pending litigation may be all the treatment that is necessary. However, to be effective as a therapeutic tool, such settlement must not be delayed too long.

For both dissociative and conversion hysterical neurosis, prognosis is better when the disorder is acute and has a definite relationship to stress, as in this patient.

11. (False) This problem has not diminished and may increase.

Malingering must be differentiated from several other conditions. The most difficult differentiation is from hysterical neurosis, although many other medical conditions can be mimicked, or feigned, by a malingerer.

Most important in that differentiation are the following: (1) Malingering is on a conscious level, whereas hysterical neurosis is not, although it may seem to be so. (2) The malingerer is seeking secondary gain, whereas the hysterical neurotic is not, although that, again, may be very uncertain in some patients. If it is questionable, the patient probably should be given the benefit of the doubt. (3) True malingering is a serious personality disorder, whereas neurosis of any type is not likely to be serious, except to the extent of discomfort and dysfunction involved. One reason that malingering is serious is that it is often a conscious mechanism for protection from a major emotional crisis.

In differentiating malingering from other diseases, it is not sufficient for the clinician to think in terms of bizarre or atypical symptoms and signs. A characteristic of the most successful malingerer is that he has studied the matter and knows exactly what symptoms and signs to "produce" on cue. Thus, the term malingering should be restricted to acts designed to deceive. A common example is a person addicted to drugs, who appears at an emergency department (the usual place) or a physician's office attempting to obtain drugs to feed his habit. He will know exactly how to simulate pain, anxiety, depression, or whatever symptom is needed to provide him with the drug to which he is addicted.

This type of problem is likely to increase, since disease simulation, using both manikins and computers, is now being widely used for teaching of, and self-instruction by, professional personnel. Non-medical persons are able to obtain such materials and "practice their act," just as professional actors and actresses are used in bona fide continuing medical education demonstrations, symposia, and seminars. The problem becomes even more difficult if, for example, the patient has a physical defect, such as an abnormal electrocardiogram, which at least initially tends to reinforce his claim of acute chest pain. One clue to such illness is that the patient "arranges" his scenario so that under the particular circumstances, the physician finds it difficult or impossible to corroborate his history, such as that of previous treatments. Another example is the patient who deliberately and repeatedly opens or contaminates a laceration or ulcer in order to prevent it from healing.

There is no universally satisfactory approach to management of such patients. If possible, they should be prevented from harming themselves or others, both physically and economically. Seeking admission to a hospital under false pretenses is a misdemeanor in many jurisdictions. Possibly, the answer to the problem of malingering will come when we find the answer to other antisocial acts. In any case, medication is not indicated in most patients unless they have concurrent illnesses. Psychiatric referral, although it may be indicated, is not likely to be helpful in most malingerers.

12. (A, C, D, E) Types of personality disorders include hysterical, inadequate, antisocial, passive-aggressive, paranoid, obsessive-compulsive, schizoid, asthenic, explosive, and cyclothymic (alternating swings between elation and depression). Although each of the types of personality disorders has its own constellation of symptoms and signs, they share certain features that usually make them unmistakable. In general, all patients with personality disorders show immaturity (C) on a chronic basis, not just as a regression in the presence of undue stress, such as a physical illness. It is almost as if developmental arrest had occurred early in life (A) and has persisted. Indeed, that concept of developmental arrest is one of the most acceptable theories on the cause of personality disorder, although the cause of the arrest in an individual patient is generally unknown.

Personality disorders affect both sexes, not males predominantly (B). The conflict is more between the patient and his environment than within himself (intrapsychic).

It is very important to distinguish personality disorders from neuroses. That importance has to do with the response to treatment and the prognosis. Although neuroses can be life-long afflictions, they often respond to superficial psychotherapy, including medications. On the other hand, personality disorders, also life-long problems, usually do not respond to any therapeutic approaches presently known (E). Encounter groups are useful for some patients with personality disorders, since there they can learn that they are not alone in their stressful relations with others, or in their immature reactions, such as drug abuse and alcoholism.

Hospitalization is not likely to be helpful, although it may be sought by the patient for secondary gain, such as when he is in trouble with civil authorities. One exception to that rule is the "borderline patient" who, under stress, temporarily exhibits psychotic ideation and behavior. A short period of hospitalization may be helpful while the diagnosis is clarified and treatment is evaluated. Such patients can usually be returned to at least their former level of functioning.

One characteristic of persons with a personality disorder is that they try to relieve their anxiety by immediate and impulsive action, with essentially no delay between stimulus and response. They are unable to postpone gratification of their desires, and they are afraid they will miss some satisfaction or thrill if they do not act immediately. Such action leads to poor marital adjustment, sexual promiscuity, vagrancy, and chronic unemployment. Those persons are usually quite intelligent, but do not hesitate to "use" people to attain their own desires, and they actively resist any obstruction of their efforts. They have few, if any, feelings of guilt or pangs of conscience.

Patients with personality disorders have a very low tolerance for anxiety or pain, making treatment even more difficult, since a therapeutic relationship tends to engender anxiety. Such patients are rarely able to confront the fact that much of their discomfort and difficulty in life arises from within themselves and not from what others do to them, or fail to do for them.

It almost goes without saying that many of the patients treated in emergency departments have one or the other types of personality disorder.

13. (False) Although, in general, the diagnosis of personality disorders means that other mental illnesses have been ruled out, those disorders are not mutually exclusive. It is common, for example, to see patients with personality disorders who have also developed neurotic symptoms. The diagnosis is largely based on the predominant features, as in the case of the neuroses, where there is considerable overlap of symptoms.

However, the personality disorders do not seem to be on a continuum with either the neuroses or the psychoses. That is, for example, a patient who has a schizoid personality disorder will not automatically develop schizophrenia in time.

::

CASE 47: PARANOID SCHIZOPHRENIA

HISTORY:

A 48-year-old man reported to the emergency department because of drowsiness and numbness in his arms and legs. The symptoms had begun after he had started taking chlorpromazine and trifluoperazine, which had been prescribed by his psychiatrist one week earlier. At that visit, he had complained that his wife and others were giving him an unknown medication, possibly to harm him, and had expressed other paranoid ideas. His diagnosis was paranoid schizophrenia, for which he had been treated originally five months earlier.

Although his wife thought - and the patient stated - that he had been taking his antipsychotic medication regularly, it was unlikely that he had been doing so.

The results of the general and mental-status examinations were normal, except that he was agitated and had pressured speech, constant circumstantial rambling, delusions of persecution, and ideas of reference. He expressed no suicidal or homicidal ideation. He refused to be admitted to the hospital. He was given an appointment to see his psychiatrist in two weeks for follow-up care. Perphenazine, 4 mg three times daily, was started; and the other medications were discontinued. He was not seen again in the emergency department.

QUESTIONS:

1. TRUE OR FALSE: The term schizophrenia is correctly used as a synonym for psychosis.

2. Which of the following statements are true regarding schizophrenia?
   A. It is primarily a disease of males and usually has an onset in the fourth and fifth decades of life.
   B. The diagnosis is almost always easy to make and is clear-cut.
   C. Onset is always insidious.
   D. Spontaneous remissions never occur.
   E. Acute exacerbations of chronic schizophrenia are fairly common.
   F. Serious medical illness may present in confusing and atypical ways in schizophrenic patients.

3. In addition to the previously mentioned, which of the following are diagnostic features of schizophrenia?
   A. There are disturbances of thinking, mood and behavior.
   B. The sensorium is relatively clear.
   C. Orientation and memory are always severely impaired.
   D. Delusions and hallucinations, usually auditory, are commonly present.
   E. The diagnosis can be made on the basis of recently developed laboratory tests.

4. Differential diagnosis in such a patient should include which of the following?
   A. Organic brain syndrome and other acute confusional states
   B. Paranoid neurosis
   C. Malingering
   D. Manic-depressive psychosis
   E. All of the above

5. Of the following types of schizophrenia, which two are probably the most important to know and recognize in the emergency department?
   A. Undifferentiated
   B. Paranoid
   C. Catatonic
   D. Childhood

6. TRUE OR FALSE: Schizophrenia can sometimes be treated with the minor tranquilizers.

ANSWERS AND COMMENTS:

1. (False) Schizophrenia is not a synonym for psychosis, but only the name for one type of psychosis. However, because schizophrenia is the most common type of functional psychosis, it will be the subject of most of the following answers.

The other major type of functional psychosis comprises the affective disorders, that is, disorders of mood or feeling, the most serious of which is manic-depressive psychosis. With lithium carbonate now available for control of both the manic and depressive phases, it is vital that the diagnosis of that condition be made as early as possible so treatment can be started.

Toxic psychoses are discussed briefly in question and answer 4.

2. (E, F) (A) Schizophrenia occurs no more frequently in male

than in female patients. Schizophrenia infrequently becomes manifest after age 40 years, as it apparently did in this patient, although paranoid schizophrenia often begins later than the other types (see answer 5). Rather, the onset is usually in late adolescence or young adulthood. Most patients have shown some schizoid personality traits for months or years before the unmistakable signs and symptoms of schizophrenia appear. Those usually consist of withdrawal from family and friends; decline in academic achievement despite a previously good (even excellent) school record; preoccupation with deep, usually unsolvable, philosophical or religious questions; and multiple neurotic complaints, such as obsessions and compulsions. The childhood form of schizophrenia, while rare, is often first suspected in the emergency department. It usually begins before puberty. Any child who is having serious school or behavior problems in the pre-teens or teens should have a mental-status examination and may require psychiatric consultation with that possibility in mind.

(B) The diagnosis is usually straightforward in the fully developed disease, but certain criteria must be met, since a diagnosis of schizophrenia has serious connotations, both medical and social (see question and answer 3). In the emergency department setting, making the diagnosis can be very difficult.

(C) Although schizophrenia usually begins insidiously, that is not the only pattern. In some patients, onset is acute, with the rapid and dramatic appearance of psychomotor excitement, delusions, hallucinations, and marked alterations in mood.

(D) Spontaneous remissions do occur in chronic schizophrenic reactions, especially in the first one to two years after onset. However, they are by no means the rule.

(E) Acute exacerbations are not infrequent in the course of chronic schizophrenia, usually occurring in the patient who surreptitiously discontinues his medication. That is an all-too-common problem, even if a responsible person - as in this patient's case, his wife - attempts to see that the patient takes the medication regularly.

(F) Serious medical or surgical illness may present in bizarre ways in schizophrenic patients. Appendicitis, for example, may have to be suspected on grounds other than the usual right lower quadrant pain. Exploratory laparotomy may be indicated on less than convincing grounds in the schizophrenic patient, and other abdominal diseases may also present in a bizarre fashion. However, objective signs, such as abdominal tenderness or distention, leukocytosis and roentgenological findings of organic disease are no different from those in other patients.

3. (A, B, D) Unfortunately, there are no pathognomonic symptoms or signs of schizophrenia. It is always necessary to rule out organic disease, and the term functional, as applied to schizophrenia, indicates that that has been done (see answer 4). In the emergency department setting, any patient whose chief complaint is, "I want to see a psychiatrist" or whose family says, "He needs to see a psychiatrist" should have a screening-type physical examination before psychiatric consultation. The exception would be the occasional patient who refuses that approach, or who is so agitated - or depressed - that the physical examination must be deferred until after the psychiatric evaluation and appropriate initial treatment have been accomplished.

Schizophrenia is primarily a thought disorder, as opposed to manic-depressive psychosis (see answer 4), which is an affective (mood or feeling) disorder.

Although the severity varies, all patients with schizophrenic reactions have a relatively clear sensorium (B) but characteristic disturbances of thinking, mood and behavior (A). The thought disorder is manifested in speech, writing and drawing. There is always misinterpretation of reality (disturbed thinking), with looseness of associations, in which several ideas will be strung together in illogical fashion. Most patients have frank delusions (false beliefs) and hallucinations (false sense perceptions) (D). The ideas of reference that this patient exhibited are misinterpretations of events, seen or heard, as referring to the patient. They often are interpreted as having derogatory intent, also clearly present in this patient. The mood is inappropriate for the situation, and there is frequently a flat, apathetic affect. The behavioral disturbances are outgrowths of the psychomotor excitement found in some patients, usually at or near the time of onset of the symptom complex (see answer 5).

Orientation and memory are almost never impaired (C) in schizophrenic patients.

The cause of schizophrenia is unknown, and there are no characteristic physical findings. Unfortunately, no laboratory tests (E) are available for confirmation of the diagnosis of schizophrenia. The diagnosis must still be made on the basis of history, interview and direct examination of the patient's mental status. Certain psychological tests are helpful in confirming the diagnosis, but they are largely extensions and refinements of the mental-status examination.

4. (E) All. (A) Organic brain syndrome and other confusional states are differentiated from schizophrenia by the presence of a clouded sensorium in the former conditions. Organic brain syndrome compromises higher cerebral function, including all of the cognitive functions, especially memory, and in particular, memory for recent events. Such impairment leads to disorientation as to time and place (not usually found in schizophrenia), as well as to impaired thinking and a decrease in logical reasoning. It cannot be emphasized too often that the schizophrenic patient almost always has a clear sensorium despite his lack of contact with reality in other ways.

Organic brain syndrome presents either as a slowly progressive course or an acute confusional state, the latter also called "delirium." Delirium may be precipitated by toxic states, such as that due to drugs, acute head injury, or abnormal metabolic states.

One of the several toxic conditions that simulate schizophrenia is amphetamine intoxication, one of the resemblances being the presence of auditory hallucinations. The prognosis for amphetamine abuse is vastly better than that for schizophrenia. Thus, extreme care is required in making the diagnosis of functional (nonorganic) psychosis. Studies to rule out toxic conditions should be undertaken, and a period of observation in the hospital is usually indicated. The finding of amphetamine in a patient's urine confirms the condition, although it does not rule out the possibility that the patient may be a schizophrenic who uses (but has not abused the use of) amphetamines. Fortunately, the toxic symptoms disappear rapidly after the drug is withdrawn.

As to diagnosis of the organic brain syndrome, a change in personality is often the only unusual sign noted by the patient's family. Naturally, that is more likely to be true for the slowly progressive organic brain syndrome. Personality changes include deterioration in personal habits, the use of poor judgment in family decisions or business deals, uncharacteristic vulgarity of speech, even highly unusual and offensive sexual behavior. A history of recent personality change should always arouse suspicion of an organic process.

The emotional disturbances of organic brain syndrome are of a wide range, best characterized as emotional lability; reactive depression; paranoid states; and painful distress with crying, either for no reason at all, or for not being able to perform during the mental-status examination.

Dementia, one form of organic brain syndrome, is manifested by a progressive, global (total), cognitive impairment. Some authors prefer to consider dementia as deterioration of intellectual ability and consider two categories: treatable forms, such as those caused by chronic cerebral anoxia, electrolyte imbalance, or hypoglycemia; and untreatable forms, such as presenile dementia (Alzheimer's disease), senile dementia, and dementias caused by alcoholic encephalopathy, multiple sclerosis, or Pick's disease.

(B) Paranoid neurosis can be differentiated by the absence of true delusions and hallucinations.

(C) Malingering is not likely to be confused with schizophrenia, although, as indicated in Case 46, malingerers can simulate almost any illness.

(D) Differentiation from a manic-depressive psychosis may prove to be difficult, since there may be significant mood alterations, delusions, and hallucinations in both. A family history of manic-depression rules strongly in favor of that diagnosis. On the other hand, a family history of schizophrenia rules strongly in favor of that disorder.

It is in the occasional schizophrenic patient who has marked depressive alteration in mood that confusion with the depressive phase of manic-depressive psychosis arises. Similarly, a schizophrenic patient's marked agitation may, on superficial examination, be confused with mania or hypomania, the latter term indicating a slightly lesser degree of mania. The reason it is so important to differentiate the two conditions is that the treatment is entirely different.

5. (B, C) It is most important for the emergency department physician to recognize paranoid and catatonic types in particular, since each of those may have an acute onset in relation to another illness. For example, the paranoid type can begin while the patient is suffering from withdrawal from chronic alcoholism. The paranoid type is easy to miss if the physician fails to think of it, particularly since the age of onset is several years older than that of most types of schizophrenia, as in this patient. Also, in such a patient, there is frequently no positive family history and no history of schizoid traits. The patient's behavior is unpredictable, and may be based on explosive hostility and

aggressiveness for which the emergency department staff may not be prepared.

The catatonic type can also have an acute onset under the same circumstances as the paranoid type. However, it is then characterized by motor abnormalities with excitement, excessive activity and, at times, aggressiveness, rather than the more usual clinical picture of stupor, mutism, and waxy flexibility (the patient usually leaves his extremities the way the examiner places them, even if in awkward positions, for minutes to hours).

In each of those types of schizophrenia, it is obviously imperative that the emergency physician suspect the diagnosis early, obtain consultation, and initiate treatment as soon as possible, to prevent harm to the patient and to those who are trying to help him.

Another reason these two types of schizophrenia are important is that phencyclidine (PCP, "angel dust") use can mimic both types, with the symptoms lasting for weeks or months after withdrawal, instead of only a few days.

(A) Chronic undifferentiated schizophrenia, especially the variant called pseudoneurotic type, may be confused for months, even years, with various types of neuroses. Since many such patients are seen only in emergency departments and consistently refuse appointments for consultation and follow-up care, the diagnosis must be suspected in any patient whose clinical picture does not fit other conditions, especially the neuroses. Unless the physician has a high index of suspicion, the diagnosis can be missed, even when the hospital record reveals several emergency department visits with similar complaints and findings. Obviously, most such patients are suffering from neurosis rather than psychosis, but the latter, more serious condition must be considered. Neuroses do not slowly evolve into schizophrenia of any subtype, but the diagnosis of schizophrenia of the pseudoneurotic type gradually reveals itself to the alert clinician.

(D) Childhood schizophrenia was mentioned earlier as being suspected in some adolescents with behavioral problems. While being careful not to stigmatize the patient, one should pursue any leads that suggest abnormal thought processes, as suggested by bizarre behavior.

6. (False) Schizophrenia should never be treated with the minor

tranquilizers, such as chlordiazepoxide or diazepam. If such treatment is attempted, the patient's problem will almost never be brought under control or will slip from adequate maintenance to an acute exacerbation, requiring reinstitution of treatment with antipsychotic (neuroleptic) drugs. The only safe and effective drugs to use for the schizophrenic patient is an antipsychotic drug, usually a phenothiazine, used along with active, supportive psychotherapy, preferably by a psychiatrist.

Since there was some question as to whether this patient had been taking his medication regularly, the psychiatric consultant thought it would be better to change the medication, at least temporarily. The phenothiazines are all similar in their action, although a particular one may be better tolerated and more effective and therefore more acceptable to a patient than others.

It should be added that certain features indicate a relatively good prognosis; the most important of which are an acute onset and a clear precipitating factor.

Once the diagnosis is made, the treatment is relatively simple, although control, rather than cure, is the goal for almost all patients.

::

GENERAL REFERENCES

Adams, R.D. and Victor, M.: Principles of Neurology. New York: McGraw-Hill Book Co., 1977.

AMA Drug Evaluations (3rd Ed.): Prepared by the AMA Department of Drugs, in cooperation with the American Society for Clinical Pharmacology and Therapeutics. Littleton, Mass.: Publishing Sciences Group, Inc., 1977.

Ansari, A. and Burch, G.E.: Influence of hot environments on the cardiovascular system. Arch. Intern. Med. 123:371-378, 1969.

Bachus, B.F. and Snider, G.L.: The bronchodilator effects of aerosolized terbutaline. A controlled, double-blind study. JAMA 238:2277-2281, 1977.

Baird, H.W., et al.: Getting to know the epilepsies. Patient Care (April 15):102-136, 1977.

Becker, C.E., et al.: Alcohol as a Drug: A Curriculum on Pharmacology, Neurology and Toxicology. New York: Medcom Press, 1974.

Boyd, A.E., III and Beller, G.A.: Heat exhaustion and respiratory alkalosis. Ann. Intern. Med. 83:835, 1975.

Chung, E.K. (Ed.): Quick Reference to Cardiovascular Diseases. Philadelphia: J.B. Lippincott Co., 1977.

Cranley, J.J., et al.: The diagnosis of deep venous thrombosis. Arch. Surg. 111:34-36, 1976.

Dagradi, A.E.: Management of major gastrointestinal hemorrhage. Mt. Sinai J. Med. N.Y. 43:338-350, 1976.

Duff, J.H.: Cardiovascular changes in sepsis. Heart-Lung 5:772-776, 1976.

Dunlap, E.A. (Ed.): Gordon's Medical Management of Ocular Disease, 2nd Edition. Hagerstown: Harper and Row, 1976.

Goldberger, E.: The Treatment of Cardiac Emergencies. St. Louis: C.V. Mosby Co., 1974.

Gombos, G.M.: Handbook of Ophthalmologic Emergencies, 2nd Edition. Garden City: Medical Examination Publishing Co., Inc., 1977.

Goodman, L.A. and Gilman, A.: The Pharmacological Basis of Therapeutics, 5th Edition. New York: Macmillan Publishing Co., 1975.

Gosselin, R.E., et al.: Clinical Toxicology of Commercial Products: Acute Poisoning, 4th Edition. Baltimore: Williams and Wilkins Co., 1975.

Handbook of Common Poisonings in Children: U.S. Department of Health, Education and Welfare, H.E.W. Publication No. (F.D.A.) 76-7004, 1976.

Karliner, J.S.: Dopamine for cardiogenic shock. J.A.M.A. 226:1218, 1973.

Kendig, E.L., Jr. and Chernick, V. (Eds.): Disorders of the Respiratory Tract in Children, 3rd Edition. Philadelphia: W.B. Saunders Co., 1977.

Knochel, J.P., et al.: Heat stress, exercise, and muscle injury: effects on urate metabolism and renal function. Ann. Intern. Med. 81:321-328, 1974.

Malt, R.A.: Control of massive upper gastrointestinal hemorrhage. N. Eng. J. Med. 286:1043-1046, 1972.

Margolis, J.R. and Wagner, G.S.: Coronary Care: Arrhythmias in Acute Myocardial Infarction. New York: American Heart Association, 1976.

Marriott, H.J.L.: Practical Electrocardiography, 5th Edition. Baltimore: Williams and Wilkins Co., 1972.

Menguy, R.: Diagnosis and management of upper gastrointestinal bleeding. South. Med. J. 69:225-229, 1976.

Moser, K.M.: Pulmonary embolism. Am. Rev. Resp. Dis. 115:829-850, 1977.

Physicians' Desk Reference to Pharmaceutical Specialties and

Biologicals (31st Ed.): Oradell, N.J.: Medical Economics Company, 1977.

Schwartz, G.R., et al.: (Eds.): Principles and Practice of Emergency Medicine, Philadelphia: W.B. Saunders Co., 1978.

Scoggin, C.H., et al.: Status asthmaticus. A nine-year experience. J.A.M.A. 238:1158-1162, 1977.

Shibel, E.M. and Moser, K.M.: Respiratory Emergencies. St. Louis: C.V. Mosby Co., 1977.

Shubin, H. and Weil, M.H.: Bacterial shock. JAMA 235: 421-424, 1976.

Smith, P.R., et al.: A comparative study of subcutaneously administered terbutaline and epinephrine in the treatment of acute bronchial asthma. Chest 71:129-134, 1977.

Solomon, G.E. and Plum, F.: Clinical Management of Seizures: A Guide for the Physician. Philadelphia: W.B. Saunders Co., 1976.

Trunkey, D., et al.: Monitoring resuscitation of primates from hemorrhagic and septic shock. J.A.C.E.P. 5:249-252, 1976.

VanArsdel, P.P., Jr. and Paul, G.H.: Drug therapy in the management of asthma. Ann. Intern. Med. 87:68-74, 1977.

Vaughan, D. and Asbury, T.: General Ophthalmology, 8th Edition. Los Altos: Lange Medical Publications, 1977.

Victor, M., et al.: The Wernicke-Korsakoff Syndrome. Philadelphia: F.A. Davis Co., 1972.

Webb-Johnson, D.C. and Andrews, J.L., Jr.: Bronchodilator therapy. N. Eng. J. Med. 297:476-482, 758-764, 1977.

Weber, C.T., et al.: Left ventricular dysfunction following acute myocardial infarction. Am. J. Med. 54:697, 1973.

Weiner, H.L. and Levitt, L.P.: Neurology for the House Officer. Baltimore: Williams and Wilkins Co., 1974.

Wilkins, E.W., Jr., et al.: (Eds.): MGH Textbook of Emergency Medicine. Baltimore: Williams and Wilkins Co., 1978.

Williams, J.W.: Venous thrombosis and pulmonary embolism. Surg. Gynecol. Obstet. 141:626-631, 1975.

Winsor, T.: The Electrocardiogram in Myocardial Infarction. Ciba Clinical Symposia, illustrated by Netter, F.H. Summit, N.J.: Ciba Pharmaceutical Co., 1977.

INDEX